# Flowers that Heal

OTHER BOOKS BY JUDY GRIFFIN, Ph.D.

*Mother Nature's Herbal*
*Mother Nature's Kitchen*
*Herbs for Health and Beauty*
*How to Master Special Diets*
*Slice of Life Diet and Nutrition Handbook*
*Romancing the Rose*
*The Healing Flowers*
*Around the World with Herbs*

# Flowers that Heal

## AROMAS, HERBS, ESSENCES, & OTHER SECRETS OF THE FAIRIES

*By* JUDY GRIFFIN, Ph.D.

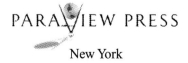

PARAVIEW PRESS

New York

The information in this book is not meant to diagnose or treat disease. The recipes are not substitutes for medication. Please consult with a healthcare provider.

Book and cover design by smythtype
Cover art: *Garden on Water Street* by Timothy R. Thies
Oil, 24" X 18"
www.sover.net
All rights reserved © 2002


ISBN: 1-931044-35-X

Library of Congress Catalog Card Number: 2002104651

*This book is dedicated to all the winged heroes of the garden,
and the grandmother I haven't met, Carmella Monzo DiTorrice.
May she grow in peace with the fairies she wanted to write about.*

# Table of Contents

# Preface

I remember the time when I was a child: the whole world was alive and glowing. Trees, plants and their flowers were my friends who danced with me in the moonlight and sparkled with dew in the sunlight. The flowers bloomed just for me and communicated special messages that made me giggle with delight. Plants were as real to me as people. I called them each by a special name and told them all my troubles as I reached over to sniff their beautiful fragrances and gaze at their dazzling colors.

I instinctively knew that flowers could "see" us and understand how I felt and what I was thinking about. Every flower was infinitely compassionate and loving, for flowers know nothing of destruction, brutality, or even judgment. They are part of a unique communication exuded throughout creation that sounds like a very high-pitched hum. Their song has rhythm that is pleasantly warm and jolly. I can remember dancing to their music and feeling as light as a fairy.

Then, my time with the flowers grew shorter. I hardly had time to stop and talk to anyone. I was always in a hurry, and the flowers had little to say. Then came a time when the flowers grew silent and without emotion. I would often wonder if the flowers still sang.

I began to rediscover the world of Mother Nature's flower essences, herbs, and essential oils while suffering from Crohn's disease. I had recently been diagnosed with cancer. I was scared, in pain, and in need of support. My answer to prayer was an inner message to work with flowers. All I really wanted was to get out of pain, but I made a promise to share everything I learned with others. Immediately afterwards, every time I walked near a plant, I received the information that I now share with you in the following pages. For more than eighteen years, much of this information has been researched and proven in clinics and private medical practices worldwide.

For every impossible or incurable situation, there is a flower essence to help us bloom. Flowers not only correct the imbalance in the personality's needs and expectations, but they also support us by opening our hearts.

When I work in my gardens, I enter a world where flowers talk and nature sings. I choose flowers that bloom even under stress from an inner joy, which expresses the wonders of Nature.

Each flower has a unique message and healing quality that can be captured into an essence at the peak time of its bloom. The energy of the flowers becomes available as the bloom opens fully. The best essences are made from flowers that are disease free, perfectly shaped, and that emit the most auric light from the center. They should be organically grown in seasons, nurtured, and chosen from an abundance of full blooms. Most of the blooms should be left untouched, attracting beneficial insects such as bees, wasps, and butterflies. The balance of Nature should be left undisturbed.

I have discovered that the experience of gardening is well worth the time and effort. Flowering plants are wonderful teachers and have taught me many songs and tunes I have heard only in gardens. The flowers also speak from the heart of all creation. They communicate the sadness they see in our eyes and catalyze the potential of what we are yet to be. They heal wounds from the deepest part of the psyche, reminding us with their beauty that all true healing comes from the heart.

During the past twenty years, I have worked therapeutically with flower essences, essential oils, herbs, and nutrition as a clinical herbalist, aromatherapist, teacher, counselor, and international lecturer. Certified in Texas as a horticulturist, I organically grow and produce quality products. I have learned that plants grown in the adverse climatic conditions of my environment enhance the immune response of the flowers, forcing them to bloom under stress just as we who thrive to achieve self-actualization do. As we search within for understanding and wisdom, Mother Nature will nurture us with the healing quality of homegrown plants and flowers.

Flower essences and essential oils have been an integral part of traditional healing since ancient times and are making their way into modern medicine as an adjunct to pharmaceuticals.

What is most important in healing from the heart is that we take responsibility for individual health and seek support on every level. Health includes taking responsibility for our own emotions, feelings, creativity, and expression. An integrated personality will then receive illumination from the spirit to express the heart's desire and to share all the treasures of the heart.

# Introduction

Mother Nature's Flower Fairies invite you to enter a world in miniature where flowers heal and fairies rule. Since the beginning of the Land of Thyme, fairies have learned to use flowers for every type of healing: for people, pets, knights in shining armor, and yes, even for fairies. Flowers have a universal charm that opens the heart of those who grow, receive, and admire them. Their aroma, color, shape, and texture integrate all the senses into a rainbow of emotional splendor known to every fairy as "healing from the heart."

Healing from the heart comes from a place deep within composed of all-embracing love. It shines like a light reflecting eternal peace and illumination of the spirit. This unconditional love is nurtured by good deeds and developed through compassion. There are no limitations, and every living being will be blessed through participation.

Mother Nature's Flower Fairies live their lives wrapped in the security of loving acceptance. They experience every moment of life knowing and experiencing the love that continually creates through Nature. By stepping into their world we can learn how to bring love into ours. We'll find fairies of every nature, size, and shape, each developing their character by utilizing their talents and learning to create new ones. They live in the Land of Thyme, a community where every being is accepted just the way they are: big, little, overweight, or hyperactive. Fairies, beneficial insects, gods, and Mother Nature herself are appreciated as equals. Creative change sprouts from this type of love, as the community evolves and develops to a higher level. The fairies change and blend into a community integrated by work, play, and self-development.

What do Flower Fairies possibly need to learn? They already understand how flowers grow and make every garden magical, but they are still learning how to take care of their health through relaxation techniques, "aromafairapy," herbs, color and chakra balancing, diet, exercise, and making the world ever more beautiful with the artistic, healing uses of flowers. Everyone living in the Land of Thyme will experience healing from the heart.

As you read this fairy tale, healing from the heart will begin for you as it did for me twenty years ago. As a result, you will experience the healing power of flowers as Mother Nature sings a lullaby to awaken your heart's desires.

# CHAPTER 1

# The Beginning

## The World According to Fairies and Flowers

*"Come away O human child!*
*To the waters and the wild,*
*With a faery, hand in hand,*
*For the world's more full of weeping*
*than you can understand."*
William Butler Yeats, 1889

Long ago when the world was young, even before the dawn of Father Time, Mother Nature dusted the earth and seas with what is commonly known as fairies. These precious nymphs, sprites, and mermaids are continuously born from the harmony of Creation and carried by the gentle east wind, Eurus, on angels' wings. When you sit under the embrace of an old oak tree, you may soon hear the warm lullaby of the angels' song:

*Little Fairy, fair and slim*
*Flowers soon will cover him.*
*Fairy fine, fairy gay,*
*Fairy now will come to stay . . .*

And they did! The fairies soon opened their wings and dived into the ocean or glided into the giant establishment known as the Forest of Conifers. In the dark reaches of this ancient forest, Father Frost held an icy embrace threatening death to the helpless travelers.

Here, pine trees were at the height of their power, snatching all the sunshine as it shimmered into the forest. These evergreen trees were very rich and they were determined to rule the forest. The tallest ones were so dense and thick that they blocked the friendly sunshine from illuminating the forest floor. In fact, it was so dark and cold on the ground that few memories of the beauty and wonder of Mother Nature remained there.

If any complaints reached the ruling conifers, they were sure to shower pinecones indiscriminately on the inhabitants below. Even worse were the messy pine needles covering the fertile soil, preventing new seeds and blankets of grass from flourishing.

The fairies could hardly find a decent flower petal to lean on, much less to make a home. They would have never been able to slide through the pine needles if the dragonflies had not shown the way. The survivors arrived at the forest floor, tired and powdered with pine pollen. They had to learn to sneeze to clear their sinuses. The sounds of *kachoo!* echoed into the forest, causing the earthworms to burrow deep into the soil and cover their ears, for the forest and its creatures were used to only silence. The fairies soon learned to adapt to the forest. They searched their surroundings for clues of a "Flower Creation Myth" they had heard long ago.

Hidden in the silence of the forest is the memory of the "Flower Creation Myth," how and why angiosperms learned to bloom. Here is the whole story, unaltered and handed down to many generations of flowers ever since. Not a day goes by in the flora world without the following story being related to the next generation.

Long ago flowering plants known as "angiosperms" evolved blooms to attract pollinators to help continue the species. They lived in dense pine forests covering the landmasses. They found little room to grow and very little light filtered down to them through the conifers. The angiosperms faced extinction in a seemingly impossible situation.

The conifers were no help. They kept dropping pinecones on the angiosperms at the least appropriate moments. If a pollinator did happen to find his way through the dimly lit forest, he was likely to be rendered unconscious by a hail of pinecones followed by the biting rain of needles.

The angiosperms felt very abandoned. They couldn't express creativity in their own land. They were hungry for sunshine, good times, and some friends. They couldn't even call up an earthworm from the densely covered forest floor or invite a newly released butterfly for a dewdrop. And the newly swarmed bees said, "Forget it, we can't form colonies in a hailstorm of pinecones. Besides, no one will want to eat honey made from sterile flowers. We couldn't support the queen through such economic hardships. We need sunshine and fields of flowers to produce golden honey for the hive and a sweet royal jelly to feed the queen."

Well, what's a timid angiosperm supposed to do? Try as they might, they couldn't produce a bloom. The best they could do was to cough up a few pine needles and sneeze out the drifting pine dust. Their only choice was to fold their leaves around them and go within. One brave flower began to think aloud. "There has to be a way out of this situation," the flower said. "We all have to learn to bloom as one. We must produce varieties that bloom in every color and every circumstance. If we can produce good seed, future generations of flowers can even catch a wind to another land. But first we must produce pollen so we can communicate with each other, and fragrance and color to attract every known pollinator."

The angiosperms were all humming as one; one goal, many varieties, and a strong desire to make it happen.

But they soon realized that wasn't enough. It seems that they needed help from Mother Nature herself.

However, Mother Nature was a little perplexed by the whole situation. She had great expectations for the flower kingdom, but the environment was not cooperating with her vision. She decided to hold a conference with the governing Elements.

She talked it over with the Sun and the Moon, the Wind and the Rain. They all felt they had given it their best, but the conifer forests were really hogging the show. They even invented Thunder to scare the pine trees from reaching to the stars! It didn't work. The stars had to pull up the sky to keep the conifers from bombarding the constellations with pinecones.

This gave Mother Nature an idea. She would call on the Star gods to produce a goddess and teach the angiosperms how to bloom in adverse situations. After all, she hadn't become the Matron of Nature without a little coaxing. And she believed she had friends in high places.

## The Flowering of the World

*We are all children of*
*A brilliantly colored flower, A flaming flower.*
Ramon Medina Silva, Huichol Artist

On the way to the Star gods, Mother Nature stopped in to see Apollo. It had been some time since they'd seen each other, but for Apollo nothing had changed. He still had a great attraction to older women, and Mother Nature knew how to take advantage of the situation. Apollo was practicing his archery skills before traveling to Delphi, an ancient city in Greece. Here he planned to battle the serpent, Python, who was blocking his prophecies broadcast at the Delphic Oracle. Mother Nature situated herself and her robes in such a fashion that Apollo dropped his bow and picked up his lyre to strum her favorite song. *I am Nature, the Universal Mother, and Mistress of all Elements.* (Apuleius, 2nd Century)

And, Mother Nature returned in song. *Fill me with beauty so I may share it with others.*

She took this opportunity to speak to Apollo of their beautiful daughter, Flora. Mother Nature quickly summed up the plight of the angiosperms and requested Apollo's permission to retrieve her from apprenticeship to teach flowers how to bloom under stress.

Flora had all the makings of a great Gaean goddess. From Apollo she received the gifts of healing, courage, wisdom, and, of course, beauty. From her mother she received tenacity, diversity, good will, and, of course, beauty. Bored with the Star gods, Flora was eager to prove herself. She felt in her heart that she had a brighter future than the stars had to offer. She had been waiting for an opportunity like this. Teaching flowers to bloom under stress couldn't be more difficult than positioning stars in constellations. She'd already exhausted every animal in the alphabet and was finding the job to be quite tedious.

Together, Apollo and Mother Nature traveled to visit Cronos, son of the Earth and Sky and ruler of the Titans. To these primordial deities, death came gently. They remained on earth as beneficial spirits, just the type of friends that could encourage flowers to bloom. With permission from Cronos, Mother Nature could enjoin angiosperms with the beneficial spirits to diversify, travel to many lands, bloom under stress, and transform every difficulty into a challenge.

"How will they do this?" asked Apollo.

Mother Nature replied, "In my domain, everyone in creation was born equipped with an inherent light that could ignite empowerment. The electromagnetic energy, or chakras, fueled by that light, would attract the beneficial spirits already inhabiting the earth. Together all of Nature can become self-healing. Each family will help raise the consciousness of the others that follow. The Celestial Mermaid brings the underwater palace of crystals and minerals to the River goddess who enlivens the soil for all flowers and plants to flourish and to nourish those who live off the land. Every part of creation is interconnected with multiple layers of awareness that awaken, honor, and preserve all life forms."

*All things share the same breath . . .*
*the perfumed flowers are our sisters, the deer, the horse,*
*the great eagle, these are our brothers.*
Chief Seattle, 1854

Infused with a spirit of cooperation, Cronos was more than happy to share the beneficial spirits. He promptly played his heavenly chimes to awaken the supernatural qualities of his earth-friendly spirits to join the light and sound within and around the lonely angiosperms.

And what about Flora? What will she do to help creation? She was last seen digging her way out of a black hole retrieving a lost star.

Apollo sent Hermes, patron of travelers, to persuade Flora to join them at the Palace of the gods. As it turned out, this was the easiest job Hermes would ever do. He spoke two words — "Let's go!" — and Flora was by his side.

Back at the palace, Cronos welcomed Flora and shared his gifts of the spirit. Flora was given the gift of abundance, the gift of fertility to reseed the land, the knowledge to live without sickness and sorrow, and the wisdom to bloom under stress. Flora was also given an assignment to prove her ability to champion flowering plants. She was to create a vision of fulfillment for the angiosperms and new ways to attract pollinators and beneficial insects. Most importantly, she must find a way to get close to the heart of humankind, the latest project Mother Nature was working on. The challenge would be to bypass the judgmental intellect that made them think about everything before they could feel.

Flora knew that the souls of flowers are closely related to humans. She dreamed of raising the consciousness of flowering plants to reflect the inner nature of humans. Flowers, however, would hold the vision of triumph through every crisis of evolution. After existing in the pine forests all these years, angiosperms certainly understood what it was like to break through limitations and bloom. Flora could use these talents to transport humans beyond everyday concerns and transcend their differences to live in harmony with Nature.

Of course, Flora would need help to orchestrate her vast vision. She first called Adonis, god of Adornment, to create flowers of every color. (Originally, flowers were only white. Surely, creating brightly colored flowers would attract pollinators.) Flowers were then standardized with five petals. Adonis was asked to make new molds for petals of every shape, size, and texture. This would confuse and repel predator insects that live on the flowers' life juices and spread disease. Adonis was so pleased with his work that he exclaimed that he'd like to be a flower in his next life, foretelling his future of being changed into an anemone.

Next Flora called the goddess of Beauty, Precious, known today as the butterfly. Precious returned from rescuing the freezing fairies from the frozen conifer forests, sheltering them with her wings and transforming them into new life. Her special talent was her song, transforming the ordinary into the extraordinary and creating joy through the ritual of dance. She would coax the flowers into opening and teach them to renew themselves by producing seeds. Her lullaby would bring the fairies to tears. The fairies decided to stay and direct sunlight into the plants to produce more photosynthesis, creating repeat bloomers.

Precious became so busy that she decided to reproduce herself into a species of butterflies. She wrapped her cloak tightly around her body and wove a multitude of butterflies, each with unique markings. These soon became a transworld airline for the fairies that dispersed flower seeds in every land. The colors, stripes, and markings on the butterflies directed the fairies to their destinations. Nonstop flights wore solid colors, warm colors went south, blues overseas, and stripes went over the Himalayas to the Orient.

But how could flowers attract humans? People seemed pleased with the colors and varieties, but they didn't quite get close enough or stay long enough for the flowers to warm their hearts and catalyze the higher centers of their consciousness.

To find the solution, Flora traveled to the top of Khunlum, the earthly home of the Lord of the Sky. The peaks emitted vapors exhaled by all living nature. Here she found the beautiful Xochiquetzal, the goddess of Delight, residing in joy and self-love, dancing in the moonlight. She could hear echoes of the ancient Mayan chant communicating with the goddess and the hummingbirds dancing to their tune.

> *You alone bestow intoxicating flowers,*
> *precious flowers.*
> *You are the singer within the house of springtime.*
> *You make the people happy.*
> Nezahualcoyotl c. 1450 C.E.

The scent Flora inhaled was like no other she had ever experienced. It reminded her of cool water and felt soothing to her emotions. Immediately she understood how to join the souls of flowers and humans. She would ask Xochiquetzal to add her array of heavenly scents to flowers and link the spiritual to the physical nature.

She took all the essences of the colors, scents, and varieties to the goddess of the Dawn, Illumination, who created rainbows to link heaven and earth. The flowers' gift of transformation would bring a peaceful coexistence and interdependence with all Nature. For their reward, each flower was given a special gift and potential to share with humankind. Illumination told Flora she would be given the opportunity to learn more about the aromatic and spiritual nature of flowers in the near future.

In the meantime, the angiosperm aromatic flowers thrived and reproduced throughout the land.

The conifers were amazed and intrigued by all the vivid color and variety developing in their forest. They didn't even recognize the angiosperms as they called down to them, "Are you a god?"

"No," replied the flowers in unison.

"Are you an angel?"

"No," replied the flowers again.

"Well, then, are you a new breed of fairies?"

"No," replied the flowers. They smiled as they replied as one, "I bloom; therefore, I am."

# CHAPTER 2

# A Fairy Feast
## Nutritious Recipes for Health-Conscious Fairies

Things have really changed since the beginning of time. Fairies no longer float to earth on angel wings. In fact, fairly recently Mother Nature decided that since life on earth began in a garden, fairies should also spring from the good earth. The fairies didn't especially like it. They became prone to headaches and searched in vain for good adjusters and yoga instructors. In the meantime, the earthworms had to reroute their highways to construct a road with an exit into the topsoil, which brought the fairies into the warm sunshine. They didn't like this, and quickly dove back into the safety of darkness. They just never knew what might be growing in the outer limits!

Earth fairies were quite happy to be in the sunshine. Although they chattered at length about the good ol' days, they understood why Mother Nature chose to bind them to the earth.

So, the fairies spent their free time trying to get into shape. They climbed up the bindweed and swung from the tendrils to strengthen their arms. Next, there were broad jumps over the toadstools. Then, they hurdled over the monkey grass. Most of the fairies didn't make it and spent the rest of the day crawling through the monkey grass to return to their camp situated underneath a cobweb. Life was really hard. Where were the angels when they needed them? The fairies were too tired to hear their lullaby at night:

> *Our revels now are ended . . .*
> *we are such stuffe*
> *As dreams are made on; and our little life*
> *Is rounded with a sleepe.*
> > *The Tempest:* Act IV, Scene I
> > William Shakespeare, 1564–1616

Earth fairies tended to have a wee problem with their weight. They evolved into a little heavier breed than the heaven-sent ones. They had more jovial personalities, of course: they were much jollier and a little more nervous than their air-borne cousins, which could be why they ate more. Earth fairies also ate more when they felt tired, anxious, depressed, afraid, alone, festive, unappreciated, overworked, and just before a full moon. Those suffering from a pre-moon syndrome even raided anthills for something spicy to eat with their chocolates.

All those snacks added up to some pretty tight-fitting leotards with seams stretched to the max. When they wore zippered jeans, they had to pull them closed with pliers; although the fairies gladly made the sacrifice to be in high style, they agreed that the androgynous extra-round, one-size-fits-all styles looked the best on them.

They were Mother Nature's darlings and she loved them all! However, she realized the fairies would build more muscle if they could trim off a little of the extra-round parts and replace them with lean ones. This would also allow them to get back into their original wings and discard the extra-strength reinforced ones hanging in their closets.

Even the flowers complained about the earth fairies being as wide as they were tall. The fairies were so out of shape, the flowers had to produce more leaves and limbs in order for the fairies to climb to their petals. The flowers were often rudely awakened in the early hours by a chubby fairy falling into a dewdrop, producing a big splash and creating shockwaves of waterfalls from their leaves. The fairies blamed their weight on high-altitude sickness, but Flora knew better. She was just beginning to learn about the power of aromatherapy, but she knew all about diet and nutrition. Flora was the type of goddess who practiced what she preached. Her perfect figure was as lean as her diet.

Birthed during the fairy boomer years, Flora was a pioneer for health and fitness. The way things were growing in the gardens, she would either have to create larger flowers or smaller fairies. She also knew Mother Nature would be too lenient with the fairies' diet, so she called a play day celebration and invited all the fairies before anyone heard of her plans. She used every bit of her persuasion to arrange for a spectacular day — a cool breeze, light fog, and occasional mist. She chose a location where the magnolia and Rose of Sharon trees lent a quiet rusticity and lots of nooks and crannies for the fairies to play in. She decorated with rosemary and curry to remind them of a holiday and all the love it brings. Flora really worked hard to set just the right mood for this festive occasion, planting fragrant flowers and herbs near the table settings to release their power of persuasion and lure the fairies to her low-fat feast.

Then she called in the insect population to help cater the food. The ants were a little cautious, but they came around after a while. Flora wanted to present a healthy feast and introduce dietary suggestions to set free the magic of metabolism and set the fairies free from unwanted pounds. She was very idealistic in those days; she did not realize the fairies enjoyed eating, especially high-calorie foods. Flora was convinced the fairies only needed education and a perfect role model, like her, to become lean once more.

The turnout was better than Flora expected. Fairies arrived on caterpillar buses and inchworms. Luckier fairies called up an accommodating bumblebee or dragonfly. Hummingbirds brought in fairy families from all over the Land of Thyme and every Transworld Butterfly ticket was sold!

Flora made sure the fairy folk were not disappointed. She uncovered a feast of favorite fairy food that made the fairies gasp in unison and the butterflies flap with joy. She announced that every entrée was based on the low-fat, high fiber, healthy New Millennium Fairy Diet. An ominous silence fell over the crowd. Fairies thought only humans went on diets so they could enjoy gaining all their weight (and more) back again! The fairies were reluctant to try new recipes, hesitating to line up for a taste. Flora was puzzled as she watched the unresponsive crowd avoid eye contact with her as she asked the fairies to get in line to sample the low-fat food.

Suddenly, there was a shriek and cry for help from the forest. Sure enough, it was Nimbus, the heaviest fairy in the Land of Thyme. Presently, he was stuck between a nook and a cranny with a very sheepish grin on his face. He was probably looking for a beehive to raid, but would never admit it. Nimbus's story was that he rescued a baby bird from the clutches of a fierce eagle and was hurled to the ground by the bird of prey. However, neither the baby bird nor the eagle was ever found, yet Nimbus was very obviously stuck in a place where his backside was too broad to fit.

It took several fairies twenty minutes to push Nimbus's larger half through the nook and then the cranny. The crowd stood around as all crowds do. Flora covered as much food as she could, and then hung up fresh sprigs of basil flowers and tansy flowers to keep the flies at a distance. They would have their turn after everyone finished. Flora was quite perturbed that the feast wasn't going the way she planned. The fairies were more interested in Nimbus's backside than eating healthy. She waited impatiently for the fairies to return. *This is no way to treat a goddess,* she pouted.

When the ordeal ended, Nimbus was first in line. He took a taste of several dishes before proclaiming the low-fat feast delicious! There was a short cheer and then a hush came over the crowd. Flora could hear fairy whispers but she couldn't understand what the fairies were saying. Suddenly, Nimbus pulled her close and whispered something in her ear.

"Ah, yes," she announced. "There will be no edible flowers at this feast!"

The crowd went wild cheering and throwing their fairy hats in the air. The sunflowers came to the table and shook their nutritious seeds over the green bean entrée, and several herbs donated leaves for seasoning while the garlics peeled off cloves for the sauces. After sampling several dishes, the fairies were asked to vote for the best recipes to be served again at festive occasions. Flora made sure every fairy turned in a ballot before calling in Spider, a reporter for the *Fairy Morning News,* to type the menus for publication. Photos of sunflowers dancing with chubby fairies made the front page of the Sunday paper.

Flora had high hopes of changing the fairy diet forever with this low-fat feast. Little did she know there was much more to do and learn about healing before she accomplished her assignment.

The following entrees won the Tasters' Choice Awards, becoming regulars in the New Millennium Low-Fat Fairy Diet. Flora included low-fat, vegetarian entrees as well as meat dishes, and selected a variety of healthy menus to tempt every taste bud.

## VEGETARIAN SELECTIONS

### NIMBUS'S FAVORITE PAPAYA SALAD

Serve with a teaspoon of fresh lemon thyme sprinkled over the salad to attract the fairies. (Nimbus will be right by your side as you prepare this dish). The papaya and pineapple help digest meats and proteins served during the meal.

**Ingredients**
  2 cups papaya cubes
  1 cup fresh pineapple cubes
  1 cup orange segments, seeds removed
  1 large banana, cubed or sliced
  fresh lime or lemon juice to taste
  ¼ cup toasted coconut

Combine all ingredients. Cover and chill for one hour. Serves four.

**Nutritional value per serving:**
  Carbohydrates: 22.5 grams
  Protein: 2.5 grams
  Fat: 1.0 gram
  Sodium: 0
  Calories: 80

# VEGETARIAN LOW-FAT LASAGNA

Serve this with a cool glass of spearmint lemon verbena tea (recipe below). The fairies asked that the fat grams be deleted so they could enjoy their meal without any guilt. Flora ignored their request.

## Ingredients

1 teaspoon extra virgin olive oil
3 quarts of water to boil
½ pound of lasagna noodles
1 pound low-fat cottage cheese or part-skim ricotta
30-ounce jar low-salt spaghetti sauce
4 ounces low-fat mozzarella, shredded
¼ cup grated Parmesan cheese
1 teaspoon each of dried basil, oregano, marjoram, and parsley

Heat oven to 350°. Boil water and oil in a large pot. Cook noodles about ten minutes; drain. Cover the bottom of an 8x8 pan with noodles. Cut to fit. Spread ricotta cheese, and then sauce, over noodles. Then add more noodles, sauce, mozzarella, and Parmesan. Bake at 350° for thirty minutes. Serves four.

## Nutritional value per serving:

Carbohydrates: 41 grams
Protein: 22.0 grams
Fat: 28 grams
Sodium: approximately 45 mg
Calories: 355

# SPEARMINT LEMON VERBENA TEA

Enjoy a glass of herbal iced tea that actually tastes good!

## Ingredients

6 tablespoons chopped fresh spearmint leaves and stems
2 tablespoons fresh lemon verbena leaves
4 cups water

Boil water for fifteen minutes, covered. Strain. Add two tablespoons of fresh lemon verbena leaves and refrigerate. Serve over ice.

**Variation:** Lemon grass may be substituted for lemon verbena. Steep two tablespoons with spearmint leaves and strain before refrigerating. Serves four thirsty fairies.

## AVOCADO BUTTER

The fairies served this with crackers. Nimbus recommends the avocado butter for the maximum amount of calories per bite.

**Ingredients**
- 1 ripe, mashed medium avocado
- ½ cup water
- 1 or 2 tablespoons lemon juice
- garlic or onion flakes to taste
- paprika sprinkled on top to taste
- finely minced fresh basil leaves (optional)

Spread thinly on a cracker. One tablespoon per serving. Serves five to six. Two crackers equal one serving. Flora recommends Melba toast (recipe on page 129) as a low-calorie, low-fat choice of crackers, which the fairies ignore, much to her displeasure.

**Nutritional value per serving:**
- Carbohydrates: 12 grams
- Protein: 4 grams
- Fat: 14 grams
- Sodium: 1 mg
- Calories: 40

# Sesame Garlic Dressing

Sesame seeds are high in protein and rich in flavor. Serve on veggies or salads. Use it as a dip for fresh veggies or as a seasoning for cooked greens or beans with rice.

## Ingredients
2 tablespoons extra virgin olive oil
1 clove garlic, peeled
2 tablespoons lemon juice
1 tablespoon Tahini (ground sesame butter. Recipe on page 119.)
2 tablespoons water
½ teaspoon (dried) oregano
½ teaspoon (fresh) parsley or cilantro, finely minced

Blend all ingredients at high speed in a blender for one minute.
One tablespoon per serving. Serves four.

## Nutritional value per serving:
Carbohydrates: 4 grams
Protein: 2 grams
Fat: 15 grams
Sodium: 10 mg
Calories: 38

# Tamari Dressing

Blend and serve on veggies, salads, grains, and lentils to add an Oriental flavor to your cuisine.

## Ingredients
1 tablespoon extra virgin olive oil
1 tablespoon Tahini
2 tablespoons water
1 tablespoon lime juice
1 tablespoon tamari
onions or garlic to taste

Puree all ingredients in a blender for one minute. One tablespoon per serving. Serves four.

**Nutritional value per serving:**
    Carbohydrates: 8 grams
    Protein: 2 grams
    Fat: 23 grams
    Sodium: 42 mg
    Calories: 37

## SUNFLOWERED GREEN BEANS

Save room for a generous serving of this high-protein dish.

**Ingredients**
    1 pound green beans
    2 cups cold water
    ¼ cup toasted sunflower seeds
    2 tablespoons chopped parsley
    1 clove minced garlic
    juice from 2 lemons
    freshly ground pepper to taste
    ½ cup pine nuts

Cut off ends of beans and wash beans thoroughly. Bring two cups of water to a boil in saucepan. Place beans in steamer basket over boiling water and cover. Cook over medium heat for eight to ten minutes or until beans are bright green but still crisp. Meanwhile, place pine nuts in small skillet and toast until brown on medium heat. Shake skillet frequently so the nuts do not burn. Remove and wrap the nuts in paper towels to absorb any oils. Chop parsley and garlic together. Mix with lemon juice and a grind or two of fresh pepper. When beans are ready, drain in a colander, place them in a warm bowl, and toss with the lemon mixture. Garnish with sunflower seeds and serve with a crunchy salad. Serves four.

**Nutritional value per serving:**
    Carbohydrates: 4.5 grams
    Protein: 22.5 grams
    Fat: 9.5 grams
    Sodium: 36 mg.
    Calories: 202

## PEAR SHERBET

The grand finale is this exquisite pear sherbet. Nimbus hopes you're too full to finish and will share yours with him!

**Ingredients**
>   1 egg white, beaten until stiff
>   1/3 cup non-fat dry milk
>   1/3 cup cold water
>   2 large ice cubes, shaved in a blender
>   2 teaspoons pure vanilla extract
>   2 tablespoons unsweetened pear juice
>   2 ripe pears, cored, peeled, and sliced

To the beaten egg white, add all ingredients except the sliced pears. Beat until thick and pour the mixture into an ice tray. Freeze for one to two hours until ready to serve. Spoon over sliced pears. Canned pears can be substituted for fresh pears.

**Nutritional value per serving:**
>   Carbohydrates: 16 grams
>   Protein: 3 grams
>   Fat: 0 grams
>   Sodium: 40 mg.
>   Calories: 76

# FREE-RANGE MEAT SELECTIONS AND DISHES THAT GO WELL WITH THEM

The earth fairies evolved into a distinct breed that thrived on a diet including a few dairy products and meat. The following menus were selected from the range, free of hormones, chemicals, and antibiotics. Nimbus enjoyed the vegetarian as well as the free-range selections.

Fairies prefer range-fed chicken and beef and offered a selection of each at the feast. Nimbus selected both, of course.

## CHICKEN BREASTS WITH TARRAGON MUSTARD

**Ingredients**
- 1 pound skinless, boneless chicken breasts cut into 4 pieces
- 1 tablespoon fresh tarragon or 2 teaspoons dried
- 1 teaspoon fresh lemon juice
- ¼ cup Dijon mustard
- cayenne pepper, to taste
- 1 lemon, sliced
- 1 tablespoon chopped fresh parsley

Place chicken breasts between two sheets of wax paper and pound with a mallet to flatten. Mix together the tarragon, lemon juice, mustard, and pepper (to taste) into a mayonnaise consistency. Coat the chicken pieces. Preheat broiler and place the breasts about four inches from heat. Broil until mustard begins to bubble (about five to six minutes); then turn and grill other side. Remove before mustard begins to burn. Top each piece with a lemon slice sprinkled with parsley. Serves four.

**Nutritional value per serving:**
- Carbohydrates: 4 grams
- Protein: 28 grams
- Fat: 3.5 grams
- Sodium: 253 mg.
- Calories: 160

# VEAL SCALOPPINI

Nimbus was very disappointed when he found no scallops in this entrée.

**Ingredients**
- 1 teaspoon olive oil
- 1 medium onion, finely chopped
- 1 pound veal scaloppini, sliced very thin
- 2 cloves garlic, minced
- 2 tablespoons chopped parsley
- ¼ teaspoon freshly ground pepper
- ½ cup red wine
- 1 cup tomato juice (low sodium) or spaghetti sauce
- 1 lemon, scored and sliced thin
- 6 sprigs parsley

Heat oil in a large non-stick skillet and brown the chopped onion. Remove onion from the pan and set aside. Brown veal slices quickly on each side. Add garlic, chopped parsley, cooked onion, pepper, and then wine. Simmer for two minutes over high heat and add tomato juice. Lower heat setting and simmer over low heat for about five minutes. If the sauce needs further reduction, remove the veal and cook the sauce until thick. Serve veal with the sauce at once. Garnish with slices of lemon and parsley sprigs. Serves four.

**Nutritional value per serving:**
- Carbohydrates: 9 grams
- Protein: 24 grams
- Fat: 11.5 grams
- Sodium: 205 mg.
- Calories: 236

# EGG SOUP

This low-calorie soup can be substituted for a vegetable or meat entrée and invites a second helping.

## Ingredients

4 cups chicken broth
1 tablespoon chopped fresh sage (or 1½ teaspoon dried)
1 cup cooked small pasta
2 eggs (use only 1 yolk)
1 teaspoon finely chopped (fresh) parsley
⅛ teaspoon fresh pepper
1 tablespoon lemon juice
1 tablespoon grated Romano cheese

Bring chicken broth and sage to a boil in saucepan. Add cooked pasta to the broth and stir. Bring back to a boil. Lightly heat together the eggs, parsley, pepper, lemon juice, and cheese. Add to this one-quarter cup of the hot broth. Just before serving, whisk this mixture into the soup. Serve in warm bowls. Serves four.

## Nutritional value per serving:

Carbohydrates: 11 grams
Protein: 4.5 grams
Fat: 2 grams
Sodium: 16 mg.
Calories: 80

# BROILED FRUIT

Flora served a light dessert with the meat entrées because fairies prefer a light touch to complete a robust meal.

## Ingredients

½ cup peeled and cubed fresh pineapple
1 banana cut into 1-inch slices
1 orange peeled, sectioned, and seeded
1 teaspoon ground cinnamon
¼ cup orange liqueur (simmered about 3 minutes) or orange juice

Thread fruit on skewers, alternating pineapple, banana, and orange. Sprinkle fruit with cinnamon and place in a foil-lined pan. Broil until lightly browned (about three to five minutes). Remove from skewers and spoon orange liqueur (or orange juice) over each serving. Serves four.

**Nutritional value per serving:**
Carbohydrates: 18 grams
Protein: 1 gram
Fat: 0 grams
Sodium: 1 mg.
Calories: 76

## COFFEE ICE

This recipe was the talk of the fairy feast. Several fairies begged Flora for this recipe, and asked for seconds!

**Ingredients**
3 cups espresso coffee of your choice
3 drops almond extract
1 drop pure vanilla extract
2 tablespoons chopped almonds
1 tablespoon minced lemon verbena

Mix coffee with almond and vanilla extracts and pour into a metal ice tray. Place in freezer about two hours before serving. Stir with a fork every twenty minutes to break up crystals. Repeat just before serving. Divide among four sherbet glasses. Top with crushed almonds and a sprinkle of lemon verbena. Serves four.

**Nutritional value per serving:**
Carbohydrates: 1 gram
Protein: 0
Fat: 0
Sodium: 0
Calories: 4

## SPARTAN FAIRY SELECTIONS

The Spartan sector of the fairy realm selected a high-protein shake to help them build muscle. They laughed Nimbus out of this line. They were getting ready for the Operation Fairy Storm Rescue Mission and their bodies were as lean as their diet.

## SOY SHAKE

High protein, low calorie, low fat, no salt. Nimbus quickly lost interest in this drink.

**Ingredients**

1 cup water
1 tablespoon soy protein powder
2 tablespoons carob powder or unsweetened cocoa
1 cup low-fat soymilk (1%)
½ cup cracked ice
1 banana (frozen) or 1 cup of fruit of your choice
1 teaspoon honey, fructose, or maple syrup
½ teaspoon vanilla extract

Blend water, soy powder, and carob on high speed until well mixed. Add soymilk, ice, banana or fruit, honey, vanilla, and blend for one minute at high speed. Makes two and a half cups, approximately four servings.

**Nutritional value per serving:**

Carbohydrates: 251 grams
Protein: 14 grams
Fat: 2 grams
Sodium: 30 mg
Calories: 110

# Fairy Children's Sweet Recipes

## Watermelon Ice

Nimbus made it back for dessert. He was first in line for this frozen treat.

### Ingredients
    4 cups watermelon peeled, seeded, and cubed
    4 ice cubes
    2 tablespoons concentrated frozen apple juice

Puree watermelon in a blender with ice cubes and apple juice concentrate. Pour the liquid into an ice tray and place in the freezer. After thirty minutes, stir to break up crystals and return to freezer. Repeat process until ready to serve, then stir once again. Serves four.

### Nutritional value per serving:
    Carbohydrates: 13 grams
    Protein: 1 gram
    Fat: 0 grams
    Sodium: 2 mg.
    Calories: 56

## Rice Pudding

The fairy children were given a selection of nutritious, delicious desserts. They favored creamy, easily digested selections that help them sleep well at night.

### Ingredients
    1 cup cooked brown rice
    1 small banana, mashed
    ½ cup non-fat milk
    1 teaspoon vanilla extract
    ½ teaspoon ground cinnamon
    ½ teaspoon freshly grated nutmeg
    ¼ cup frozen concentrated apple juice
    1 teaspoon raisins
    2 egg whites, beaten stiff

Mix all ingredients together except the egg whites. After blending, fold in egg whites and pour into a baking pan. Bake in the middle of a preheated 350° oven until the top is brown and pudding is set (about one hour). Serves four.

**Nutritional value per serving:**
Carbohydrates: 20 grams
Protein: 4 grams
Fat: 0 grams
Sodium: 146 mg.
Calories: 96

To the top of each serving, add one scoop of soy whipped cream. The recipe follows.

## SOY WHIPPED CREAM

This is a delicious high-protein treat to add to pudding and fruit desserts.

**Ingredients**
½ cup soymilk
¼ teaspoon vanilla
½ cup safflower oil
1 tablespoon honey or fructose

Blend soymilk and vanilla at medium speed. Gradually add oil until the mixture becomes very thick. Blend in honey to make one cup. For best results, use chilled beaters. Serves four.

**Nutritional value per serving:**
Carbohydrates: 6 grams
Protein: 4 grams
Fat: 40 grams
Sodium: 2 mg.
Calories: 125

# PEACHES MELBA

This elegant dessert is low in fat and high in protein, a favorite for both children and parents.

## Ingredients
4 large ripe peaches
1 cup raspberries
½ cup part-skim ricotta cheese
1 tablespoon grape juice

Blanch peaches by dropping them into boiling water for thirty seconds. Remove them and run under cold water until the skins peel off easily. Cut in half, discard pits, and place two peach halves on each of four individual dessert dishes. Puree raspberries with ricotta cheese and grape juice, reserving two tablespoons of whole berries for a special topping. Spoon puree over the peaches, top with a few berries, and serve cold. Serves four.

## Nutritional value per serving:
Carbohydrates: 22 grams
Protein: 5 grams
Fat: 3 grams
Sodium: 41 mg.
Calories: 135

# PEACH PUDDING

Fairy children thrive on peaches and pudding! This dessert may also be molded and served as a fruit salad.

## Ingredients
1 package unflavored gelatin
¼ cup cold water
2 cups peeled and mashed fresh peaches
1 cup plain low-fat yogurt
1 teaspoon pure vanilla extract
4 teaspoons concentrated frozen orange juice
1 tablespoon grated orange rind

Sprinkle gelatin over cold water. Stir over low heat until dissolved. Set aside and let cool. In a medium bowl, mix together all remaining ingredients except orange rind. Add the cooled gelatin. Cover the bowl and set in a freezer until firm (one to two hours), but not frozen solid. Garnish with orange rind. Serve in individual dessert glasses. Serves six to eight.

**Nutritional value per serving:**

Carbohydrates: 16 grams
Protein: 5 grams
Fat: 1 gram
Sodium: 41 mg.
Calories: 93

CHAPTER 3

# Operation Fairy Storm
## Physical and Mental Stress Reducers

*A world without flowers is like a face without a smile.*

After the feast, the Spartan fairies worked out while Nimbus burped and slept. The plans for Operation Fairy Storm were formulated in a nearby garden. Everyone was given an assignment. The time was quickly approaching to rescue the fairies trapped at the Roswell, a secret military outpost in the desert. Every fairy knew the plan and each had a role. The flower fairies thought of an environmentally safe way to overtake the camouflaged giant knights who were guarding the Roswell. Mother Nature approved. Flora consulted the flower fairies and prepared the gardens for production. Radio operations were assigned to the crickets. They practiced chirping in unison, sending out various frequencies throughout the night.

Hawks flew missions to map the territory. Detailed plans were made for the journey. How long would it take and what supplies would be necessary for the crew? The quickest and safest route was posted on a bulletin board for the crew chief. A lone eagle flew reconnaissance high above the waterless beachhead at the Roswell. He was careful not to be detected by the huge, shiny satellite dish pointed at the sky. The eagle flew away before he was caught. Back at the base, he gave the word: "All clear. Fairies, prepare to storm!"

There was a flurry in the garden. The flowers were now in full bloom. Garden fairies hand-picked spike and French lavender blooms while devas prepared a distillation unit to make essential oils and flower essences. The flowers were happy to donate their best blooms, those filled with relaxing essential oils and essences to enhance cooperation between plants and people.

Sage was the next to bolt into bloom, offering its purple flowers for distillation. Their essence would enhance friendship and the ability for individuals to value one another. Sage essential oil is a muscle relaxer that blends well with lavender. Together they would relax their foes for a non-violent takeover at the Roswell.

These combinations are the main ingredients in the environmentally safe Agent Aroma bomb designated to free the fairies at the Roswell. Yarrow flower essence was added to increase the potency of the Agent Aroma bomb. A blend called Harmony was added to ensure a peaceful entrance. In case of viral warfare, antiseptic interceptor missiles containing thyme, eucalyptus, and silver lace essences and essential oils would be prepared. Since the fairies didn't know if the giant knights would bite, the crew was sprayed with a dilution of lemon grass essential oil repellant. Since lemon grass works on insects, it should also repel the giant knights!

## All's Quiet on the Fairy Front

The time had come for the fairies to execute their mission. The fighting force was prepared for takeoff. The fairies gathered to send them off, equipped with hankies to catch their tears. A fairy ring was formed atop mushrooms to silently affirm a safe landing and return. The remaining flowers bowed in reverence as the bees prepared to fly overhead in a twenty-one-stinger salute. The valiant Fairy Navy SEALs winked at each other as they were given a few drops of Indian paintbrush essence by their crew chief to ensure success. Their hearts were open, their minds were pure, and their souls devoted. They marched on, confident of victory.

Everyone gathered at the airstrip. A special flight had been prepared for this occasion. All the fairies and flowers gasped in unison as a Phoenix taxied into a field of wild oats. Every color imaginable shimmered in the sunlight as the Phoenix moved into position. A wing slowly lowered for the crew to board. The crowd cheered wildly as the Fairy Navy SEALs were lifted onto the wing by hummingbirds. The Phoenix shook its feathers and slowly positioned itself for takeoff. All the interceptor missiles and the Agent Aroma Blend bombs were loaded. With a graceful leap, the crew was airborne!

The Phoenix was a fabulous creature. Its head was as bright as the sun, and its body as luminous as the moon. The wings were guided by the wind, sustained by the power of the life force. Clouds formed around it to offer heavenly protection and parted to provide direction. The ride was smooth and effortless.

Inside, the fairy crew was busy going over their plan and checking their gear. Only the Phoenix knew something was wrong. There was a drag and pull coming from the tail. Fearing infiltration, the Phoenix finally called the crew chief and relayed the problem. It felt like a large weight on his tail, and it was beginning to move!

The chief quickly moved to the back of the immortal bird armed with his garden tools, ready to defend his men and his mission. He immediately saw what the Phoenix had felt. There was a large mass wriggling under the canvas. The chief heard a loud slurping noise. He hoped it wasn't one of those disgusting gargoyles that enjoyed eating fairies for fun. He threw some vanilla essence in the air for protection and slowly prodded the canvas with his pitchfork. There was a familiar-sounding shriek as the canvas unbundled. "Oh, my stars, Nimbus, what are you doing here?" cried the chief. "We're on a secret garden mission on Fairy Force One! You're not supposed to be here, Nimbus. You're in the tank division of Ground Force!"

Nimbus looked puzzled and was quite concerned about the stinging feeling he felt when he tried to sit. "Ouch! I've been hit! Mayday! Mayday!" Nimbus cried, ignoring the crew chief's question.

"Nimbus, that was my pitchfork. Now, tell me how you got here." The chief sat down beside Nimbus and patiently waited for his answer, shaking his head in disbelief.

"Well, uh, I was looking for a large place to take a nap and before I knew it, I was being lifted into the heavens," Nimbus replied, looking rather guilty.

Just then the chief noticed a large pile of wrappers. "Nimbus, what are all of these empty containers? Where's all our rations?" asked the chief, looking around him with wide eyes, his patience quickly disappearing.

Nimbus hiccupped and blushed. "I was looking for something to coat my stomach. Too much acid, you know. I have a fear of heights. I think I'm going to faint!" Nimbus moaned as he placed his head between his knees, never offering an answer to the chief.

"Nimbus, you drank all of our ginseng elixir!" screamed the chief. "You have enough heat to ignite a rocket! Your face is turning bright red and you're dripping with sweat," cried the chief, as he jumped to his feet.

Suddenly, Nimbus felt exactly what the chief described. He felt the rush of heat from the ginseng elixir as his head began to pound. He turned to the chief. "Oh, chief, you've got to help me!" he pleaded. "My shoulders are crawling up to my ears and I can feel every fat cell moving in my body!"

"Okay, okay," replied the chief as he began to think.

The chief had an idea. He would use Nimbus as a living tank to storm the doors at the Roswell. The giant knights would think he was a fire-breathing dragon and fall back. "Wait right here, Nimbus, and let me call the crew to beam up Agent Aroma."

The crew appeared from every corner of the Phoenix. As they worked, they gawked at red-faced Nimbus.

"What kind of detox is he doing, chief?" asked one of the crew. "He looks like he's been in one of those Native American sweat lodges!"

"Are you having any visions yet, Nimbus?" asked another crewmember.

There was no reply. Nimbus was breathing hard now as the Phoenix began its descent. The crew was mopping the sweat from the floor and getting ready to follow behind him. They were as strong as Nimbus was wide, a powerful force to be reckoned with!

## The Roswell

Meanwhile, at the Roswell, the giant knights were discussing last night's lottery winners. The garden nymph scouts heard the giants calling out numbers as they moved cautiously into place. Were the fairies to be auctioned? Could the Fairy Navy SEALs rescue them in time? The nymph scouts scurried into place, trembling with apprehension, as the hawks delivering them dove out of sight.

Suddenly, the Phoenix landed and prepared to lower a wing. The crew chief called for a clearance and slowly aimed his pitchfork. "Sorry, Nimbus," he said. "I promise to recommend a violet heart award and free tickets to the local all-you-can-eat diner." Then, the chief poked Nimbus with his garden pitchfork where he was jiggling the most.

"Yeeooowww!" cried Nimbus, in searing pain. "Enemy fire! Let me out of here!" Nimbus steamed out of the Phoenix with the flight crew right behind him, pitchforks ready to make sure he stayed on course. The rescue mission was about to commence.

The Fairy SEALs cried, "On to victory, fairies. Remember the Roswell!"

Nimbus's ears were so full of the ginseng rush that he could hardly hear his own screams. He produced a cloud of sand as he moved forward, shrieking "Yeeooowww!" Back at the Roswell, the lookout alerted the captain of what appeared to be a desert windstorm.

"Captain, look at that twister in the desert!" called out the Roswell's lookout. "It looks like it's headed our way! Better call the weather bureau and send out a plane. We could throw out some chemicals to disperse it. Listen to it howl!"

As the door to the Roswell opened for the weather team to head out, they realized it was too late. Just as the door opened its widest, Nimbus flew in and crashed to the floor. Kaboom! Nimbus fell hard and heavily, producing enough steam to disperse a fine mist throughout the room. The impact of the fall ignited the Agent Aroma bomb simultaneously. The combination was both relaxing and sedative. Even the Fairy SEALs dropped their garden tools and swooned into a euphoric sleep, followed by the fearless giant knights.

In an instant, everyone was fast asleep, except Nimbus, who was examining his backside for shrapnel and catching his breath. Suddenly, he heard a faint cry for help from a giant knight. Hoping he would offer food for ransom, Nimbus shuffled toward him, dragging the remnants of Agent Aroma behind him.

The giant pointed in the direction of the cells that held the fairies in captivity. "Get him out of here," he whispered. "He's been driving all of us nuts!" With that, the giant tossed the keys to Nimbus and drifted off to sleep.

Nimbus was still hoping the keys were to a giant refrigerator or, better yet, a bakery, when he heard a loud noise in the direction the giant had pointed.

"Get me out of here!" cried a shrill voice. "Hey, are you one of those blimps that advertise used car dealerships?" Nimbus was too sore to be insulted.

"Well, climb on down from that cell and help me find some food," he replied. "I feel my blood sugar falling. I won't make it much longer now." Nimbus jiggled the keys until the door opened. The hyper fairy kept right on talking while Nimbus opened his cell.

"Sure looks like you could stand to lose a little weight," he continued. "What are those little holes in the back of your leotard? You know, for the first time in my life I feel sort of normal! I think I'll sit down for a minute. Ah, this feels good! I always wondered what it would feel like to sit down. Is that a happy face I see on the back of your pants? Looks more like a grinning Cheshire cat it's so stretched. You know, chubby, that funny smell you're dragging around sure calms me down." The hyper fairy smiled at Nimbus, while he chattered as though they were old friends.

Nimbus smiled politely back to the chatterbox fairy. Suddenly, a very strange feeling came over him, too. He was not hungry! The more he inhaled the aroma cloud following him around, the more he felt his appetite slip away. Maybe he was dying! No, fairies didn't really die, he thought to himself; they were given blinking lights and carried into the heavens to become stars. No one has located a light big enough for him yet, and the angels put a rider in his contract naming Nimbus a high-risk fairy. Oh well. He'd rather eat than blink anyway, at least until this bomb came behind him and changed his ways. With luck, it wouldn't last much longer, but right now Nimbus couldn't even think about food.

## Nimbus Falls in Love

Instead of looking for food, Nimbus walked from cage to cage, unlocking doors so the captives could escape as they awakened. All of a sudden, his eyes were drawn to the most beautiful sight he had seen since discovering a seven-layer chocolate cake with caramel frosting. It was a fairy, clad in a lavender dress with ice cream cones printed on it. Lavender ice cream! Now that's something Nimbus hadn't tried before. But instead of his stomach growling, he felt his heart chakra bubble like a carbonated drink.

As his eyes danced over every inch of her gorgeous body, Nimbus mused. She was lovely, a perfect ten, and everything he had ever dreamed of in a woman. Large, full, and heavy! The sight of her made his heart thump wildly. Oh, what a complement she would be for his kitchen. No one could be that heavy without possessing exquisite cooking skills. He intuitively sensed she could really clean her plate, too.

Nimbus forgot all about the kitchen and that noisy hyper-fairy and sat down beside her. He fantasized about holding her hand through a seven-course meal. And what might this lovely Madonna's name be? He leaned over and read her inmate tag sewn over a particularly large ice cream cone. "Ah, yes, of course. Her name is Sweet Tooth! Lovely name, lovely woman!"

Sweet Tooth began to stir. She smelled chocolate on Nimbus, who always kept some on him for emergencies. Her dreamy eyes slowly opened. She smiled at Nimbus and asked, "Are you a sugar-woofer?"

"Why, yes," he replied, and quickly searched for his knapsack for something sweet. His pants were too tight to carry candy in his pockets. He had tried it once and still harbored memories of many long hours trying to get out the candy. Nimbus didn't want to keep Sweet Tooth waiting. This was his chance to make a favorable impression on her!

He reached into his knapsack and dug out a handful of chocolates. He watched in awe as she ate every one. Oh well, for some reason he wasn't hungry. Anyway, he was thoroughly enjoying every moment of her graceful hand-to-mouth movements.

"Is there any more?" she asked as she licked her dainty fingertips. Nimbus stood up, reaching out his hand to her. This was his chance to bring her into his arms!

"Come with me, lovely lady, to a land of milk chocolate. I'll provide you with every chocolate known to Fairyland. You'll never be in want of chocolate as long as we're together," Nimbus announced proudly.

This was just the commitment Sweet Tooth had been waiting for. She smiled sweetly and offered her hand to him. They joined hands and walked down a long corridor toward the kitchen together. They had a long life of meals to share and so many desserts! Surely this was heaven on earth!

The new couple sampled desserts in the kitchen and spent hours talking and comparing dietary preferences. Sweet Tooth was not only an accomplished cook, but also a very delightful person. Her charm and beauty secured a place in Nimbus's heart that would grow into a fruitful romance.

While Nimbus was in the kitchen stealing a kiss, the fairies and giants awakened. Immediately, fairy medics prepared aroma blends to soothe every need and complaint. After recuperating from the effects of the bomb, the giants realized the fairies were not a product of germ warfare or alien origin, but a compassionate breed of elementals. The fairies were quickly released from the Roswell and allowed to return to the Land of Thyme after a show of arms and a twenty-one-gun salute from the grateful giant knights.

## The Return

The Phoenix groaned as it slowly gained speed. The extra passengers filled the seats to maximum occupancy. The fairies and their rescuers were in a festive mood as they returned home. Medics continued to massage the passengers who were stressed by the flight.

Only one passenger was working hard the entire flight — the budding journalist, Spider, on his first assignment. All eight legs were busy typing what would later be published as "The Secret Chronicles of Operation Fairy Storm." Every aroma blend, tea, and recipe was carefully documented for future use as only a reporter, such as Spider, could do. Spider could never be as important as a flower fairy, but he was determined to be the best reporter in the Land of Thyme.

## THE SECRET CHRONICLES OF OPERATION FAIRY STORM

The following blends are taken from "The Secret Chronicles of Operation Fairy Storm." Proceed with caution before using them, and do not — I repeat, *do not* — administer ginseng elixir with the Agent Aroma blend!

### AGENT AROMA BLEND

Although the exact blend cannot be divulged due to top-secret garden security, the following one is acceptable for insomnia, stress, hyperactivity, food cravings (except possibly lavender ice cream), and muscle tension. This blend is also safe for children and pets. (Avoid eye contact.)

To each cup of warmed bottled water, add the following essences and spray into the air, or apply two drops on the temples and neck for immediate relaxation.

10 drops lavender essential oil

5 drops sage essential oil *(Salvia officinalis)*

2 drops each of the following floral water essences prepared by distillation of fresh, blooming herbs: French lavender, spike lavender, purple garden sage, and yarrow.

**Note:** This blend can be added to an aroma lamp to disperse scent throughout the room.

**Variations:** For a knockout massage oil, blend the above essences and essential oils in two ounces of a carrier oil, such as jojoba, canola, sweet almond oil or equal amounts of the three. Pour into a dark glass bottle with a plastic screw top. Allow one to three hours of curing before applying. Set the bottle in a pan of warm water three to five minutes before massaging. Store any unused blend in a dark bottle with an airtight screw top.

For back pain, an excellent carrier oil can be prepared with the yellow flowers of St. John's wort *(Hypernicum perforatum)*. The spring blooms can be gathered daily from an abundant source and kept covered with canola oil in a glass bottle for three weeks. Use a wide, sterile glass jar, and macerate (crush) six flowers in two ounces of oil. After three weeks, strain all plant material very well. Store in a cool place in a dark glass bottle for up to six months. Essential oils and flower essences may be added after straining. Shake well before using. For acute back pain, see a physician. See also "How to Massage a Fairy" at the end of this chapter

### ANTISEPTIC ANTIVIRAL BLEND

The following is an antiseptic blend used by Fairy SEALs for germ warfare. The blend may be dispersed in interceptor missiles or through a room humidifier for maximum efficiency. It's a killer blend during cold and flu seasons.

    1 cup distilled or bottled water
    7 drops thyme essential oil
    5 drops eucalyptus essential oil (especially if asthma or upper respiratory infections are a concern)
    4 drops sage essential oil
    2 drops silver lace flower essence
    1 drop of yarrow flower essence (optional, for extra potency)

Blend ingredients and spray or disperse in the room.

**Variation:** This blend can also be added to a cup of canola oil or a carrier oil of your choice and applied to the back thoracic area. Several drops may be rubbed into the chest.

### HEAT EXHAUSTION BLEND FOR NIMBUS

This blend is very refreshing during hot summer days. It can also be used to increase alertness during the day.

    1 cup bottled water
    5 drops spearmint essential oil
    5 drops lemon grass essential oil
    Spray around the face and neck. Avoid eye contact and abrased skin.

## TIRED ACHY FOOT BATH

The rescue team was treated for blisters and sore feet with the following essences.

    1 cup of warmed bottled water
    5 drops lemon balm and lavender essential oils
    2 drops rosemary essence


## LEMON GRASS MOSQUITO AND ANT REPELLENT

The following aroma blend keeps the fairies free of mosquito and ant bites all year. Mosquitoes just hate the taste of lemon on their dinner. Apply immediately before gardening or going outdoors. Heavy oils like sesame and olive oil sedate the skin and stay on longer. Reapply every two hours or when you hear a singing, buzz-diving noise around you. This blend also repels ants and it's safe for children and pets, but avoid eye contact.

    2 ounces of sesame oil or olive oil
    10 drops lemon grass essential oil

**Note:** Growing lemon-scented herbs in the garden, patio, and lawn will also repel mosquitoes. The fairies recommend lemon basil, lemon thyme, and lemon grass.

    **Variation:** For an effective flea repellent, add five drops of eucalyptus to the above blend, and rub onto your pets before playtime. Fairies generally jump higher than fleas. (Well, except Nimbus.)


## Insect Repellent Ointment

This blend was combined for Nimbus because it spreads over large areas. It's a general insect repellant for those who attract more bugs than fairies when enjoying the great outdoors!

    4 ounces coconut oil
    2 teaspoons of beeswax
    10 drops lemon grass essential oil
    5 drops eucalyptus oil
    5 drops tea tree oil or thyme essential oil
    2 drops neroli, pennyroyal, or oregano essential oil

Melt the coconut oil and beeswax in a double boiler. Remove from heat and pour into a four-ounce sterile jar. Allow to cool, stirring twice to assure consistency. Perforate the mixture with a fork and add the essential oils (already blended). Seal with a screw-top lid. Allow to blend for thirty minutes to one hour before scaring the bugs away.

## SUNBURN

When the sun nipped the fairy scouts' noses, they used this blend.
 1 cup cold bottled water
 1 tablespoon vinegar
 6 drops lavender essential oil
 3 drops chamomile essential oil
 2 drops yarrow essences

Apply with a clean cloth or cotton ball. Fairy wings are especially sensitive to the sun. If necessary, reapply every thirty minutes until the sting of the sunburn fades.

## GINSENG ELIXIR

The following is the energizing tonic used by the Fairy SEALs during maneuvers. Nimbus does not recommend it! Neither is it recommended for those who abstain from a low-fat diet and enjoy their extra padding. It may raise metabolism and lower fat cell production.

To 2 cups distilled or bottled water, simmer the following ginsengs for one hour:
 2 tablespoons chopped root American ginseng *(Panax quinquefolium)*
 2 tablespoons Siberian ginseng *(Eleutherococcus senticosus)*
 5 jujube red dates *(Zizyphus jujube)* to relax and smooth muscles, avoiding tight shoulders and headaches.

Remove from heat and allow the tea to cool before straining. Serve warm and sip slowly. Serves two.

 **Note:** If hypertension or inflammatory intestinal disease exists, or headaches and tight shoulders result from ginseng drinks, substitute one ounce of foti *(Polygonum multiflora)* for ginseng. Foti is also safe for women on estrogen blockers and men taking estrogen to reduce prostatic cancer occurrence. However, it's best to check with your health care provider before drinking an herbal elixir.

## OVEREXERTION

If the Ginseng Elixir is too stimulating, make a tea of fresh gardenia or honeysuckle blossoms instead. Steep for ten minutes and strain before serving on ice.

1 cup boiled water
1 gardenia flower or 8 honeysuckle blossoms

Variation: An essential oil blend consisting of two drops each of basil and lavender and two drops of stock essence (a flower essence) can be diluted in four ounces of water and applied to the face with a cotton ball.

## WAKEUP FAIRY DUST

Sprinkle the Wakeup Fairy Dust in shoes or wear in a tiny muslin bag placed in a shirt pocket. Combine the following ingredients and stir:

1 tablespoon sea salt
2 tablespoons cornstarch
3 drops peppermint essential oil
1 drop lemon grass or lime essential oil

## BE ALERT TEA

Upon awakening, the following tea can be served.

1 cup boiled water
1 teaspoon of green tea
1 teaspoon of candy mint, orange mint, or peppermint leaves

Cover and steep for five minutes, then strain and sip during the *Good Day Fairy News and Talk Show* from 7 to 9 a.m. on the Sunrise Channel!

**Note:** Green and black teas contain caffeine and are not recommended for those with fibrocystic breast disease, hypertension, insomnia, and anxiety.

After the smoke had cleared and re-entry was safe, a team of fairy medics was sent in to help other newly released captives. After looking around, the fairies decided they would also help the sleeping giants, but helping the fairies came first! They would awaken sooner than the giant knights since they are more ethereal and aided with a special fairy dust sprinkled by the reconnaissance scouts.

## POST-TRAUMATIC STRESS BLEND

For those fairies feeling a little insecure or suffering from post-traumatic stress syndrome, the following blend was applied to the heart chakra center.

    1 ounce jojoba carrier oil
    2 drops vanilla essential oil
    2 drops vanilla flower essence
    2 drops wisteria flower essence
    2 drops begonia flower essence
    1 drop white hyacinth flower essence
    1 drop each of rosemary essential oil and rosemary flower essence

Store in a clean, dark bottle and shake well before applying two drops to the heart center twice daily.

## FAIRY EYE-OPENER HERB TEA

Fairies prefer this tea while watching early-morning cartoons.

    1 cup boiled water
    1 teaspoon fresh or dried chamomile flowers
    ½ teaspoon spearmint leaves

Cover and steep for five minutes. Strain. Add one-half of a teaspoon of tupelo honey and stir well.

## MUSCLE AND WING TENSION BLEND

Nimbus used this blend the day after carrying the Agent Aroma bomb around the Roswell. For muscle stiffness and tension, add the following essential oils and essences to several ounces of peanut oil or canola oil or a lotion of your choice.

3 ounces of oil or lotion
3 drops peppermint essential oil
1 drop ginger essential oil
2 drops pine essence

Allow to cure one to three hours before applying topically. Smooth onto arms and legs and briskly rub the tight muscles.

## I CAN'T BELIEVE I'M SEEING FAIRIES BLEND

When the giant knights finally awakened, they required treatment for shock. A bouquet of harmonious essences was sprayed to acclimate them with the natural elements.

To create this blend, dilute two drops each of a blend of rose and vanilla essences in two ounces of bottled water. Add two drops of white hyacinth flower essence. Using an atomizer, spray on the hair and neck until the head clears.

## LAVENDER ICE CREAM CUSTARD

After the giant knights finished rubbing their eyes in disbelief, they were served this treat from Sweet Tooth's kitchen recipes. The following recipe is just enough for Nimbus, so be sure to make an extra batch for guests.

**Ingredients**
¾ cup sugar or ⅓ cup fructose
2 tablespoons cornstarch
1 egg
1 cup lavender infusion: Steep three tablespoons lavender flowers (fresh or dried) in one cup of boiled water, covered, for five minutes. Strain.
1 cup heavy cream or soy cream

Blend the sugar or fructose, cornstarch, and egg at high speed for one minute in a blender. Pour all ingredients into a pan and cook over low heat until thickened, stirring constantly. Refrigerate to reach room temperature. Beat cream or soy cream until it forms stiff peaks. Fold into custard. Garnish with a few lavender flowers and freeze until firm. Serves two, or one giant appetite!

## How to Massage a Fairy

For a therapeutic massage, consult a licensed fairy masseuse.

Fairies enjoy a gentle touch. They benefit from some basic massage strokes with a romantic blend of aromatic essential oils.

Choose a warm, quiet room. Turn down the lights and play some relaxing music. Fairies are shy and need time alone to take off their wings and things and dive underneath clean covers.

Provide a firm table with padded covering or a futon placed on the floor. Cover the table with a clean sheet. Place an aromatherapy blend on a nearby table in a small bowl of heated water.

Wash your hands in warm water and towel dry them. Rub them together to make sure they are warm.

Begin with the feet. Bathe and dry them before applying a small amount of oil. Place one hand on the sole of the foot, the other hand on top of the foot. Work the oil on to and between each toe. Then move on to the ball of the foot, using your thumbs to work in the oil. The arches are a little tender. Soft strokes will reduce tension. Use a little more oil on the sole of the foot since it tends to be drier. Rub the top of the feet before moving up to the ankles. Massage around the ankles with your thumbs, and then move onto the calves.

Gently squeeze the calves as you massage them and increase circulation. Work up to the back of the knees with firm strokes.

Continue to the top of the legs with firm, brushing strokes. Slowly work more oil into cellulite with a kneading motion.

Carefully turn the fairy, keeping him draped with a clean wrap. Massage the other side of each leg, stroking sideways to the top with alternating hands. Keep upward strokes firm, downward ones light. Knees can be massaged with circular movements using the thumbs.

Fairies especially enjoy a brisk backrub. Position the fairy on his stomach with his arms cradling his head. Lightly touch the base of the spine and head simultaneously to establish a rapport with the energy pattern. Fairy and masseuse should relax and breathe together a few times.

Lightly cover the entire back with oil. Be sure to get under the wings. Use the thumbs to make circular movements on the neck, staying clear of the vertebrae. Lightly squeeze the trapezius muscles descending from the neck, sliding your hands over the shoulders and down the little arms. Hands and fingers enjoy some attention, so work down to the tiny fingertips.

Begin again at the base of the neck and slide your hands across the shoulders. Rub down both sides of the back with circular motions, never touching the spine. Use slow, rhythmic movements. Place your thumbs above the hips and make an outward curve over the hipbone. Complete the massage by using long, slow strokes over the entire back. Have you ever heard a fairy snore?

## BLEND FOR RHEUMATIC PAIN

When fairy wings begin to creak, this blend gives a lift to their wings.

    1 cup sesame oil, canola oil, or St. John's Wort oil
    7 drops eucalyptus essential oil
    5 drops rosemary essential oil
    4 drops peppermint essential oil
    2 drops zinnia and yarrow essences, for an extra lift

Massage the blend into unbroken skin and apply a hot pack.

Relaxation is a wonderful way to allow the body to heal itself. Even fairies become stressed at times. To learn more about relaxation, the fairies study "aromafairapy." Their favorite teacher is none other than Sweet Tooth, the lovely fairy who stole Nimbus's heart.

---

### WHEN TO AVOID MASSAGE
- Do not massage when back pain is severe, or after an operation.
- Do not massage a fairy with fever or during an acute illness.
- Do not massage if cancer is a possibility. Check with a physician first.
- Do not cause discomfort.
- Do not massage after a sauna or hot bath when the body is eliminating through the pores.
- Do not massage after mealtime. Wait one hour.
- Do not massage any injured area.
- If the fairy is very tiny, consider practicing on Nimbus first for a larger surface.

# CHAPTER 4

# Aromafairapy
## Blending Essential Oils

*"Earth laughs in flowers."*
Ralph Waldo Emerson

## A Lecture from Sweet Tooth

Sweet Tooth, besides being an excellent cook, is a professional beautician who specializes in flower petals. The name of her business is Pretty Petals™. During her several years of clinical practice, she has become quite accomplished in the use of herbs and flowers for beauty and skincare.

Now that the Roswell had been captured, the fairies were busy planting native herbs and flowers, and Sweet Tooth was summoned to help nurture them. While they worked, the attending fairies asked Sweet Tooth to share her knowledge about skincare. Sweet Tooth had beautiful, soft porcelain skin like vanilla custard.

"Our face mirrors our health and attitudes," she said, her sweet voice rising above the hum of the crowd. "The Chinese believe we inherit the face of an angel until thirty. After thirty, we inherit the face we deserve!" Everyone laughed and Sweet Tooth continued, content that the audience was relaxed.

"The skin is a dynamic organ that regenerates every twenty-eight days as the moon cycles. It is the body's largest detoxifying organ, extending cellular longevity by breaking down chemicals, toxins, and environmental pollutants. Our skin also initiates immune-stimulating thymic cell production. This affects organ function, increasing lymphatic drainage and the elasticity of connective tissue. Beautiful skin can indicate a healthy immune system!"

Sweet Tooth paused to make sure the fairies were following her lecture. Then, she cleared her throat and continued.

"Essential oils, flower essences, and therapeutic herbs awaken this vital energy. They soften the skin, preserve hydration, and reduce fungal, viral, and bacterial invasion. Aromatic compounds balance the central nervous system. They enhance stress management by reducing insomnia, depression, anxiety, tension, and muscular aches, while increasing circulation. The skin responds beautifully to chemical-free, organically grown plant products."

The fairies nodded in agreement as they shifted on their leaf cushions.

"Each plant has a unique color, aroma, texture, genetic memory, and therapeutic quality inherent in its cells. In aromatic plants, these are concentrated as volatile oils. They are alcohols, which evaporate into the air. Floral and citrus scents have a floral molecule shape and are referred to in perfumery as 'high notes.' Mints, spices, and woody scents are wedge-shaped and referred to as 'middle notes.' Resins like myrrh, vanilla, amber, and sandalwood are round and are called 'low notes.' These are often blended in aromatherapy to create a scent that lasts for hours. High notes awaken the highest centers of the cortical brain and dissipate quickly. Middle notes bring in a mysterious quality to a blend and offer a long-lasting scent. Low notes hold the scent so it dissipates slowly. When we smell these scents, they can change our mood, reduce stress, and affect our perception of life.

"We can also use essential oils to make perfumes. Creating a unique perfume is called a 'signature scent.' Always use a dark sterile dram bottle that is thoroughly dry. Perfumes spoil in a dusty or damp bottle. Measure essential oils in drops. One teaspoon is equivalent to sixty drops!"

A curious fairy interrupted Sweet Tooth. "What is an essential oil and how is it made?" she asked.

Sweet Tooth blushed, and then chuckled. "Of course, I assumed everyone already knew these things! Essential oils are steam distilled from pounds of fragrant herbs and flowers during their peak season. The flowers or leaves are ground to expose these volatile oils and combined with distilled water. Then the plant mixture is cooked in a thick glass container that's attached to a glass elbow and a glass condensing tube. During the heating process, the condensation produces fragrant, healing water, called a hydrolate, and a small amount of essential oil, which floats on top. The essential oil is separated by hexane, a solvent, or by hand using a glass separator. I prefer and only use natural separation, free from chemicals that may offend sensitive fairies."

"What is a volatile oil?" asked several of the fairies in unison.

"A volatile oil is the fragrant aroma contained in an essential oil," replied Sweet Tooth. "Volatile means that the molecules of fragrance evaporate quickly into the air as they are released from the plant. They can rise faster and higher than a fairy!"

The fairy audience oohed and aahed at the thought of anything faster than a fairy. As the crowd became silent, one fairy asked, "Why don't fairies smell like essential oils or their fragrant water?"

"Actually, we do have a unique smell," replied Sweet Tooth, intrigued by the questions of her curious listeners. "Actually, every organic living thing or being has a unique scent they carry throughout life. The scent originates genetically, like a peach or apple. In fairies, and even the giants at the Roswell, the scent enhances social, reproductive and parental behavior. The people and experiences we attract are often determined by our unique odor."

With that thought, everyone turned and stared at Nimbus for several reasons. First, Nimbus turned bright red, then grinned from ear to ear as his eyes met Sweet Tooth's and glowed with delight.

Sweet Tooth blushed as she smiled and turned to the audience to continue her lecture.

"Let's learn how to make fairy scents and essential oil blends," said Sweet Tooth, as the fairies flew circles around her before settling near the demonstration table. She held a small, dark bottle high above the crowd and began to lecture.

Here's a combination that will lift you even higher than your wings do.

In a 1 dram dark-colored bottle, add:

20 drops rose essential oil

10 drops geranium essential oil

2 drops lemon balm essential oil

4 drops sandalwood essential oil

Fill the bottle with distilled water and cap tightly. Allow the perfume to cure for a few days, protected from bright light. Apply the perfume to warm skin so the body's heat will lift the aroma: Wear the blend behind the ears, on the temples, throat, or between the breasts.

## Carrier Oils

"Carrier oils are used to dilute essential oil blends, especially for massage and therapeutic uses. Carrier oils soften the skin and promote elasticity." Sweet Tooth handed out the following information on large maple leaves. Here are examples of the most popular ones used alone or in essential oil blends.

## Carrier Oils for Essential Oil Dilutions and Blends

• **Jojoba Oil** is derived from the nut of a desert plant. It is an ancient healing agent of the Native Americans, used for eye and throat infections and numerous skin afflictions, such as psoriasis and eczema. It does not oxidize and will not spoil. Jojoba has a natural emulsifying ability, excellent for handmade creams, and it's a natural sunscreen, sun-proof fairy screen of 4 (SPF). As a cold-pressed oil, it nourishes all skin types and contains vitamin E. Jojoba oil is odorless and combines well with essential oils and fragrances. Jojoba oil penetrates the skin and hair very rapidly.

• **St. John's Wort Oil** (*Hypernicum perforatum*) is an excellent choice for massage, burns, and wounds. Pick fresh flowers from an abundant source and steep in canola oil for three weeks before straining. Canola oil is a good source of essential fatty acids that nurture the skin and reduce inflammation. Calendula flowers can be substituted for St. John's wort flowers. Calendula oil is traditionally used to reduce inflamed skin and wrinkles around the eyes.

Note: Steep two grams of flowers in one ounce of canola oil. *Hypernicum perforatum* will turn the color of the oil red.

• **Olive Oil** (cold pressed) is a disinfectant healing oil helpful for wounds, rheumatism, and infections. It benefits dry skin and hair and blends well with tree resins such as pine, sandalwood, and vanilla. It is a heavier oil that does not deeply penetrate the skin's surface.

• **Coconut Oil** is stable to 76° and then melts. Coconut oil improves rehydration of the skin and is excellent for massage. It is safe for babies' skin and often is used in blends with other carrier oils to enhance mature skin.

• **Aloe Vera Gel** can also be used to create harmonious blends. The fresh gel is best. Add two drops of grapefruit seed oil to reduce oxidation. Aloe vera gel tightens the skin, maintains moisture, and stimulates circulation. Aloe also treats burns, eczema, and psoriasis, combining well with St. John's wort oil for treating wounds and burns.

• **Wheat Germ Oil** is a natural preservative high in vitamin E. A small amount of oil is derived from pounds of wheat kernels. The oil is especially beneficial for dry and aging skin. It is usually diluted into another carrier oil to extend shelf life by adding twenty percent to another oil and essential oil blend. It becomes rancid when exposed to air, so refrigeration is necessary to extend its shelf life.

• **Sweet Almond Oil** has been used since ancient Roman times to nourish the skin and heal wounds. It aids every skin type, especially dry, sensitive skin. Almond oil is preferred for its penetrating properties.

• **Hazelnut Oil** is used for damaged, dry, and burned skin. It blends well with sandalwood, rosewood, and sweet, exotic fragrances such as ylang ylang.

• **Evening Primrose Oil** (*Oenothera biennis*) reduces acne, psoriasis, dermatitis, and anxiety. It is used orally and in aromatherapy massage oils. The tiny seeds of the yellow evening-blooming flower are high in omega 6 essential fatty acids and linoleic acid, and are a hormone regulator. One half teaspoon of primrose oil can be added to two teaspoons of carrier oil, or it can be applied directly to a skin problem.

• **Borage Oil** is extracted from the seeds of the blue flowering borage, or "starflower." It is higher than evening primrose oil in essential fatty acids and less expensive. The oil is often blended with evening primrose oil, using twice as much borage oil for massage and stress-relieving formulas. It is most beneficial for aging skin.

**Note:** Use at least ten drops of essential oils for every ounce of carrier oil. The blends will last six to eight months when stored away from heat in a dark glass bottle.

## Hydrolates

"What can we do with the water that condenses from essential oil distillation?" asked one of the fairies.

Sweet Tooth paused and began to explain hydrolates.

"Hydrolates are the aqueous by-products of steam-distilled essential oils. They contain minute amounts of essential oils and can be taken internally, as well as worn externally. I often splash a favorite scented water on my face after washing. In medieval times, hydrolates were used as compresses to treat eye problems such as conjunctivitis. Rose, lavender, and rosemary hydrolates were often used for this purpose. Many hydrolates, such as lemon grass, lemon balm, neroli, and lemon verbena, make excellent skin toners. Others, such as chamomile, yarrow, sandalwood, and lavender, are especially beneficial due to their anti-inflammatory properties."

Sweet Tooth continued:

"In Renaissance times, hydrolates were used medicinally. They were considered more effective than essential oils for ailments:

• **Rose Water** decongests the liver and gallbladder, relieving heartburn, nausea, and poor fat digestion.

• **Lavender Water** was used as an antibiotic for the intestines and to stimulate the immune system to abate cancerous growths. It can be applied topically to the abdomen or directly on a growth. It can also be used to cure warts.

• **Chamomile Water** was used for colic and intestinal problems. Dill seed and fennel seed hydrolates were also used for these ailments. The hydrolates can be applied to the abdomen as a warm compress or sipped as teas. One or two ounces for an adult is sufficient after meals.

• **Lemon Balm Hydrolate** was used to relieve stress and overexertion. (Nimbus could have used some to sedate the effects of the Ginseng Elixir.)

• **Orange Water** was given at the onset of a cold and as a heart tonic for chest pains. The water was distilled from fresh orange rinds. Two ounces were taken to abate a cold.

• **Sage Water** was applied to the face to decongest the sinuses and relieve facial swelling and numbness. It can be sipped like a flavored water or tea to reduce sinus congestion and promote better digestion. Some prefer to use it topically due to its strong flavor.

• **Grapefruit Water**, distilled from rinds, cleansed the intestines and normalized low-blood pressure. It was not used for people with high blood pressure or migraine headaches. It was believed to make them worse. Two ounces can be sipped as a tea once a day.

• **Lime Water** was used to reduce flatulence and stimulate metabolism, increase energy, and reduce weight. A few ounces were sipped upon rising. Sweet Tooth chuckled. "I obviously haven't tried it."

• **Marjoram Hydrolate** lowers high blood pressure by dilating blood vessels. It was used to calm excessive sexual desires and promote menstruation. Marjoram oil and water are not used during pregnancy or for those who bleed easily because of its ability to dilate blood vessels. It can be applied to the face and neck or a few ounces may be sipped as a tea once daily.

During the lecture, the fairies were sitting on the end of their seats, their wings on a low hum. Nimbus's eyes were crossed. Sweet Tooth was wearing a rose-colored blouse that reminded him of marmalade. Hearing her informative lecture made his heart swell with love and admiration. Her mannerisms and presentation were as sweet as her name.

Mother Nature was attending the lecture. She thought her heart would burst with pride. Flora was hoping to teach Sweet Tooth that fat-free did not mean "all the fat you could eat." She gave up momentarily when she saw Sweet Tooth taking a chocolate break to get her blood sugar up before resuming the lecture. This gave Flora an idea. She soon disappeared to formulate her plan.

## How To Use Essential Oils

During the break, the fairies asked Sweet Tooth for more ideas on using essential oils. She licked the last drop of chocolate from her fingers, and launched into a new explanation.

## Aroma

Lamps are a simple, subtle way to transform a room into a place with magical healing qualities. An aroma lamp is a ceramic or glass container using a small amount of water heated by a candle. Add five to fifteen drops of essential oil to the warm water and allow the fragrance to fill the room. Choose one or a blend of two or three essential oils, such as lavender, lemon balm, and sage.

- Relaxing aromas for the home include lavender, sage, sandalwood, geranium, chamomile, lemon balm, and clary sage.
- At work, use aromas to enhance concentration, such as lemon grass, lime, tangerine, lemon verbena, or peppermint.
- Children enjoy vanilla, lavender, tangerine, and lemon balm in a playroom or bedroom. Lavender will help children sleep or reduce hyperactivity.
- Air fresheners and disinfectants include thyme, eucalyptus, lemon grass, rosemary, hyssop, tea tree, sage, lavender, and pine. They're great during the flu and cold season and are quite energizing.
- The essential oils of lemon grass, eucalyptus, geranium, wintergreen, and cedar repel insects. Apply a dilution on unbroken skin or release the scent into the air with an aroma lamp.
- Favorites for meditation are sandalwood, frankincense, and patchouli.

"If you don't have an aroma lamp, here are some other ways to use aromatherapy," smiled Sweet Tooth. "Aromas can be added to a bowl of heated water, a humidifier, or dabbed on a warm light bulb. A few drops of essential oil can enhance the atmosphere in a room within minutes. We can change our mood by the aroma we choose."

## Saunas

Essential oils can be combined with water and poured over warm sauna stones. Just dilute five drops in two cups of warm water and pour it over warm stones to facilitate detoxification. Favorites include eucalyptus, pine, lemon grass, thyme, cedar and tea tree. These aromas are also antiseptic and reduce viral and fungal growth while stimulating phagocytosis, the white blood cells that dispose of invading bacteria.

## Compresses

Warm compresses can be applied to the face or an ailing body. Dilute four drops of essential oils in one and a half cups of warm water. Saturate a clean cloth with the aromatic water and apply to the neck and face. Lavender, basil, sandalwood, and rosemary are especially beneficial. Cold compresses may be prepared to reduce headaches or recent traumatic injury by adding essential oils to chilled water.

## Sitz Baths

Sitz baths can be used to alleviate many common ailments. In a shallow tub of water, add fifteen drops of essential oils dispersed in a tablespoon of honey. The following recipes are historical treatments used to reduce symptoms.

For abdominal and menstrual cramps, use basil, chamomile, and marjoram. If pregnancy is not possible, use lavender or sage to reduce discomfort.

Rosemary and peppermint increase circulation and reduce tension after a stressful day.

To reduce insomnia, dilute clary sage, lavender, and sandalwood in a shallow tub of water.

Thyme, tea tree, and eucalyptus can be used to treat athlete's foot and external fungal problems that affect the skin and nails.

Lemon grass and lemon balm refresh the spirit, stimulate energy and increase mental alertness.

Pennyroyal and oregano help heal sprained ankles and bruises. Stimulating essential oils such as these are not recommended for pregnant women.

Ginger can be used to warm the body, increase circulation and open the pores. It can be used to abate the onset of a flu or cold, reduce arthritic and rheumatic pain and promote detoxification through the skin. Hypertensive fairies, pregnant women, and those experiencing heavy menses should avoid ginger baths.

## Foot Baths

"Gee, I could use some healing oils to soothe my sore feet after tilling the garden. Can any relaxing oils be used in a foot bath for an old fairy with aching feet?" inquired an elderly gardener fairy.

"Why, yes," replied Sweet Tooth. "I recommend fifteen drops of a combination of the following essential oils: four drops of rosemary, four drops of lemon balm, five drops of lavender, and two drops of clary sage for tired fairy feet. Soak in a shallow pan of warm water for fifteen to twenty minutes and your feet will feel as light as your wings!"

"Do you have any suggestions for varicose veins from poor circulation? My legs suffer after a full day of flying around the flowers. All my blood seems to stay in my wings," an old timer called out from the back of the fairy audience.

"Hmmm," pondered Sweet Tooth while tapping her manicured finger on two beautifully formed lips. "Oh! I know! Take a sitz bath with ten drops of each of lemon balm and yarrow. That will soothe the veins. Then add a few drops of pine essential oil to increase circulation. Remember to soak twenty to thirty minutes, since longer baths can drain your energy.

"Of course," continued Sweet Tooth, "a combination of basil and sandalwood is excellent for meditation and calming the emotions. I would use ten drops of sandalwood and five drops of basil because sandalwood opens the heart and basil calms the mind."

"Wow! I like the idea of meditating in water. It reminds me of the natural birthing process!" exclaimed a fairy mother. "Can essential oil baths stimulate milk flow for nursing mothers?"

"Why, yes," answered Sweet Tooth. "European fairies use fennel or dill essential oils to stimulate milk production and add a few drops of sage essential oil to promote the let-down response allowing the milk to flow. They enjoy the essential oils in a bath or sometimes they simply smell the aromas several times a day before nursing."

## Therapeutic Uses

"What other ailments do the European fairies use essential oils for?" asked a studious fairy who was rapidly taking notes.

For cystitis and bladder irritation, dilute five drops of lavender and clary sage in a tablespoon of honey and add it to a warm bath.

For abdominal cramps or delayed menses, combine eight drops of marjoram, five drops of rosemary, and two drops of chamomile. An alternative blend is six drops of oregano and four drops of pennyroyal.

Remember to avoid marjoram, chamomile, and pennyroyal if pregnancy is a possibility. Consult with your doctor first."

"Is there any way to tell if your body will respond well to an essential oil or blend?" asked the studious fairy.

"Good question," smiled Sweet Tooth. "I always ask the recipient to test the aroma by passing it under their nose first. A brief sniff will allow the body to respond. If the odor is offensive, I make a different blend or ask the fairy to choose a scent they enjoy."

"What if I want to immerse my whole body in a tub or aromatic water?" asked a fairy who was flying over Sweet Tooth to attract her attention. "Should I make a blend using a carrier oil and add it to a tub of warm water?"

"For a full body bath, aromatherapists use cream or honey as an emulsifier," replied Sweet Tooth as she cocked her head to one side and looked up at a fairy flying just above her head. "However, I have used honey when cream was not available. Both honey and cream rehydrate the skin. For every two to four tablespoons of cream or honey, add ten drops of essential oils to set a mood for relaxation and pleasure."

"Can we use honey and cream in the same bath?" asked the flying fairy.

"Oh, yes," she replied. "Use two tablespoons each of honey and cream. Be sure to add the essential oil mixture after the bath is drawn. Otherwise, the essential oils evaporate quickly. We want to experience them on the body as well as an aroma floating in the air."

Suddenly, a tiny fairy stood atop a beautiful purple echinacea coneflower and shouted, "What about a love aroma to attract a lover? I'm so little no one can even see me to ask me out! Maybe I can attract a handsome fairy with an aromatherapy blend."

The crowd clapped and cheered, calling out to Sweet Tooth for a love aroma.

Sweet Tooth giggled as she waited for the crowd to settle down. She had her favorite combination in mind as she reached into her cosmetic bag, threw out several candy wrappers, and pulled out four little brown bottles. Each bottle contained a different fragrance. A combination of each would charm the wings off a butterfly.

"Here's a combination to attract a lover," said Sweet Tooth, as she held up each dark brown bottle.

To 1 dram of jojoba oil, add:

5 drops rose oil, distilled from fresh blooms

2 drops lavender oil

1 drop sandalwood oil (Mysore of sandalwood essential oil is the best grade)

Then, add 2 drops gardenia flower enfleurage fragrance.

She blended the combination as she talked.

"Allow to cure for three hours before applying to your throat and heart. Curing is just another way to allow the combination to blend into a unique aroma."

The fairies each took a sniff as she passed around the combination. Everyone agreed it would attract a lover, or at least some beneficial insects! Nimbus was at the end of the line and left the bottle open as he continued to day-dream about you-know-who. The alluring scent brought a swarm of friendly bees that were racing to locate the origin of this lovely fragrance. When Nimbus saw the bees headed his way, he grabbed the bottle and started running. He ran as fast as his chubby little legs could carry him. The only sound was Nimbus's legs rubbing together as he ran. The bees were right behind him. They had no idea a fairy could run so fast!

In his haste, Nimbus spilled the whole dram of aromas on himself. He was breathing hard from running and quickly sniffed the fragrance in such a large dose that he was soon seeing stars. He imagined the bees to be cupids until one finally caught up to him. "Yeeeooowww!" Nimbus blindly ran into a large object that was blocking his exit. It was Sweet Tooth, bending over to smell a new plant surreptitiously left by Flora. Nimbus was taken by her beauty. He stood beside her, dazed, massaging his stinging backside.

As Sweet Tooth stood up, Nimbus's heart chakra opened wide, very wide, and he blurted, "Sweet Tooth, would you marry me?"

Sweet Tooth had just had her first sniff and taste of chocolate mint and stood up, exclaiming, "Yes!"

She had no idea what Nimbus had said; she just knew she had found the ultimate culinary herb. They smiled as their eyes met. Each moved closer until their lips became as one. The combination of her chocolate mint and his rose blend made a new, unique love blend, a winning combination for both!

The fairies that were following them cheered in unison, throwing their tiny fairy caps wildly into the air. Roadside flowers were opening and closing their petals and beating the grass with their lower leaves.

The bees began buzzing a happy tune and took off to spread the news.

There are no secrets in the closely knit fairy community. They enjoy love and laughter, knowledge and gain, tears and pain as one entity.

As his romantic heart sang, Nimbus disconnected from his embrace with Sweet Tooth. He bent over and grabbed one of the many chocolate wrappers surrounding Sweet Tooth and wrapped it around her dimpled finger as an engagement ring.

A tear came down Sweet Tooth's round cheek as she ate the last of the chocolate mint leaves. She never expected to experience so much happiness in one day. Of course, she accepted Nimbus's proposal joyfully, but her mind quickly began to think of all the culinary delights she could make with chocolate mint.

There were other blends Sweet Tooth wanted to share, but, overwhelmed with love and passion, she dropped her lecture notes and headed for the kitchen, where a new world of culinary delights awaited her. Nimbus tiptoed right behind her. No one knows what happened behind closed doors, but the following list includes the recipes Sweet Tooth left behind:

## SWEET TOOTH'S SHAMPOO RECIPES

Add ten to fifteen drops of essential oils to four ounces of an unscented shampoo. Follow the chart to make appropriate choices. Use up to four essential oils to create an essential oil blend just right for your hair.

**Dry, colored or permed hair:** Geranium, rose, marigold mint
**Dandruff:** Yarrow, lemon balm, pine, sandalwood
**Itchy, scaling scalp:** Tea tree, clary sage, lavender, sandalwood
**Split ends:** Ylang ylang, orange, lemon balm, rosemary
**Hair loss:** Rosemary, lemon grass, coriander, pine
**Increase hair growth:** Rosemary, coriander, aloe vera gel
**Oily hair:** Lemon grass, sage, rosemary
**To enhance blonde hair:** Marigold mint, grapefruit, lemon grass, thyme
**To enhance brunette hair:** Sage, rosemary, peppermint
**To cover gray hair:** Coriander, sage, oregano

## CREATE YOUR OWN CONDITIONER

A conditioning treatment can be created from a flower oil or jojoba and castor oil. Add the following essential oils and allow the mixture to blend overnight. Work into the hair, especially the ends, and rinse thoroughly with cool water after thirty minutes.

2 ounces castor oil or flower oil, such as calendula or St John's wort
2 ounces jojoba oil
5 drops sandalwood essential oil
5 drops lavender essential oil
5 drops clary sage or ylang ylang essential oil for a flower fragrance

Any remaining conditioner may be stored in a dark glass bottle for up to three weeks.

**Note:** To make flower oil, steep one tablespoon of flowers in two tablespoons of warm oil for ten minutes. Mash the flowers during straining.

## ROSE OIL LIQUID SOAP

Pure castile soap combined with rose oil makes an exquisite showering soap as light as fairy wings.

10 tablespoons grated castile soap
4 ounces rose water or hydrolate
½ teaspoon almond oil
5 drops rose essential oil

Melt the castile soap in a double boiler, and then add the rose water or hydrolate. Immediately remove melted mixture from the heat and slowly stir in the almond oil and rose essential oil. Pour the liquid soap into a clean squirt bottle, preferably glass, and dispense in tiny amounts.

## FRUITY BATH SALTS

Allow stress to melt away in this refreshing bath.

2 cups of Epsom salts
1 cup baking powder
½ cup sea salt
3 tablespoons of fresh, finely chopped orange or tangerine peel
6 drops of orange or tangerine essential oil

Combine the Epsom salts, baking powder, and sea salt and mix well. Then add the orange or tangerine peel and the essential oil. Combine and cap tightly in a glass jar. Allow to cure at least three hours before adding one or two cups to a bath of warm water.

# CHOCOLATE MINT AROMATHERAPY FROM THE KITCHEN

While the fairies showered in the nearby garden fountains to try out some of the aromatherapy recipes, Sweet Tooth emerged from the kitchen with a new culinary aroma recipe. Nimbus followed right behind his new love with a spoon in hand.

## CHOCOLATE MINT AND ROSE SORBET

For those who would like to taste what Sweet Tooth was creating in the kitchen, try this for aromatherapy.

**Ingredients**
- 4 ounces superfine sugar
- 1 cup chocolate mint tea, room temperature*
- 2 lemons, juiced, and grate the rind
- 1 cup chocolate mint leaves blended with the chocolate mint tea in a blender
- 1 egg white, beaten stiff
- 1 cup distilled rose water

Dissolve sugar in one cup of rose water over low heat. Add lemon rind and simmer for five minutes. Remove from heat, stir in blended chocolate mint leaves, and refrigerate until cool. Add lemon juice and freeze in a plastic container until crystals begin to form. Fold in the stiffly beaten egg white and freeze until firm. Serve in chilled champagne glasses with a few chocolate mint leaves to garnish and one drop of rose oil atop each sorbet. (Distilled rose essential oil is safe to ingest.)

* To make chocolate mint tea, steep two teaspoons of fresh leaves in one cup of boiled water for five minutes.

## A Visit to the Rose Garden

While Sweet Tooth cooked and smooched with Nimbus in the kitchen, the rose fairy, Rosie, invited the other fairies to tour the antique rose garden later in the evening. The fairies were delighted that so many roses were in bloom.

"The roses look especially lovely this year, Rosie. Could you tell us more about the origin of roses and how to use these lovely flowers blooming in profusion today?" asked one of the touring fairies. The other fairies encouraged her by clapping their wings as they gathered around Rosie.

Rosie blushed as she climbed above the crowd and perched atop a newly opened rose. She cleared her throat and began her lecture, feeling a little insecure.

"Roses have flourished since prehistoric times, even before homo sapiens. The first roses had five petals, except *Rosa sericea,* a four-petal rose. They reproduced from seed and produced a variety of scents and colors to attract pollinators."

"Why do the old roses have such big thorns?" asked one of the younger fairies.

"To repel predator insects and small animals who would feed on their tender buds," replied Rosie, smiling.

"Didn't roses always live in gardens?" asked a baby fairy.

"Why, no," replied Rosie. "Roses are believed to be wild plants that originated in the northern hemisphere, specifically, Europe, Asia, America and the Middle East."

"So when did roses come to live in a garden?" asked the young fairy.

"Probably around five thousand years ago in China," replied Rosie, "as early as 500 B.C."

"Ooohh," signed the fairies in unison.

"Roses are almost as old as Mother Nature," piped one of the young fairy gardeners.

"Shh!" hushed one of the old timers. "You know she doesn't like us to talk about her age."

"Well, then, tell us what the ancient gardeners did with the roses," replied the novice gardener, changing the subject.

"Ancient cultures first produced flower essences as enfleurages," Rosie continued. "Fresh flowers were repeatedly soaked to saturate a medium, such as animal fat. I use the humectant properties of vegetable glycerin to pull off the flavors, scent, and catalyzing properties of highly scented flowers. My process takes one to three years to extract the fragrant healing properties. When applied to the skin, body temperature will produce a subtle scent and a chemical action, catalyzing healing from within us. These may help people, pets, or beneficial environmental elements like fairies!"

"What do enfleurages do and how do they heal us?" asked the fairy gardener.

"As a healing agent, enfleurages sedate and soothe the skin," Rosie replied. "They may be safely applied to smooth skin such as the face, or to open wounds or inflamed skin. Their action is slowly released over a period of six to eight hours. Enfleurages are applied undiluted directly to the skin. They are especially soothing for children, pets, and people."

"Can anyone benefit from an enfleurage fragrance?" asked the novice gardener.

"Yes," replied Rosie. "Their scent is very subtle and non-offensive to chemically sensitive men and women. The scent of an enfleurage immediately affects the brain through our sense of smell. The brain then signals hormones to be released into the bloodstream and throughout the nervous system to allow the whole body to respond to the scent. Some scents stimulate us, such as lilac and white ginger, while others sedate us, like curry and lemon balm."

"But what about rose enfleurages? What do they do?" asked one of the fairies as he snuggled into a rose bud.

"Enfleurages are made from antique roses," explained Rosie. "They carry the original scents of the most ancient flowers. Antique roses are also called old roses. Their blooms look different from hybrid roses. Antiques often have flat, open blooms or cabbage-looking roses. Their parentage is either unknown or dated before 1865."

"That's not very old," exclaimed an old timer. "My parentage dates back to the beginning of the Land of Thyme!"

Both the roses and the fairies giggled with delight. No one else could imagine being so old, except Mother Nature, and she never talks about her age!

Rosie waited to attract everyone's attention before continuing. "Antique roses carry a scent that attracts friends and lovers into your life. Enfleurages are a simple way to wear the scent that best suits your needs."

"Give us some examples, Rosie," cried the small crowd of fairies.

"Okay," she replied as she pointed to a nearby rose. "This beautiful pink cabbage rose is Alfredo de Damas. It has a fragrance that attracts romantic love from others."

The fairies became quite attentive when romance and lovers were mentioned.

"I want that one," sighed a dreamy fairy.

Rosie chuckled as she moved to the next rose. "This salmon and yellow beauty is Fortune's Double Yellow. It has a very subtle scent that dispels loneliness and reduces anxiety about a lover."

"Maybe I need that one, too!" exclaimed the dreamy fairy. The audience laughed.

"You need to have a lover first," explained an old timer as he patted the wishful fairy on the shoulder.

The tiny fairy shook his head in agreement and followed the crowd to the next bush.

Against a fence a huge, vining rose stood draped in creamy, large flowers. The scent of gardenia filled the air.

"This is the gardenia rose," Rosie explained. "It attracts long-term love relationships."

"How did that big rose vine get here all the way from China?" asked a young fairy.

"They were brought over in ships by seafaring adventurers who held gardening close to their heart," smiled Rosie.

"Well, I definitely need that enfleurage," said the dreamy fairy as he inhaled the magical scent. "Will it help to just smell the rose?" asked the tiny fellow.

"Oh yes, please do smell them. The rose will surely find its way to your heart," Rosie replied as she invited them all closer.

The fairies filed past the many blooms, smelling each one before progressing to the next. They all looked a little dreamy as they were escorted to a bushy rose covered with bright pink blooms.

"This is Old Blush, another rose brought to the West from China." Rosie smiled proudly as the fairies all commented on the rose's many blooms. "This is a repeat-blooming rose. "Only Father Frost can coax Old Blush into resting," explained Rosie, as she walked past the bush.

Old Blush took the opportunity to bow as the fairies applauded. Rosie laughed. "Old Blush has a tea rose fragrance that increases energy and enthusiasm," she continued. "It is believed to warm the cold heart of a lover."

The fairies mumbled as they turned to each other and nodded. The dreamy fairy looked puzzled.

"Rosie, how can a lover have a cold heart? What does that mean? Is he dead?" queried the tiny fellow.

Rosie looked down and had nothing to say. Finally, she answered, "Well, that's what somebody told me," she stammered.

Old Blush stood nearby shaking its leaves and stems from left to right in response to Rosie's answer.

An old timer thought he understood the underlying problem and stepped forward to approach Rosie.

"Young lady," he chided, "you have to leave the past behind and any foolish lover who left you." He lifted his hand to Rosie's cheek as she began to cry.

The fairies gasped empathetically and gathered around Rosie to support her. Rosie's tears fell in puddles around their pixie feet.

"Don't cry, Rosie, please, don't cry!" they begged her.

Rosie was quite embarrassed. Her cheeks were turning crimson as she brushed the tears away and tried to smile.

Before she could answer, the dreamy, romantic fairy elbowed his way through the crowd to take Rosie by the hand. She could hardly see the lad through the blur of tears swelling in her eyes.

"Rosie," he began, caressing her tiny finger. "My fairy godmother once told me I'd meet a beautiful fairy with rosy cheeks and dewy eyes. Would you like to walk the gardens with me this evening?"

Rosie's cheeks burned brightly as she nodded in reply.

The fairies moved closer, peering over each other's shoulders at the potential couple. Suddenly, a gust of wind showered everyone with tiny pure-white petals. A light violet scent filled the air as the towering twenty-foot Lady Banksia vine called out to Rosie.

"What about me?" the vine called out. "Don't forget about me! I'm known as the Banksia rose and you can make an enfleurage out of me, too! What am I good for, Rosie?"

Rosie smiled as the fairies looked up and up and up to the top of the violet-scented rose, amazed at its height and beauty.

"Lady Eubanksia encourages trust in love relationships, and this is the end of my lecture." Rosie laughed as she accepted the arm of her new suitor.

As the couple walked away arm in arm, the fairies stood around shuffling their feet, not sure what to do with themselves. Slowly, the crowd began to disperse into the night.

One of the fairies walked up to the old timer and asked, "Isn't he a little young for her?"

"Love knows no age," the old timer replied softly as they walked into a moonlit path. "Love speaks to the heart through constancy, commitment, and respect. Where love grows, passion is sure to follow."

The old timer's voice trailed off into the distance as he walked toward his home with his newfound friend.

## How Essential Oils Are Produced

Many aromatherapists prefer distillation, as it has been used to produce fine essential oils for thousands of years. The oldest distillation unit is five thousand years old, found in the Indus Valley of present-day Pakistan. The ancient cultures believed aromatic oils to be sacred, a link between the spiritual and physical realms because they possessed smell, an invisible, spiritual presence, and a physical nature as a liquid or resin. The process of distilling was believed to correlate to inner, conscious growth and transmutation of the lower senses such as greed and lust.

Essential oils are extracted by one of the following methods and used with complementary medicines, cosmetics, perfumes, and worship.

Distillation is the most common method of releasing essential oils. Plant, leaves and/or flowers are stripped from the stems and ground to a paste at the time they produce the most oil. For example, the rose only produces oil when it blooms in early spring.

Once blended with distilled water, the plant material is poured into a glass container and boiled to soften the tissues. This causes the essential oil to be released and to condense. Both water and essential oil condense into a liquid as they pass through a glass pipe surrounded by cold flowing water. The oil and liquid drip into a glass vessel and separate. The essential oil, being more viscous, floats on top of the water and can be drawn off by a glass separator. The remaining liquid is used as floral water, such as rose water and held in ten percent alcohol.

Essential oils of delicate flowers, such as carnation and jasmine, are made by solvent, absolute extraction. The flowers are mixed in a volatile chemical solvent, hexane, until the solvent penetrates the flowers and pulls out the essential oil and resinous properties. This liquid is poured into another container and very gently heated until the volatile solvent vaporizes. The remaining extract is called a concrète. The concrète is then mixed with 190 proof, pure alcohol, which separates the residual wax from the absolute, containing the essential oil. The final product is sold as an absolute essential oil. Most rose oil is obtained as an absolute, because steam distillation is costly. Thousands of rose petals will produce less than an ounce of essential oil by steam distillation.

Citrus oils are expressed from the outer rinds of fruits, such as orange, lemon, and grapefruit. The rinds are squeezed, or expressed, in machines to produce essential oils.

Today, many large companies are using nitrogen or carbon dioxide to extract essential oils under high pressure. No solvents or distillation are used. The process is very expensive, but yields unadulterated oil.

## What Every Fairy Should Know About Aromatherapy

Essential oils have been used by ancient cultures for medicine, cosmetics, perfumes, and ritual worship. They are the oldest psychoactive substances known to man.

Essential oils contain many naturally occurring chemicals and components, producing a unique physical, mental, emotional, and spiritual effect.

Smell has the most impact on our emotions. The olfactory nerve, which relates to the sense of smell, is the sense organ that connects the external world to the brain and has the greatest influence on how we feel.

Smell is associated with memory and the sense of well-being. Specific aromas reduce stress and enhance relaxation, creativity, alertness, and productivity in repetitive tasks. Aromatic odors can be detected indoors at levels of twenty parts per trillion.

According to clinicians, the healing qualities of aromas are not apparent in synthetic, "nature-identical" chemical reproductions of essential oils.

Essential oils can become more effective the more they are used as the body learns to respond to each aroma.

Store essential oils away from light, heat and air. Cap tightly to avoid oxidation and alteration of the aroma. Use a dark-colored glass bottle with a plastic screw top. Avoid rubber inserts, since essential oils will destroy them.

Use a patch test on the arm to try out an essential oil blend. Wait one hour before applying a blend to other parts of the body.

Essential oils may take from thirty minutes to fourteen hours before traces of aroma molecules are voided in the urine.

If irritation occurs, rinse with cold water for twenty minutes. Always avoid the eyes when applying oils. If eye contact is made, rinse with cold water or proceed to an emergency medical clinic.

Use half doses for children under twelve; one-quarter doses on babies. Children respond best to relaxing blends such as lavender and vanilla.

Avoid using essential oils and aromas if a medical physician diagnoses cardiac fibrillation.

Check with your fairy midwife or doctor before using essential oils during pregnancy. Best selections include rose, lavender, sandalwood, vanilla, and lemon balm.

# CHAPTER 5

# Pet Scents

## Aromatherapy and Herbs for Animals

*"All my hurts my garden spade can heal."*
Ralph Waldo Emerson (1803–1882)

### Collie Seeks a Cure for Itching

The next morning everyone was back to work in the gardens. Nimbus had been assigned to the herb gardens, where he was hard at work. He was hoping to reduce his appetite by working near the lavender blooms. Sniffing the odor made him dream of Sweet Tooth and lavender ice cream. The number of bees in the garden distracted his daydream, making him feel a little anxious about his past run-in with them.

As Nimbus worked hard to keep his backside away from the bees, a local pet approached him.

"Hey, Nimbus," called Collie, "I heard there was an aromatherapy lecture here last night. Were any blends for pets mentioned?"

"Well," stammered Nimbus. "I don't think so. I was so taken by Sweet Tooth's beauty I forgot to take notes."

"Wow! You've really been bitten by the love bug," laughed the collie.

"Actually, I got stung by a bee, but it all worked out okay because Sweet Tooth agreed to marry me," Nimbus explained as he worked.

"Well, congratulations, you lucky fairy! This is one ceremony I don't want to miss!" Collie exclaimed. "Hey, since you're really close to Sweet Tooth, do you think you could ask her for some blends for pets like me? I've got a case of fleas that keeps me awake itching at night."

"I'm so sorry you're itching. Gee, with the army of ants that lives nearby I wouldn't expect fleas to be a problem," Nimbus replied.

"Well, I intend to go see the fairy healer and clean up my diet, but I just thought you might put in a good word for us pets to Sweet Tooth. We'd like to use aromatherapy, too. I'm tired of smelling like a dog and itching like a monkey," he laughed.

"I'll see Sweet Tooth at lunch today. We've planned a picnic in a secret garden all alone," Nimbus grinned sheepishly.

Suddenly, out of thin air, a fairy buzzed by and interrupted the conversation.

"Wow! A picnic! Can I go, too, Nimbus?" the buzzing fairy asked.

"Who is this energetic little guy? I've never seen a fairy flap his wings so fast and talk at the same time," remarked the collie.

"This is my gardening partner, Vinnie," Nimbus explained. "He's a little on the hyper side. We both benefit from the relaxing effects of lavender, so we've been assigned to the same garden. Just pinch some lavender buds and leaves to release their relaxing aroma and he'll come down to earth."

Thump! Vinnie landed in the garden relaxed and smiling.

"Now, what about this picnic? I love to eat, too. I think I'm getting hungry right now," said Vinnie as he looked around for the food.

"Good grief. I think I've seen it all, now. A hyper fairy," laughed Collie.

Nimbus turned to Vinnie and pleaded, "Vinnie, there's no food here now, but I promise to bring you extra helpings if you stay here and take care of the garden while I spend some time alone with Sweet Tooth."

"Well sure, Nimbus. You're always looking out for me. I'll be glad to help you, but you have to tell me what to do while you're gone."

"You can swat the fleas off my back with one of those lavender blooms," interrupted the collie. "It'll keep you and me calm until Nimbus returns with some essential oil blends. Ah! That feels good!" the collie moaned softly as Vinnie attacked his fleas with a lavender bloom.

Within a few hours, Nimbus returned to the garden waving his notes in the air as he talked.

"I have it, I have it, Collie. Here are some ideas for pet scents."

Nimbus's face was covered in chocolate lipstick kisses. He was too excited to notice Collie and Vinnie giggling and pointing to his face.

"Look, here!" he continued. "We can dilute five drops of eucalyptus essential oil in one cup of water and spray it on your coat. Or we can dilute the essential oil in vegetable oil and rub it all over your fur. Smells pretty good, huh, Collie?"

"Sure does! I can see the fleas jumping off of me as we speak! Did Sweet Tooth have anything that will sedate the itching?"

"Sure! She told me lavender oil will stop the itching and help you relax," replied Nimbus.

"Is lavender oil good for anything else?" asked Vinnie.

"Bee stings!" Nimbus guarded his backside as they all began laughing and walking into the garden.

"Do you know the fairy healer, Collie? I might want to go to her if I have another run-in with a bee."

"First of all, Nimbus, the fairy healer is male. Secondly, I've only seen him work on small animals, like pets."

"Does he treat pets for bee stings, too?"

"Well, no," laughed Collie, as he laid down in the shade. Vinnie sat next to him and dug into a large lunchbox packed by Nimbus and Sweet Tooth. "He sure is quiet when he has something to eat," observed Collie.

Nimbus chuckled as he sat down gingerly.

Collie stretched out between Vinnie and Nimbus and began to tell them his story.

## Collie's Story of Jason and His Remedies for Pets and Owners

"During gardening breaks, a fairy named Jason — which means 'the healer' — became friends with many of the neighborhood pets. His nature gave him a special rapport with the animals and they soon confided in him. He would not only listen, but would also make every attempt to help them with their problems. This led him to learn natural pet care. He gathered supplies, remedies, and wisdom from fairies and plants and applied his knowledge to help his pet friends in need.

"During his leisure time, he gathered plants from nearby gardens to make compresses, teas, and tonics for the ailing animals. The animals loved him and they mentioned him often to their fairy friends.

"When the garden fairies heard that Jason was a healer, they were quite surprised! The community had accepted Jason as a loner and left him alone. He was often seen walking in the gardens talking to plants and his animal companions and did not interact with the fairy community that often. The fairies knew very little about Jason's expertise or private life and mused about what they remembered.

"When Jason's former nanny learned of Jason's healing abilities, she recalled her memories of the child.

"Jason's a healer?" Nanny exclaimed with surprise. "I never saw him do anything but sleep," she laughed. "Every time he slept, he grew out of his shoes! That child had the biggest feet I ever cared for! I wonder how he learned about healing with herbs and flowers?" Nanny pondered.

"Maybe he learns in his sleep because he sure helped me out of a bind when I had heart worms. He gave me raw garlic every day and a flower essence made from an amaryllis. I never tested positive again!" explained the cocker spaniel. "It took a month or two before I knew I was healed. Jason continues to feed me a little raw garlic daily to keep me healthy."

The Siamese cat came forward to tell his story. "I had diabetes. Jason fed me a multigrain diet and cooked vegetables. He made an herbal tea with one teaspoon each of *Rehmannia glutinosa* and *Polygonum multiflorum,* and a one-quarter inch slice of licorice root, steeped in one cup of water for fifteen minutes. It looks dark, but tastes very good. He added a few drops of primrose essence in the tea and fed a cup to me with a dropper three times daily. I ate one teaspoon of brewer's yeast with my three small daily meals. I quit losing weight and felt much better in just a few moons," meowed the Siamese.

Then a Doberman walked to the forefront of the circle. "I had cancer. Before it became advanced, Jason started giving me a combination of lilac, Blue Danube aster, and gaillardia flower essences. Then he made a Bulgarian recipe. Jason mashed five and one-quarter ounces of aloe leaves in a wooden dish and mixed them with eight and three-quarters ounces of spring honey and twelve and one-quarter ounces of red wine. He poured the mixture in a dark glass bottle and refrigerated it for five days. He always strained and filtered the tea, and gave me one teaspoon to drink fifteen minutes before breakfast and lunch. I became stronger with each sunrise and now I am cancer-free. The recipe is an old Bulgarian folk recipe used by pet owners centuries ago. After I became stronger, Jason put me on a low-fat vegetarian diet, and I drank a tea brewed from the tops of stinging nettle. I watched as he steeped one heaping teaspoon in one cup of boiled water for ten minutes and strained. Jason poured a tablespoon in my water or fed it to me with an eyedropper. Look at me now," cried the Doberman. "I'm healthy!"

After the Doberman sat back down, another dog told how Jason helped him. "I had periodontal gum disease. Jason made a paste of one teaspoon of goldenseal root, one teaspoon of aloe, and one-quarter teaspoon of myrrh to apply to my gums daily. He just rubbed the paste directly on my gums and I was healed within one moon cycle."

Next, a shy pig wiggled to the front of the fairy circle. "When I fell, Jason wrapped my leg with yarrow leaves and it stopped bleeding! Then he bruised comfrey leaves in warm water and wrapped my leg to reduce my bruising. He applied a blend of essences and essential oils to remove trauma and help heal any hemorrhaging. I healed very quickly, and I loved Jason's compassionate touch," squealed the pet pig as he settled into a nearby puddle.

The fairies became very pensive and quiet until a Husky broke the silence.

"Achoo! Where are my aromas and essences for allergies? Jason gave me a combination of two drops of lemon balm and five drops of lavender in one ounce of jojoba oil. I wore it on my temples and down my neck. Just wearing it calmed my sneezing. He added a few drops of lantana and snapdragon flower essences to calm my immune response. And when my ears get waxy, he warms an oil made from calendula and mullein flowers. After he strains it, he adds a few drops of lavender or sage essential oil. That feels good! Then, he crushes a 500 mg vitamin C tablet in my food for an antihistamine. I believe in Jason and his natural cures!" exclaimed the Husky as he waddled to the back of the gathering.

Finally, a beautiful Persian kitten walked to the forefront of the circle swishing her tail as she addressed the group. "My skin breaks out. Jason calls it eczema. I get red patches of skin that itch and itch! Then, my hair falls out. I have rosy bald spots that itch and then bleed when I scratch. When I went to see Jason, he took one look at my skin and went to work. First, he made an infusion by steeping two tablespoons of gotu kola leaves, one tablespoon of fresh coriander seeds crushed with a mortar and pestle, and two teaspoons of rosemary leaves simmered in one cup of St. John's wort oil. He said canola or sweet almond oil can be used as a substitute. After fifteen minutes, Jason strained out the herbs and while it was still warm, applied it to my skin. It sure felt good. He even made a gentle shampoo from herbs. Now my fur has grown back long and luxurious."

## Gentle Pet Shampoo

The kitten smiled proudly as she produced a recipe for a mild shampoo that Jason wrote for her owner.

"Cut and bruise ten soapwort stems, six inches long," she read. "Bring to a boil in two cups of distilled water, cover, and simmer for twenty minutes. Add two tablespoons each of nettle tops and gotu kola leaves. Steep, covered, for ten minutes. Then, strain and bottle.

"When I asked him to add aromatherapy to my shampoo, he added two drops of lavender essential oil so I can attract a mate when I walk in the park. Lavender essential oil is kind to my hair and skin," meowed the kitten. "I'll let you know when I find a mate!"

Just then a very aggressive German shepherd joined the circle. Everyone scattered. Jason walked over to pet the shepherd. They had made friends some time ago, when Jason fed the shepherd until he could locate an owner. Shepherd mellowed from Jason's touch and confided in him.

"Jason, I don't understand it. Everyone leaves when I come out to play."

"Well, Shepherd, you're easily excitable and play very rough," Jason explained calmly. "Fairies don't like dog bites and you hog the toys from the other animals, too. When you bark and growl, it blows the fairy dust away. Why don't you let me help you? I will make you a calming essence of essential oils and flower essences."

As the animals watched from a distance, Jason diluted five drops of lavender essential oil, two drops of vanilla, and two drops of verbena flower essence into one cup of water. He sprayed his hand and applied it to the shepherd by petting him. Shepherd quit pacing and settled down beside Jason, who was just stretching out to take a nap.

## Calming Pet Blend

Jason uses one drop of this calming pet blend for every three pounds of weight.

    1 cup water
    ½ teaspoon valerian root
    1 tablespoon passionflower vine or skullcap leaves, fresh or dried

Simmer a half-teaspoon of valerian root in the water for fifteen minutes. Remove from heat. Add the passionflower vine or skullcap leaves, fresh or dried. A combination of the two can also be used. Cover and steep for ten minutes, and strain. Add ten drops in the water bowl or dispense directly into the side of the mouth with a dropper.

While Jason snoozed, Collie found more recipes crumpled in his pocket. Any leftovers are safe for pet owners, too!

## Calendula and Mullein Flower Ear Oil

Here's a soothing oil for inflamed or itching ears.

    1 tablespoon each of calendula and mullein flowers, or 2 tablespoons of 1
        flower
    ½ cup sweet almond oil, canola oil, or olive oil

Simmer the flowers in the oil for five minutes. Allow to steep, covered, for ten minutes longer before straining into a sterile, dark glass bottle. Apply two to five drops in each itchy ear. Warm the oil first by placing the bottle in a bowl of hot water for several minutes and apply the warm oil on a cotton ball before inserting into the ear.

## Cystitis

Cats are especially troubled with bladder problems. Here is a home remedy to help prevent or resolve any problems.

    1 tablespoon marshmallow root (*Althea officinalis*)
    2 cups bottled water
    1 tablespoon dandelion leaves (and/or chicory leaves)
    1 teaspoon red raspberry leaves
    2 drops begonia essence

Simmer the marshmallow root in the bottled water for fifteen minutes. Remove from heat. Add the dandelion leaves (and/or chicory leaves) and the red raspberry leaves. Steep, covered, for ten minutes. Strain. Add the two drops of begonia essence before dispensing. Dilute fifteen drops in a bowl of water or dispense fifteen drops directly into the side of the mouth with a dropper.

## Periodontal Disease

For bleeding or infected gums, rub this mixture directly onto the gums.

1 tablespoon goldenseal root powder
1 tablespoon aloe vera gel
¼ teaspoon of myrrh powder

Make a paste of the above ingredients and apply twice daily and for an additional ten days after symptoms abate.

## Immune Enhancer

Use this remedy to fight infection.

Dilute fifteen drops of echinacea root tincture in one ounce of distilled water. Dispense directly into the side of the mouth with a dropper three times daily, up to fifteen drops in one serving. Add 300 mg of powdered vitamin C daily for animals over three pounds. This can be sprinkled in the one ounce of echinacea tincture to be administered throughout the day.

There are two ways to make a tincture of echinacea. Note that two- to three-year-old echinacea roots may be used. Varieties include: purpura, augustofolia, or pallida roots. Only roots two to three years old have an appreciable amount of antibiotic properties.

• The most effective method is to soak two ounces of fresh or dried root in two cups of brandy, vodka, or gin for three weeks. Use a clean Mason jar with a tight-fitting lid. Strain the mixture after three weeks and dispense fifteen drops daily in water.
• Or, simmer two ounces of root in two cups of water for thirty minutes, covered. Strain and add two-thirds of a cup of brandy, vodka, or gin to prevent mold, or freeze the liquid in ice cube trays without adding the alcohol. To serve, defrost one cube daily and dispense fifteen drops three times daily. Refrigerate leftovers.

**Note:** Owners may use one teaspoon of echinacea tincture up to three times daily to enhance immune function at the onset of a cold or flu. Using it continuously will weaken natural immune responses. Discontinue use after seven to ten days or less.

## BLOATING AND FLUID RETENTION

For a safe, mild diuretic, make a tea of fresh dandelion leaves. It will also cleanse the kidneys and liver to alleviate the reoccurrence of symptoms.

Steep one tablespoon of fresh dandelion leaves in one cup of boiled water, covered, for ten minutes. Strain and dispense fifteen drops for every ten pounds. The tea can be directly dispensed into the side of the mouth with a dropper for pets. People and fairies prefer a cup, thank you.

## ANTISEPTIC BATH

Bathe your pet in this aromatic bath to repel fleas and ticks. Teach your kitten to appreciate a bath as early as possible to avoid frantic paw prints on your mirror.

An aroma sitz bath can be prepared with four drops of cedar essential oil and two drops of pinecone flower essence in one quart of water.

## EPILEPSY

Seizures are becoming quite common in purebred dogs. The following recipe can be taken in small quantities every other day with your veterinarian's blessing if seizures plague your pet.

Black cohosh tincture (*Cimicfuga racemosa*) is most effective for seizures prepared as an alcohol-based tincture. Soak two ounces of black cohosh root in four ounces of brandy, vodka, or gin for three weeks. Strain and dispense directly into the mouth, one drop per two pounds of body weight. The dose should be doubled for large dogs. Dispense a maximum of thirty drops at one serving.

Black cohosh tincture will produce drowsiness, especially in large doses of thirty drops. Only an alcoholic tincture as described above will reduce epilepsy.

## STRESS REDUCTION

Pets experience stress as well as empathize with their owner's stress. Here's an aromatic blend that will calm the storm of stressful emotions.

1 cup water
5 drops lavender essential oil
2 drops vanilla flower essence
2 drops sandalwood essential oil

Blend the ingredients and apply twice daily to the ears and neck.

## FOR INTERNAL BLEEDING AND SHOCK

Internal bleeding can be abated with shepherd's purse (*Capsella bursa-pastoris*). Proceed to the nearest animal hospital immediately to determine the cause.

Simmer one ounce of cut dried herb in one cup of bottled water for ten minutes, covered. Strain and dispense with a dropper one-half teaspoon per ten pounds of body weight. Apply white hyacinth essence on the pet's coat every fifteen minutes for shock and trauma.

## PET BIRTH

One cup of tea daily, two to three weeks before delivery, can facilitate, or make the birthing easier. Passion flower (*Passiflora incarnata*) leaves may be substituted or combined with skullcap. Check with your pet midwife before serving. Steep one tablespoon of raspberry leaves and one teaspoon of skullcap leaves in one cup of boiled water for ten minutes. Strain and serve one tablespoon twice daily.

To enhance relaxation during birthing, combine this aroma blend.

3 drops sage essential oil
3 drops lavender essential oil
1 drop pennyroyal essential oil
4 ounces warm canola oil
2 drops vanilla orchid flower essence

Combine the sage, lavender, and pennyroyal essential oils in the warm canola oil. Add the vanilla orchid flower essence and apply to the tummy and limbs of the mother during the birthing process.

## FOR SPRAINED OR CALLUSED PAWS

Reduce swelling and pain with this soothing blend.

    1 tablespoon fresh comfrey leaves
    1 cup heated canola oil
    3 drops peppermint essential oil
    3 drops oregano essential oil
    2 drops pennyroyal essential oil

Steep the comfrey leaves in the heated canola oil for ten minutes, covered. Strain and add the peppermint, oregano, and pennyroyal essential oils. Apply gently twice daily.

## BOWEL PROBLEMS

Functional bowel problems can cause diarrhea or constipation. Use the following recipes appropriately and consult with your vet.

For constipation, simmer one ounce of dandelion root (*Taraxacum officinales*) in two cups of water for fifteen minutes. Strain. Add two drops of crossandra flower essence and dispense twenty-five drops for every ten pounds of weight. The tea may be combined with food or dispensed by mouth with a dropper. Add a few tablespoons of cooked, pureed vegetables or whole grains into the diet. Pets less than ten pounds should use five to ten drops.

For diarrhea, restrict solid foods for forty-eight hours. Steep one tablespoon of carob powder or lotus root power *(Nelumbo nucifera),* which is available at Asian supermarkets, in one cup of boiled bottle water for ten minutes. Stir and serve two tablespoons every hour until symptoms abate. The liquid may be dispensed by mouth in a syringe.

## ANEMIA

If anemia is diagnosed, the following tea can be served daily.

    2-inch square of *Rehmannia glutinosa*
    1 cup water
    1 teaspoon blackstrap molasses

Simmer the *Rehmannia glutinosa* in the water for thirty minutes. Strain. Add the blackstrap molasses and serve one tablespoon for every ten pounds of body weight. Mix with food or dispense by mouth in a syringe three times daily.

Refrigerate leftovers or serve one-half cup to listless pet owners who complain of chronic fatigue.

## ARTHRITIS

Arthritis is a chronic condition of aging that may have many causes. The following formula will alleviate symptoms and allow the body to regenerate in time.

Steep one ounce of yucca root powder and one ounce of devil's claw in two cups of brandy, vodka, or gin. Strain after three weeks. Dispense fiffteen drops per ten pounds of body weight one to three times daily until symptoms abate.

Owners may benefit from this formula if arthritic problems occur. Dilute one teaspoon three times daily in water to reduce inflammation and pain.

## HEART HEALTH

These herbs will improve circulation and tone the heart muscle.

For a healthy heart, steep one tablespoon each of hawthorn berries, gotu kola leaves, and rosehips in two cups brandy, vodka, or gin for three weeks. Strain and serve fifteen drops per ten pounds of weight in water daily.

This is a great heart tonic for owners. Dilute one teaspoon in water daily to enhance circulation.

## Nimbus Plays Cupid

After Collie shared the recipes in Jason's pockets, he fell fast asleep, enjoying a mid-afternoon nap next to his fairy friend. As Jason escaped into dreamtime, visions of the woman of his dreams floated through his head. He smiled and sighed peacefully. Dreamtime offered him security from the external world that often overwhelmed him. Sleeping was the only remedy Jason employed for his problems. He was painfully shy and felt inadequate around women, except when he dreamed, and it seemed as if Jason were sleeping more and more these days.

In contrast, the tiny fairy who wished to attract a handsome lover wasn't sleeping at all. She was busy making a love essence. As she walked through the moonlit gardens at night, the tiny fairy cried out for one who would fulfill her love essence. The aroma she wore attracted many insects. She competed with the alluring scent of the petunias and night blooming jasmine, but had no lover. Exhausted and lonely, she cried her heart out in a nearby garden, perched on a large rock.

While she sobbed, a garden snake crawled out from underneath the rock and twirled his forked tongue.

"Surely I can help you, my sweet. Tell me why such a lovely little thing cries such large tears."

"For just that reason," replied the tiny fairy in anger. "I'm so little no one can find me, even with this romantic love essence I'm wearing!"

"I see," smiled the snake. "This is very serious, but my ancient wisdom can overcome such a difficult problem," mused the snake as he scratched his molting skin on the rock. "Give me just a moment to scratch while I devise a plan of action."

"Why should I trust you?" sobbed the tiny fairy. "You're just a lowly snake. Why, you can't even fly!"

"Hey, hey," chided the snake. "We got a bad rap in a garden a long, long time ago. Things have been downhill ever since. Just give me a chance to redeem myself. I don't even know what an apple looks like, but I do have friends in high places. Believe me, I can help. Now, what's your name, little one?"

The tiny fairy began to cry again. "I don't have a name. I was so little as a baby, no one could even see me, and now I don't have a love relationship because I'm so little!"

"I got it," the snake said. "We'll just call you 'Petite.' Don't worry. I can take care of all this and you'll have the pick of all the eligible men. Just you wait and see," the snake promised as he slithered out of the garden while Petite fell fast asleep from exhaustion.

While she slept, the snake visited his only friend, Vinnie, and told him about the forlorn fairy.

Vinnie listened as he paced the garden. "Do you think I should ask Petite for a date? I don't have a girlfriend."

"Well, maybe not this time," the snake replied. "I have her hopes built up for someone really special, but I have an idea that you could help me with."

Vinnie leaned over, allowing the snake to whisper his plan in his ear. As the snake explained his plan, Vinnie's eyes grew as large as his wings. He nodded his head in agreement and announced his intention to find his only friend Nimbus to help them out. He flew swiftly toward the gardens.

It wasn't long before Vinnie found Nimbus. He figured out right where to look for him. Nimbus was enjoying the company of his new friend, Collie. They often walked the garden paths and swapped stories about the good old days. Collie usually gave Nimbus a piggyback ride home, which was pure delight for his tired wings.

In his excitement, Vinnie flew directly into their path and landed in Nimbus's lap, chattering with excitement. He soon relayed the whole story and snake's plan of action, flapping his wings as he bounced up and down in Nimbus's lap.

Nimbus listened carefully, but was too overwhelmed to answer.

"Cupid?" he stammered. "You want me to dress up like Cupid and fly over the Spartan fairies' campsite?"

The thought of Nimbus dressed up like a cherub caught Collie by surprise and he began to laugh. "All you need is a small bow and arrow," he chuckled.

"That's right! We need a bow and arrow," exclaimed Vinnie as he flew out of sight.

"What possessed Vinnie and Snake to ask me to dress up like cupid? I don't even resemble a cherub," whined Nimbus.

"They need somebody chubby and dimpled for a cupid and you fit the description," replied Collie.

"What about using a real angel?" asked Nimbus.

"They're all on holiday overtime right now. It's Mushroom Festival, you know. Besides, you always want the best for others, so you're just like an angel."

Nimbus blushed. "Well, now what about me having to fly out of a nearby tree?" he asked. "I can't fly that high and besides, the trees we planted last year are just seedlings. They bend very easily, you know."

"I know a tall pine tree in the area that would be willing to help us. My owners have a small pulley we can use to lift you up so you appear to be flying," explained Collie. "Just think of it as an adventure and trust the process."

With this, the two friends left to meet Vinnie and Snake, stopping along the way to borrow the pulley. Nimbus hesitated at the sight of the pulley, but Colley coaxed his friend into continuing.

"Just think about helping this lovely, petite fairy," reminded Collie.

Nimbus smiled weakly, nodded, and marched toward the tall pine tree, trying to imagine himself flying like an angel.

Vinnie and Snake caught up with Nimbus and Collie on their way to the pine tree. They brought with them a ruffled white sheet for Nimbus to wear and a toy bow and arrow from one of the pet owners' children. Snake, smiling wisely, produced a very large bottle of love essence to disperse over the Spartan fairy camp nearby.

As Nimbus dressed, protesting loudly, the pine tree dropped a few pinecones in disbelief.

While Nimbus struggled with the ruffles on the sheet, Collie began to hoist him into the air very slowly.

"Wait! Wait! I forgot my bow and arrow!" shouted Nimbus.

Vinnie flapped furiously to bring Nimbus the bow and arrow with the large bottle of love essence in a spray decanter. Snake and Collie cheered on Nimbus as he was lifted higher and higher, jerking and swinging with each pull. The higher he was lifted, the more he resembled a real cupid, equipped with bow and arrow and ready to advance on a lover for Petite. However, just as he aimed at the Spartan fairy camp, a cold wind began to blow in from the north. Old Man Frost was arriving with a winter storm. As the wind blew, Nimbus began to swing wildly back and forth, his bow and arrow pointing in a different direction each time. The pine tree tried its best to stand tall, but the winter wind soon shook the limbs as it howled through the campground. Nimbus defended himself vigorously against the cascading pinecones, but was unprepared for the bite of the pine needles as they pierced his tender backside.

"Ouch! Get me down from here! I'm being attacked by killer bees!" His voice was soon muffled as the ruffled sheet engulfed him.

Below, his friends clapped and shouted, "Shoot! Shoot! Shoot!"

Collie barked, "Let'er rip, Nimbus!"

Nimbus did just that. Bow, arrow, and the bottle of love essence went flying from under the ruffled sheet. The wind played a tune on the bowstring as it sailed through the air. A crowd was gathering below and soon moved toward the destination of the bottle, bow, and arrow, while Nimbus dangled helplessly dodging pine needles.

Vinnie and Collie worked quickly to bring Nimbus to safety, as Snake slithered away to awaken Petite. Collie and Vinnie assured Nimbus he'd accomplished his aim and became a hero of the garden once again. Nimbus swooned as his feet touched the ground and he collapsed into his ruffles. Vinnie flew off to find Jason, hoping to obtain a salve to heal his friend's wounds and revive him.

### Jason Falls in Love

Before Vinnie arrived, Jason was rudely awakened by a flying object. The bow and arrow narrowly missed his head as the decanter of love essence fell across his chest. The aroma filled the garden, bringing birds, bees, and, finally, Snake with Petite riding on his shiny, new skin.

Jason smiled sweetly as he inhaled the lovely aroma. It reminded him of his dreams and he felt another good sleep coming on. Before he closed his eyes, he felt, then saw, something sliding across his chest. He jumped onto his feet, yelling, "Ugh! A snake! I hate snakes!"

As Jason hopped around, Petite laughed out loud. Just then, Jason got a big whiff of her love essence. Her smile made her visible as her white teeth flashed in the sunlight. Then her love aroma filled the air.

Jason was taken aback by her smile and aroma just long enough for Snake to take cover under a rock. Jason forgot about the snake and just about everything else as his eyes met Petite's. He was sure this was the woman of his dreams. She looked a little taller in his dreams, but the scent was unmistakably hers. His smile reached from ear to ear as Jason's eyes twirled in delight. As he reached out to touch her, she flew into his hand, batting her eyelashes demurely.

It wasn't necessary. Jason was in love already. He reached out to hold her close to his heart, indulging in her scent and winsome smile.

Nearby, Snake coiled underneath a rock.

"I don't know what it is about those fairies," Snake complained to himself. "They always want to be in love with starry eyes and kissy face. Yuck! I prefer a solar-heated rock any day!"

Meanwhile, Vinnie followed his nose to locate Jason. As he came close, he flapped furiously in an effort to find him. The strong aroma of the love essence momentarily disoriented him and he landed on the tip of the arrow.

"Ouch!" Vinnie screamed. "My wing is torn and I feel wonderful! I must be back in heaven!"

"Actually, you're on my foot, jumping up and down," explained Jason. "Let me apply some comfrey salve to your wing to help it heal quickly."

"Gosh! That's a foot? I never saw one so big in all my fairy days!" Vinnie remarked. "Hey! What's that little thing on your chest?"

"I'm the woman of his dreams," chided Petite. "I've come into his life to fulfill his heart's desire." She dazzled the boys with her alluring smile.

"Gee, I feel all sticky!" Vinnie replied, looking around to see what happened to him.

Jason couldn't take his eyes off Petite and applied comfrey salve from head to toe on Vinnie, smiling dreamily all the while.

"Save some of that salve for Nimbus," reminded Vinnie. "He's been in a sword fight and sustained some minor injuries!"

"We'd better go help him!" cried Petite. "Jason, can you give Vinnie and me a ride? Vinnie's wings are stuck together and it's too cold for me to fly!"

Petite nuzzled up to Jason as she spoke. Jason nodded in agreement as he tucked Petite in his shirt pocket close to his heart and Vinnie slid down his back and attached himself to Jason's belt loop.

With that, the threesome took off into flight to help Nimbus, while Snake dreamed of love for the very first time.

## JASON'S COMFREY SALVE

Apply locally to injured fairy wings and watch them heal overnight!

    3 tablespoons fresh comfrey leaves or ounce dried root
    1 cup coconut oil
    2½ teaspoons melted beeswax

Simmer the comfrey leaves or root in the coconut oil for fifteen minutes. Remove from heat, cover, and cool. Strain, squeezing the herbs to express all the oil. Pour into a plastic jar. In a double boiler, melt beeswax over low heat and whisk two and a half teaspoons into the comfrey-coconut oil infusion. Stir several times as the mixture hardens to set the salve. Cover with plastic wrap overnight and seal the jar the following morning.

## PETITE LOVE ESSENCE

Apply two drops of this combination to each side of the neck and two drops on the heart center, and get ready for the love of your life!

    20 drops fimbriata flower essence
    10 drops autumn damask flower essence
    10 drops Champney's Pink Cluster flower essence
    10 drops Alfredo de Damas flower essence
     2 drops wisteria flower essence

In a one-dram bottle, combine the flower essences and essential oils. Add two drops of steam-distilled rose essential oil and cap tightly with a tight fitting screw cap containing a plastic insert. (Rubber inserts may deteriorate over time.)

## Healing the Body and the Mind

Nimbus recuperated from his injuries as a cupid during the late winter. The comfrey salve soothed the pine needle pinches and scratches within days. However, the wind bounced and jerked his joints and limbs in such a way that he required extra healing from Father Time. Petite blended essences and essential oils to facilitate her hero's healing, while Vinnie took over some of Nimbus's workload to allow him time to rest. As he focused on Nimbus's gardening, Vinnie somehow felt calmer. He knew just how Nimbus wanted his chores done and went about it in a fury of enthusiasm. He felt proud to help his friend. While Vinnie worked, Nimbus napped and met Collie in a nearby park to run and play. He was jogging up and down Collie's back every day to increase his physical fitness. His wings flapped as his legs pounded upon Collie's back. After a few laps, he collapsed onto a cushion of fur, panting and sweating.

"Take it easy," Collie chided. "You're supposed to be recuperating!"

"I don't understand why I haven't lost any weight," Nimbus complained. "I can still feel my seams stretch every time I bend over to touch my toes."

"Well, you've fooled me! I thought for sure you'd dropped some weight! Your body is getting firmer every day. I can see muscles peeking through the dimples on your legs."

"Why, thank you, Collie. It's still a little hard for me to see over my tummy. You know, I find it much easier to talk to you about losing weight. It's difficult to explain to a goddess like Flora that I really work hard at losing weight. Of course, I'm more determined since my wedding date is fast approaching," Nimbus said with a big grin.

"Well, first of all, I can't see over my tummy either!" Collie said. "Look at me, Nimbus. I was born to be big! Who ever saw a skinny collie?"

"Who ever saw a fat fairy?" replied Nimbus sadly.

"From the eyes of a big dog like me, you look like a normal-sized fairy. Your friends admire you for who you are not what you look like. Only an ego can judge and egos are not very impartial."

"What in the Land of Thyme is an ego?" asked Nimbus, puzzled.

"An ego is called the masque of the personality. It develops to hide fears," replied Collie.

"I must not have one, then," mused Nimbus. "I'm scared of a lot of things!"

"Well, that's not exactly right, Nimbus. The ego evolves from unresolved hurts and feelings going back to infancy."

"I don't remember *that* far back, Collie! Somebody should have told me about this before I got this old! Now I'm stuck with an ego and it doesn't *like* me!"

"An ego doesn't like whatever threatens the unresolved hurts and fears. The ego doesn't want to feel unhappy feelings. Everybody's supposed to have an ego, according to my owner. It's not all bad, I don't think."

"Where did your owner learn all about this ego thing?"

"From people called psychotherapists. They help people learn about their inner self and what motivates them to do, or not do, things, regardless of consequences."

"Oh! My inner self must like to eat a lot, because I find myself participating very often," Nimbus mused in a thoughtful voice.

"My owner learned that he used his favorite foods for comfort when he was afraid or upset. Instead of getting in touch with his feelings, he ate and paid the price when he got on the scales."

"I wonder if I can learn what makes my inner self so hungry?" wondered Nimbus. "Or what makes my body hold onto this extra weight."

"Good idea, Nimbus! That reminds me of something else I heard my owner explain. He said extra weight is an imbalance and that even disease processes may begin as an imbalance."

"Do you think I have a disease? I must sit down under some shade – I'm feeling dizzy and may faint!" moaned Nimbus, staggering towards a nearby tree.

"Sit down right here and stretch out. You're just overheated and feeling scared. My owner said the ego's greatest fear is death, and the thought of disease has you shaking inside. I didn't really mean you had a disease, Nimbus! Gee, I don't know about those things. Animals like me really don't overeat, but we have feelings and react to other's feelings when they're near us. And we can become overweight from disease, or being overfed by an owner. My owner didn't really say being overweight is a disease, just an imbalance."

"Well, I must say, my head is spinning from all this, but my curiosity is encouraging me to learn more about ego and imbalance. What do you know about being balanced?" asked Nimbus.

"Probably not much," chuckled Collie. "From the way I understand imbalance, it is a mental, emotional, or physical process that is not promoting optimal health."

"Well, Collie, you know my next question is, what is optimal health?"

"Optimal health is more than a lack of a disease. It's what is known in psychotherapy as a self-actualized individual. These people use creativity and self-acceptance to fulfill potentials, talents, goals, and harmony with nature, their family, and their community. They're also known as self-motivated achievers, who measure success by how quickly they rebound from a challenging setback. Their motivation and achievements are used to help others and solve problems for the community and planet."

"Are they fat?" Nimbus asked, quite overwhelmed by Collie's information.

"Well, I'm sure self-actualized people come in all shapes and sizes. However, my owner believes that to be self-actualized he should take the best care of his body by maintaining a healthy diet and weight."

"That sounds like something Flora would say," Nimbus murmured under his breath. "This is a lot to learn in one afternoon. First, I find out I have an ego running my inner life and making me eat too much, then I learn there are self-actualized people who are as accomplished as Flora. And she's a goddess!"

"Well, Nimbus, you already have many of the traits and social skills of a self-actualized person," said Collie kindly.

"Like what?" asked Nimbus, looking quite stunned.

"Well, you have genuine compassion and concern for others and your loving nature has even turned around someone like Vinnie!"

"Oh, I was just being a friend," said Nimbus, blushing.

"You are being self-actualized," smiled Collie. "You are self-disciplined and responsible for yourself, for nature, and for others with a great capacity to enjoy life. You just need to love yourself enough to continue to watch what you eat and stay physically fit. Then you can progress on to other goals, creative expressions, and self-fulfillment," explained Collie.

"Gee! I thought I was taking a big step by getting married! This self-actualization sounds very complicated. I don't know if I can do all the things you mentioned. I haven't even lost weight for my wedding!" moaned Nimbus.

"Here's the good news, Nimbus. My owner says self-actualization, also referred to as spiritual growth, is a step-by-step process. It happens in degrees, like a light slowly becoming bright."

"Collie, you're a genuine poet. How'd an old dog like you get so smart?" asked Nimbus.

"By degrees," laughed Collie, "and some loving friends and teachers."

"Will you introduce me to some of those teachers, Collie? I think I'd like to spend the rest of eternity becoming self-actualized," mused Nimbus. "Maybe I could look slender and muscular like the Spartan Fairy SEAL chief! I'd like to be able to flex my muscles like him. But when I tried it, all I did was sweat more."

"Yes, yes, of course, Nimbus. Calm down! You're beginning to act like Vinnie. In time, I can take you to visit and meet the teachers I know, all who have gained their knowledge from personal experiences. However, your vision of being muscular and slender is an excellent way to begin your transition. Your vision will attract to you who and what you need. Just practice *feeling* like you're already slender and muscular. The teachers will come as you need them," affirmed Collie. "And you will become your vision."

Nimbus closed his eyes to envision a lithe, muscular body as Collie carried him home.

# CHAPTER 6

# The Aesthetic Garden
## Flower Arranging and Tea Ceremonies

*"Let Nature be your teacher."*
Wadsworth, *The Table Turned*

In the fall, the fairies pruned the perennial flowers and plants to prepare them to bloom again in spring. The beds were mulched and new seedling trees were planted to extend their roots deep into the earth during the cold winter months. Now the plants, as well as the earth, were ready for the dormant months.

The fairies looked forward to some time off to pursue their personal interests and hobbies. They had requested instruction on aesthetic ways to use aromatic flowers in arrangements. Tonight they were invited to the lecture hall to hear a well-known teacher speak on Oriental flower arrangements and the ancient tea ceremony. Excitement grew as the time neared to begin the lecture.

The fairies were gathering at the lecture gardens escorted by their favorite flowers. The lecture tonight was on the Oriental wisdom of healing with flowers. The fairies were very excited as they rarely had a traveling speaker pass through the gardens these days. Time had seemed to accelerate; the workload was more stressful and on top of their busy schedule, Flora had all the fairies attending nutrition classes!

Every fairy had to pass a nutrition quiz before being assigned a flower. Rumor had it that Nimbus had flunked the test at least a dozen times. He fainted every time he saw the page in his book with a large X over jelly donuts. However, tonight Nimbus attended the lecture with Sweet Tooth on his arm and looked sharp in his gym shorts and shoes and a wee bit thinner.

Tonight the lecture would include aesthetic healing with flowers. The fairies would learn ancient stress reduction with flower arrangements and participate in an authentic Japanese tea ceremony. There would be a food-tasting ceremony, too. The fairies could hardly wait! They pulled together their cuttings and clippings to make cushions and benches for tonight's lecture.

The speaker was a panda bear that escaped from the zoo in Washington, D.C., many years ago. He hitchhiked back to his homeland in China where the bamboo was abundant, knowing he would find a new direction in life. He lived in a Buddhist monastery and learned many ways to use flowers for healing. His name was now Lao Poo, and he looked very different since first leaving the States. Lao

Poo had shaved his head and now wore a long robe. He appeared a little thinner than the fairies remembered. He probably ate less bamboo since he'd been spending so much of his time in meditation, a higher form of hibernation.

"Here he comes!" yelled a fairy near the side door.

There was a hush over the crowd as Lao Poo slowly walked into the room. It was as if he was in a trance, with his eyes half-closed and a mystical look on his face. He turned to the crowd, raising his arms to greet them.

"Tonight, I'm going to teach you how to grow peacefully and how to have beauty and simplicity in your life. The end result is health, in nature and in your heart!"

Lao Poo then began his lecture, which kept the fairies on the edge of their cushions.

## Lao Poo's Lecture:
## *Chabana:* The Art of Flower Arrangement

*Chabana* is the art of flower arrangement that originated with the ancient tea ceremony in the cultural city of Kyoto, Japan. The Zen art form transcends all cultural boundaries to enliven and enhance the atmosphere of the *chashitsu* (tea room). The flowers are living art arranged with intuitive understanding to set free the spirit of Mother Nature, as well as the arranger.

Chabana pursues the path of *Wabi* in the shadows of a busy society. Wabi takes us away from everyday concerns into the realm of nature spirits. Living in harmony with the elements and rhythm of nature brings a deep appreciation and new sensitivity to life. Turning away from materialism and experiencing beauty through the eyes of simplicity, devoid of glamour, is Wabi.

Experiencing the potential beauty in a fleeting moment of life is the aesthetic ideal of Wabi. Creating beauty in a simple, enlightened flower arrangement is Chabana. There is only one set of rules in this floral art: to seek harmony in the choice of flowers and placement of the vase. The flowers are arranged by allowing each one to take its place effortlessly. As each individual flower is viewed from the heart, their combined quiet beauty causes the viewer to shut the door of the external frenzy and seek the peace that can only be found within.

Certain flowers are unattractive for Chabana: those with strong, sweet, and overwhelming odors, like rose and gardenia, or those possessing an unpleasant-sounding name like dead nettle. These flowers might destroy the delicate mood or compete with the odor of incense burned to purify the room. Flowers that bloom all season may be forbidden because they have no peculiarity. Brightly colored flowers are avoided because they are shocking to the eye. Flowers with sharp thorns are avoided, as well as those bearing fruit.

Simple, stark beauty can be found in seasonal flowers. The cherry blossom is a favorite early springtime choice. The petals are light and delicate, the color is alluring, and they are easily blown by the wind, reminding even the Samurai warriors of their fleeting existence. This stark realization allowed the Samurai to live every moment to its fullest, recognizing beauty in simplicity.

As the March winds herald spring, bulb flowers such as daffodils begin to appear. One bashful bloom looks elegant in a tall and slender dark vase placed where the color will not excite the emotions. A feeling of regeneration evokes a refreshing sense of youth and innocence.

Summer brings heat as the quick pace of spring slows to a crawl. Under the shade of a tree, the lacy blooms of the daisy seem to dance in the sunlight. Under the moon, evening primroses open in the soft music of the night. An arrangement can be made for a daytime or nighttime Chabana for any special occasion.

On the lunar calendar, the first day of autumn is August 8. For Chabana, weeds and herbs make a harmonious display of Nature's best. Thistle, cradled in a spray of burnet leaves, gives a subtle taste of the harvest to follow. On the eve of a harvest moon, the Japanese tree "Lotus," Rose of Sharon, *Althea officinalis*, adds a sense of completion during a new moon. Use a simple, unlined vase guarded by a sprig of half-blooming crepe myrtle. To enhance water absorption, cut the stem while submerged in water or scorch the end of it to increase the longevity of the bloom.

Late fall slows the march of the growth cycle to dormancy. In many gardens, the last flowering herb is marigold mint, *Tagetes lucida*. The golden yellow petals open wide to absorb the sun during the shortened days. They make a colorful display when combined with lantana and butterfly bush cuttings placed in a brown basket deep enough to hold a wide-mouthed vase. The most colorful arrangements are often available during the shorter days of the year.

The icy frost of winter allows Nature to rest. Only the deepest roots of trees continue to burrow toward the warm center of the earth. All plants seem to be asleep, enfolded in the arms of Mother Nature. The warmth of an afternoon tea ceremony is most welcome before another cold night sets in. A dimly lit room is accented by a bamboo bottleneck vase holding the elegant camellia, supported by a forest of witch hazel branches recently wrinkled by frostbite.

The New Year is the most important celebration in Asia. The formal arrangement is made with the handsome narcissus placed in a tall, slender black vase. However, a traditional setting would include a branch of the lovely Japanese field plum, with pine and bamboo, to symbolize happiness.

Here are some ways to practice in your home allowing your room to be a special sanctuary away from the hurried world.

- Keep the stems uncrowded with no leaves resting on the mouth of the vase.
- Choose an odd number of flowers and stems.
- Use only one to three flowers in small rooms.
- Always display seasonal flowers.
- Keep flowers in water until placing in a case or basket.
- Allow the flowers to comfortably situate themselves in the container.
- Spray a mist of cold water onto the arrangement and receive their blessings for the rest of the day.

After the lecture, the fairies enjoyed a cup of tea and discussed their interest in learning more about Japanese culture. One fairy suggested an extended lecture about the Japanese tea ceremony, which Lao Poo graciously agreed to present. The fairies gathered around him and quietly waited for Lao Poo to begin.

"First," he explained, "we must learn about tea, and then we'll concentrate on the cultural roots of the ancient ceremony, where it began, and what the tea ceremony represents." The fairies nodded in agreement.

One fairy bravely asked in a meek voice, "Can you tell us about a real Japanese tea garden?"

"Of course," replied Lao Poo. "I can even teach you about the food served at a tea ceremony."

The fairies cheered and flapped their wings in unison. Food always interested the fairies.

Lao Poo held up his hands and chuckled quietly to quiet the crowd.

## *Chado:* **The Way of Tea**

"Tea was introduced to China from southern Asia more than three thousand years ago. It soon became an expression of harmony and tranquility, the first principle underlying Chinese medicine. In its debut, tea was a medicine. Tea calmed the mind and soothed the soul as it imparted a sense of mental clarity for the participant. Although tea was first given to the Imperial Court to be enjoyed only by the elite, it soon spread throughout Asia and crossed all cultural barriers to become a way of life.

"The tea plant, *Camellia sinensis,* is a native of southeast and east Asia, and has been grown extensively throughout the Orient since the fifth century. Although there are various flavors and aromas of teas, they all originate from the same plant. It is actually a tree close to fifty feet (fifteen meters) tall. Cultivation is kept under six feet (two meters) to enable harvesters to choose the best young leaves. Trained monkeys pick tea leaves grown in certain mountainous regions that are difficult for harvesters to reach. Individual location and climate, as well as harvesting and processing conditions, create the difference in taste.

"Tea is like wine. It is created under unique conditions. There are more than 250 varieties varying in price and flavor, and all are derivatives of green or black tea. Young and tender green tea leaves are picked from the top of trees before they wither. They are immediately sun-dried or put in drying rooms where currents of warm air completely dry them. The leaves produce a golden brew with a delicate bouquet. It is popular during the summer or served with stir-fried entrees. Black tea leaves are allowed to wither on the bush before gathering, rolling, fermenting, and drying. Fermentation alters the chlorophyll, changing the color from green to black. The tea has a full body and a red color. It is a favorite winter tea and often served with deep-fried food. Oolong is semi-fermented (partly dried and fermented) and produces an amber-color tea with a delicate fragrance. It is served with an evening meal or with strongly flavored food like broccoli.

"Flower teas are served at banquets or between meals. The addition of fragrant flowers in tea makes the ceremony a special occasion. Jasmine is the most popular, brewed in green tea with fresh or dried buds. The taste is delicate and very aromatic. It originates from Formosa. Lichee (Lay Jee) is a light, sweet tea from Taiwan. It is popular with the Cantonese, who serve the yellow-blossomed tea to renew friendships. Chrysanthemum leaf is served in a tea or brewed alone with rock sugar to alleviate mental fatigue. Honeysuckle is often brewed alone to cool the body during the hot summer or reduce a fever during the winter.

"Flower teas are meant to be soothing to the soul and tonic to the heart. Tea is served to further harmony within, with others, and with nature. Flowers are added to remind us of the beauty within all three."

Lao Poo paused and glanced around the audience to look for questions. The fairies were mesmerized by his lecture and quietly waited for him to continue. He cleared his throat, sipped a glass of water and smiled briefly to the fairies and flowers before he continued.

"Now that we understand the importance of tea, we can appreciate the tea ceremony. Let's begin with the origin of the tea ceremony, the four principles, and highest ideals of spiritual growth," explained Lao Poo.

As everyone in the audience relaxed onto their cushions, Nimbus squeezed Sweet Tooth's hand in excitement and anticipation. He had become very interested in spiritual growth since his initial conversation with Collie. He was hungrier for information than for his favorite foods. Sweet Tooth was very supportive and took time from her busy schedule to attend lectures with him. She nuzzled next to Nimbus and laid her perfect coiffure on his softly padded shoulder as Lao Poo began to lecture.

### *Kaiseki:* The Japanese Tea Ceremony

"*Kaiseki,* the spirit of simplicity, purity, and good taste, pervades the ceremony of tea. Over the centuries, tea embodied the highest ideals of Oriental culture. In the thirteenth century, the Zen Buddhist monks began the spirit of the ancient tea ceremony during their devotion. Simplicity and a mind emptied of all chatter initiated an aesthetic austerity for the ceremony.

"By the sixteenth century, the greatest tea master, Sen Rikyu (1522-1591), raised the tea ceremony to a fine art in Japan. Sen Rikyu is best remembered for the four principles of the ceremony: harmony (*Wa*), respect (*Kei*), purity (*Sei*), and tranquility (*Iyaku*). The highest ideals of spiritual cultivation were represented in the tea ceremony. Courtesans and laymen acquired peace of mind and meditated upon world peace while enjoying a cup of tea. Tea not only became the national drink of Oriental countries, but also their link with nature, humanity, and inner harmony.

"The Zen emphasis removed any elitist emphasis from the ceremony. Everyone could afford powdered green tea and time out from the day to find harmony with nature. The ritual still reminds us about how we live and treat one another, and what our true values in life represent. The Japanese observe the rules defined by the great tea masters of the fifteenth and sixteenth centuries. With the proper intention, the ritual can be observed in your environment. A seasonal flower, such as hibiscus, can also be added to the tea. Choose a flower by matching the flower's essence to your present emotional environment. For example, white flowers represent beginnings in life; yellow flowers encourage friendship."

Lao Poo proceeded to demonstrate the tea ceremony, step by step, as he explained each procedure.

### The Ceremony

> "If you host a tea without deviating from any of the rules . . . I will become your disciple."
> Sen Rikyu

"The tea ceremony may take place in any room of the home. The Japanese ideal is a simple hut decorated by a wall hanging and Chabana flower arrangement. Light a subtle incense or scented candle and place the brazier and kettle on bamboo mats covering the floor. As the two to three guests arrive, bring in a bamboo dipper, a teaspoon, tea caddie, cup, bowl, and any appropriate utensils. Wipe the caddie and spoon with a silk napkin, called a *fukusa*. Use the bamboo dipper to put a small quantity of hot water from the kettle into the bowl. Use a pure linen cloth, called a *chakin,* to clean the bowl, turning it round and round in your hands. Rotating the bowl is meant to clear the mind as well as ensure cleanliness. An appropriate aromatic or decorative flower may be placed nearby on a tiny round plate. With careful motions, the tea caddie is opened holding the carefully ground tea. The tea is measured by spoonfuls and mounded into the bowl. Gently tap the spoon against the rim of the bowl to focus attention on the ritual. The Japanese use a bamboo spoon to achieve just the right sound.

"Next, dip the bamboo dipper open-side down into the tea kettle holding the boiled fresh water. The kettle's song signals to the hostess that the proper temperature has been reached. Adding a dipper of cold water, on standby in a china jar, can calm a rolling boil. This is said to 'restore the youth of the water.' Place one-third of the dipper of steaming water into the tea bowl. Take the handmade whisk, or *chasen,* and whip the tea and water together into a jade-colored liquid. The hostess then lifts the bowl with a silk napkin and offers it to the first guest. Sip slowly to fully partake in the flavor and aroma. The ritual will be repeated for each guest, taking about forty to forty-five minutes. Any flowers to be added are best placed in the cup *after* whisking. A flower-only tea can be substituted if caffeine is not acceptable by adding a spoonful of fresh flower petals into a cup of boiled water. Allow the tea to steep for five to ten minutes before offering the flower tea to the guest."

## The Setting

"Certain rules are followed in Japanese homes to create the correct atmosphere for a tea ceremony. Each rule represents a step toward inner harmony and union with Nature. In a Japanese home, the guests remove their shoes before entering. They will be given a pair of fresh white socks to remind them to leave behind their busy world and begin anew as they enter. This will be an excellent opportunity to hand them an appropriate seasonal flower to reflect upon during the ceremony.

"If the ceremony is held outside of the home, a path is prepared with meticulous care. In an outside ceremony, a tea garden path, called a *roji,* is swept and sprinkled with fresh water to purify the atmosphere. A few leaves or pine needles are purposely left to keep a natural, rustic feeling. Seasonal flowers and plants present a serene environment where the six rules of Sen Rikyu are followed."

Lao Poo paused to pass the following handout to each fairy in the audience:

1. Make a tasty cup of tea
2. Lay charcoal to heat water
3. Arrange seasonal flowers as they appear in their environment; have a feeling of coolness in the summer and cozy warmth in the winter
4. Prepare ahead of time
5. Prepare for unusual weather patterns
6. Give your guests every consideration

## A Harmonious Tea Garden

Vinnie could not contain his excitement any longer. He flew out of his cushioned chair and up to the podium. Lao Poo chuckled as Vinnie flapped in front of him, requesting a plan or design for a tea garden. Lao Poo sat him on his lap as he informally described an appropriate tea garden.

"A harmonious tea garden is a blend of fantasy, color, form, and texture that allows enlightenment to occur without leaving home," Lao Poo explained. "The design should remind the viewer of a natural scene of beauty, small in size, no bigger than a tennis court. Small trees, shrubs, and seasonal aromatic flowers of several varieties should quietly guard it. Stepping-stones, bridges, running water, and soft lighting set a mood of delightful fantasy where every turn will bring a fresh scene. Rose bushes, shrubs, and trees whose leaves turn colors in the autumn will add a heightened awareness of the harvest. As the viewer travels the garden walk, the problems of the outer world fall away.

"Imagine a pebbled path lined by azaleas, wisteria, cherry, and local fruit trees weeping petals to lead the way to the tea ceremony. Approaching the tea ceremony area, the flowers become sparse as the area is shaded by the three friends of winter: pine, bamboo, and plum. Small leaf maple and native trees may be substituted in varieties of three. Native plants, such as iris, hyacinth, and morning glories, specially placed rocks, and horsetail (*Equisetum hyemale*), may enhance a feeling of austerity as the viewer approaches the tea area. Leaving the past and even beauty behind, the viewer holds the jewel in his heart."

The fairies leaned forward on their cushions, spellbound by Lao Poo's last words. He took this opportunity to request a few minutes of silence as the fairies meditated on the jewel in their hearts. After a solemn moment, he continued his lecture, describing the tea ceremony. This is what the fairies had been waiting to hear.

## Kaiseki Ryori

"The tea ceremony often includes a meal or specially prepared snacks that appeal to the guests," Lao Poo continued. "The theme of harmony is expressed in the choice of food, color, style of dishes, order served, variants of texture, flavor, and temperature of the food offered. The alluring fragrance and presentation will subtly charm the eye and nose and refresh the soul — a complete sensory experience. As the natural flavors unfold, the guest is reminded of the purpose of the tea ceremony: to create order out of chaos and bring peace and serenity, simplicity and perfection into an imperfect world. The feeling remains, even after the experience ends."

The fairies stirred in their cushions as Flora entered the room, pad and pencil in hand for notes. Lao Poo acknowledged her by bowing and offering her a cushion on the front row. Her cheeks blushed a beautiful rose color as she took her seat and Lao Poo continued.

"The choice of food follows the season, colors, flowers, and presentation. The plate arrangements may resemble a scene in nature. For example, in autumn, the theme may be viewing the harvest moon. The food may include a seasonal dish, such as chrysanthemum flower leaf salad (*shungiku*), with red perilla vinegar, moon noodles which include a lightly poached or raw egg resting on a cloud of white rice noodles, and a basic soup stock, *dashi,* with a floating fish cake to note the movement of the moon. Of course, no meal is complete without a bowl of steamed rice (*gohan*).

"In the autumn, the plates will be earthen-colored and rectangular and decorated with red maple leaves. Soup will be served in a red lacquered bowl, tightly covered to seal the aroma. Salad may be on an oblong dish, decorated with a chrysanthemum flower, grated burdock root (*gobo*), and a dime-size spot of horseradish sauce. Rice is always served in a round bowl, representing abundance, for austerity is a choice. Persimmons may be served as a promise of new life in the spring.

"In summer, the soup will be served chilled with burnet leaves as a garnish, floating in the bowl. Fresh carrots may be cut in the shape of fans to entertain the idea of coolness, and served on a glass plate with a fish or tofu dish served in the shape of a seasonal fish. Two melon balls may be served as a dessert."

Nimbus gulped loudly at the thought of so little food served at a meal. The audience rippled with laughter, knowing well what he was thinking. Lao Poo smiled, bounced Vinnie on his lap and spoke directly to Sweet Tooth, who was nuzzled against Nimbus's shoulder.

"For special occasions, a seasonal tea can be served. In springtime, cherry blossom tea is a favorite, especially with brides, who are served a cup of this tea before or after the ceremony. When added to steaming water, the blossoms blush like a bride."

Lao Poo smiled broadly as he gently moved Vinnie aside and demonstrated brewing a cup of cherry blossom tea.

## Cherry Blossom Tea

"Steep one teaspoon of salted cherry blossoms in one cup boiled water. In just a few minutes, the tea is ready to offer to the bride." The audience watched as Lao Poo turned toward Sweet Tooth to offer her the freshly brewed blushing tea. His eyebrows rose as it became apparent that Sweet Tooth and Nimbus were nowhere in sight. The crowd held its breath until the silence was broken by loud smooching underneath the cushions where Nimbus and Sweet Tooth had been sitting.

The fairies cheered and the flowers clapped in unison until the couple appeared from underneath their cushions. Nimbus's hair was disheveled and standing on end. Sweet Tooth's lipstick was smeared all over his face and neck. She reached up and politely accepted the cup of tea from Lao Poo, as he stood next to her, smiling knowingly. Nimbus, feeling the need for nourishment, quickly grabbed the cup of tea from Sweet Tooth and gulped it down. The warm tea turned his face as pink as a cherry blossom. He smiled sweetly at Lao Poo, thanking him as he returned the empty cup.

As Lao Poo walked away shaking his head and chuckling, Flora passed out the following recipes, inviting each fairy to a tasting party in the next room.

## TEA CEREMONY FOOD PREPARATION

The high art of sensual presentation and deep reverence for nature lends a visual feast for the mind's eye and food for the spirit.

### BASIC STOCK (DASHI)

The Japanese elevate nutrition to an elegant, fine art.

**Ingredients**

    5 cups water
    1 inch piece seaweed (*kombu*)
    1 tablespoon dried bonito (*katsuobushi*)

Combine water and kombu. Bring to a boil and remove from heat. Add the dried bonito. Heat almost to a boil, then remove, let settle, and strain. Serves four.

# Summer Chilled Miso

One-sixth of the daily protein requirements are met with this soup.

## Ingredients
    4 cups basic stock (*dashi*), chilled
    3 ounces miso
    salad burnet, cilantro, or parsley

Mix one cup of stock with the miso. Add the remaining stock. Garnish with burnet leaves. Serve chilled in a glass bowl.

# Autumn Chrysanthemum Leaf Salad *(Shungiku)*

*Chrysanthemum indica* leaves are used to treat skin infections and high blood pressure. It is enjoyed as a salad and eaten during harvest time as a preventative.

## Ingredients
    2 bunches of chrysanthemum leaves (wilted in hot water for 20 seconds)
    10 chopped canned gingko nuts
    1 teaspoon soy sauce
    1 teaspoon sugar
    1½ tablespoons sesame oil

Combine all ingredients. Toss and serve. Garnish with a chrysanthemum flower. Serves four.

# Perilla Leaf Vinegar

This vinegar has a beautiful cherry color and a spicy taste.

## Ingredients
    1 cup of rice vinegar or white vinegar
    5 purple perilla leaves

Bring vinegar to a simmer. Cover and remove from heat. Steep for fifteen minutes and strain into a clean glass jar. Serve on a summer salad or add a teaspoon to a fruit salad for a zesty taste. Serves four.

# Moon Noodles in Hot Broth

Moon noodles are served in autumn during the harvest.

## Ingredients
   ½ pint dashi stock
   3 tablespoons dark soy sauce
   1 tablespoon sugar
   2 tablespoons mirin*
   2 teaspoons salt
   2 young leeks or spring onions (scallions)
   14 ounces dried buckwheat or udon noodles

Simmer stock, soy sauce, sugar, mirin, salt, and scallions for five minutes. Add the noodles and continue cooking for eight to ten minutes until the noodles are soft. Serves four.

*Mirin is a sweet golden cooking wine with a low alcohol content available at specialty food stores.


# Japanese Steamed Rice (*Gohan*)

The secret to cooking rice in the Japanese manner, so that it clings together and is easy to pick up with chopsticks, is to measure the water properly and cook the rice without peeking.

## Ingredients
   2 cups Japanese rice (or other short or medium-grain rice)
   2½ cups cold water

Pour rice into a strainer and rinse with cold water until the water runs clear. Drain well. Transfer rice to a heavy, deep saucepan with a tight-fitting lid. Add the cold water. Place the saucepan over high heat and bring to a boil. Cover, reduce heat to the lowest setting, and cook for fifteen minutes. Do not remove the lid during cooking. Turn off the heat and let stand, covered, for ten minutes. Makes six cups of cooked rice.

## Nimbus Asks For Help

As the fairies sipped the soup and nibbled at their salads, Nimbus made a beeline to a very large bowl of perfectly steamed rice.

He quickly spooned the rice from the bowl into his mouth, unable to stop himself. Sweet Tooth stood beside him, nibbling a few chocolates she found at the bottom of her purse. Before Nimbus could satiate his hunger, Flora flew to the table and snatched the spoon from his hand.

"Nimbus! What are you doing? This rice is for everyone. There won't be any left if you keep helping yourself!" she scolded.

"I'm really sorry, Flora. I was so nervous and hungry, I couldn't stop myself. Just the idea that the rice bowl represented abundance made me want to eat the whole bowl!"

Nimbus's voice quivered. He felt his neck getting hot as he began to sweat. He felt embarrassed and ashamed that Flora caught him hogging the rice. Of all the people to catch him, why did it have to be Flora? By the time his face flushed a bright red, he was thinking that Flora must really hate him. He glanced down and put his hands in his pockets.

Instead, Flora smiled briefly before she threw her head back and laughed out loud. "Nimbus, don't look so guilty! You're making me feel mean! I just want to make sure there's an abundance of rice for everyone. Let me get you a bowl." As Flora attempted to fly to the serving line, Nimbus grabbed her by the hand and turned her to face him.

"Flora, you've got to help me," Nimbus begged as he swallowed his pride. "I don't like myself when I lose control. I don't remember when I start eating and I don't even feel better when I lick the bowl clean," sighed Nimbus, feeling defeated.

"Well, at least you've switched to a low-fat food," replied Flora as she stared at Sweet Tooth.

Sweet Tooth smiled demurely as she licked her manicured fingertips. Nimbus was quick to defend his lady.

"Oh, she's cut back on her chocolate. We've made a commitment to health and a long life together." Nimbus smiled broadly at the thought of spending light years romancing his true love.

Flora nodded in approval as she watched Sweet Tooth apply her lipstick. "What about using aromatherapy to reduce your appetite?" Flora asked, still staring at Sweet Tooth.

"Oh, it certainly helps," replied Nimbus quickly. "I just feel like I have more to learn about self-control so I can work towards self-actualization."

Flora's perfect lips parted in amazement. "Why, Nimbus, I never thought I'd hear that from you! Love must really be changing you!"

"Oh, yes, Flora. I never knew my heart could feel so much love for any one fairy. Every time I'm near Sweet Tooth, I fall more deeply in love." Nimbus's eyes became dewy as he spoke. "However," he continued, "I learned about self-actualization from my friend Collie. He also told me I had an ego that rules my inner world and I think that's why I eat so much. My ego is either very hungry or it doesn't really like me," explained Nimbus. He was quite amazed at how easy it was to talk to Flora. He actually felt comfortable telling her his troubles, even if she was perfect.

Flora listened, nodding her head as she reflected on what Nimbus had just said. As she rubbed her chin, she thought of how she could best help Nimbus. He stood across from her, frozen in a half smile, as he awaited her answer. Somehow he knew an important decision was about to be made. He held his breath until Flora answered him.

"Okay, Nimbus," Flora answered. "I think I know a way to help you take responsibility for your actions, but you'll have to leave the Land of Thyme temporarily."

"Where am I going?" asked Nimbus as he wiped tears from Sweet Tooth's eyes.

"To visit a working garden where flower essences and essential oils are grown and prepared. They are used to help others achieve self-actualization and conscious growth," replied Flora.

"Oh, thank you," Nimbus answered nervously, "but if I grow any more I won't be able to squeeze into my leotards."

Flora bit her lip as she tried to hide her smile. "Conscious growth is the step leading you to self-actualization, Nimbus. Your inner world will open to a spirit-filled life of self-love and service to others."

"Oh! Well that sounds good to me," smiled Nimbus, relieved that he could grow somewhere other than out. "I've been so busy eating, I didn't realize there was another way to grow!"

Nimbus cuddled Sweet Tooth in his arms, consoling her for the time they'd spend apart. As she wept softly, streams of mascara dripped from her eyes.

"Can this journey wait until after our wedding?" asked Sweet Tooth in a quivering voice.

"Why, I had every intention of your accompanying your husband after the wedding," replied Flora with a smile. "You can help with the essential oils and essence blends while you share your expertise with the gardener," Flora explained.

Nimbus and Sweet Tooth simultaneously grabbed Flora and squeezed her tightly. Flora soon disappeared into Nimbus's arms and Sweet Tooth's bosom.

When she was finally released, she was gasping for air.

"Wow! You two sure have a lot of love to share! I know you have a lot of questions about the journey, too. We can work out the details during the winter. Right now I need to hand out recipes for tea ceremony food and help Lao Poo answer questions. Come and sample some authentic Japanese food and we'll make arrangements to meet again later." With that, the trio joined hands and flew towards the tasting table.

The following recipes were shared with the fairy community. The fairies ended their evening with a moment of silent appreciation for Lao Poo as he continued on his lecture tour to faraway gardens. The flower and fairy community would remember his presentation as the finest cultural experience of the season. Lao Poo's lecture touched each of their hearts and changed their lives in a favorable way.

## A Romantic Tea Party

The lectures about the Japanese tea ceremony also inspired Sweet Tooth. She decided to have a romantic tea party and invite only Nimbus. Sweet Tooth chose a secluded area overlooking the famous Azalea Path. She picked a giant magnolia to stage her tea ceremony high in the treetops. What a beautiful view! She gathered her finest teapot and cups and prepared tea ceremony delicacies with chocolate-covered rice cakes, a low-fat substitute for a high-fat food. An angel was asked to play soft, romantic music as Sweet Tooth made the Chabana flower arrangement. A few neighboring fairies flew by to visit on the way to their next assignment and a hummingbird dropped by to bring joy for the lovers to share. Mamma Rabbit came to bless the ceremony with abundance, carrying five baby bunnies all the way to the top of the magnolia tree. A fairy lamp was lit to lead Nimbus into his lover's arms.

When all arrangements were made ready, a butterfly brought Nimbus an invitation written on a fragrant hankie belonging to Sweet Tooth.

An eagle was summoned to fly Nimbus to the treetop. The Phoenix was still out on disability after Operation Fairy Storm. Try as Nimbus might, his little fairy wings couldn't lift his chubby body to the magnolia treetop where his lover anxiously waited! He anticipated being fully recuperated from the pine tree injury in only a few more weeks. In the meantime, he needed help flying to the treetop.

Although the teapot was whistling when Nimbus finally arrived, the eagle was producing even more steam!

"Whew! I'm used to soaring to the treetops with ease, but I must say this was quite a challenge," puffed the eagle. As Nimbus dismounted, he realized he'd forgotten to bring Sweet Tooth a bouquet of freshly picked flowers. He quickly reached over to the eagle and plucked some downy feathers to present to her.

"Ouch! I'm out of here!" cried the eagle as he soared into the sun.

"Well, now! It's just the two of us," Sweet Tooth whispered as she moved toward Nimbus. The intoxicating aroma of gardenia filled the air. Her dress was made from freshly picked blooms. She wrapped herself around him in an embrace.

Nimbus began to sweat as he swooned. "I feel my blood sugar falling. Or maybe it's rising. Either way, we'd better eat," said Nimbus nervously.

The teakettle harmonized with the angel's music in the background as the couple began to dine. Sweet Tooth had brewed her famous celestial chocolate mint tea for the occasion. The lovers gazed into each other's eyes, forgetting about the angel who silently slipped away.

As the happy couple sipped and flirted, word went out to neighboring fairies who gathered underneath the benevolent magnolia to have their very own tea party. Fairies swarmed from surrounding areas for the party and hung from trees and rose bushes in all shapes and sizes. They all came to share their joy with the local animals, sip a cup of tea, and snoop on the romance upstairs in the tree.

Without warning, the wind began to blow and the trees braced for an oncoming storm. The fairies scattered for cover. They knew Mother Nature had not ordered a storm to clear the environment. The gods must be playing Star Wars again!

Suddenly, the sky turned teal and became very still.

"Oh, no! It must be one of those wild tornadoes twisting through the forest!" cried a little rabbit. "Run for cover!"

"Yeehaaaaaw!" the twister cried as it blew into the forest. The storm brought rain, then hail as big as golf balls. As the tree branches bowed in the wind, many broke and carpeted the forest.

"Yahoo!" The twister ripped through the forest and bent the trees as the wind whistled its song. The forest shook to the twister's tune. The fairies were all safe in the basements of surrounding trees, except for the two lovers who couldn't get down to safety. Eagle tried in vain to rescue them, but the storm kept him away. Everyone feared for the lives of Sweet Tooth and Nimbus as the rain continued to beat onto the forest floor. Their eyes were riveted on the magnolia tree where Sweet Tooth and Nimbus were last seen.

The magnolia withstood the storm like a southern tradition, never losing a limb to the screaming wind. Nimbus and Sweet Tooth were clinging tightly to each other on a very large branch. Nimbus whispered how fortunate it was that their tea and treats were finished before the storm blew everything away. He was holding onto Sweet Tooth and shaking. Sweet Tooth nuzzled into his arms and felt so very safe. Try as it might, the tornado couldn't even make the strong magnolia budge, but it sure scared Nimbus. The forest echoed with Nimbus's mighty screams of "Whoooah!" far into the night.

When the storm finally tired and blew away, the fairies slowly came out of their shelters. All, that is, except for Nimbus. He was still straddling a large branch of the strong magnolia, shaking like a leaf. Sweet Tooth had disengaged from Nimbus and climbed down the tree to look for help. We'll never know what happened that day up in the tree, but when Sweet Tooth crawled down the tree, she had stars in her eyes. All she said was, "That is some kind of man!"

The next morning, a special edition of the *Fairy Morning News* displayed a photo of the valiant magnolia on the front page, along with Nimbus's backside and chubby legs hugging the tree limb. Nimbus refused to make a statement as to why the back of his leotard was irreparably damaged. The flowers and fairies all gave their account of his bravery throughout the storm, although no one could quite remember what brave deed Nimbus had done. Just surviving such a terrible storm seemed valiant to the fairy community.

The fairy firefighters had engaged the whole community in rescuing Nimbus from his frozen grip around the magnolia branch. Nimbus left a permanent ring around the tree limb, not to mention shreds of his leotards. The fairies finally had to use Jason's large foot as a crane to pull Nimbus back to earth. A loud cheer greeted him as his feet touched the ground. He was visibly shaking and white as a lily, but very appreciative. Nimbus acknowledged his rescuers with a wave and a weak smile and reached over to tickle Jason's foot.

The fairies offered refreshments and everyone sat in fairy rings to rest and recount their version of the storm. Flora took this opportunity to improve her talent as a lecturer and teacher (her nutrition classes were declining in popularity).

This was Flora's big chance since the fairies were too tired to leave. So, she climbed the tallest mushroom and, after sipping cool clear water, began to lecture on how stress affects the bodies of fairies.

## Living with Stress

"The life of a garden fairy can be very stressful. We work under all conditions and inclement weather. To further conscious growth, we must take responsibility to alleviate the effects of a stressful lifestyle. Stress is responsible for the onset of 80 percent of disease. It is a silent imbalance that we can learn to control. A stressor may be environmental, mental, emotional, physical, or situational. Stress reduces biological changes known as 'adaptation.' The adrenals become exhausted, tired, and stressed out, and a fairy becomes prone to allergies, asthma, and depression. When stress puts the adrenals in a hyperphase, anxiety, hypertension, high cholesterol, and high blood sugar result. Hyperactivity is a sign of run-away adrenals. Stress and exhaustion may manifest in an inherently weak organ or kick off a disease like arthritis or ulcers.

"Tonight, we're going to focus on the adrenal response with nutrients, diet, and adaptagenic herbs, as well as simple aromatherapy techniques to facilitate relaxation. The adrenals are like car batteries that need to be recharged. Certain nutrients will reduce atrophy and shrinkage during stress, if adequate amounts are available to the cells."

Flora pulled out a chalkboard and began to write as she lectured.

## Nutrients that Reduce Stress

"Potassium loss is severe during stress. Low potassium causes cells to die. The body does not hold spare potassium because it is prevalent in nature. Foods high in potassium are oranges and juicy fruits like apples, melons, and bananas. Other sources of potassium include blackstrap molasses, sunflower seeds, almonds, raisins, potatoes, chicken, beef, pork, and fish. Herbs may include dandelion leaves, parsley, uva ursi, mints, and salad burnet added to salads or brewed as teas.

"Vitamin C increases lymphocytes in the white blood cells to reduce infection and increase antibody response. It is very similar to interferon as an antiviral and also assists connective tissues to promote elasticity. Bioflavonoids, such as the anti-inflammatory quercetin, assist vitamin C. I use it to reduce allergic tendencies. Pantothenic acid ($B_5$) works with vitamin C and the adrenals to reduce stress and increase antibodies. High-potassium foods are generally also high in vitamin C.

"Zinc is involved with many immune responses, thymic function, and vitamin A absorption. It reduces the cold virus and herpes simplex and promotes growth hormones affecting secondary sexual characteristics. Zinc is excreted rapidly when alcohol is ingested and during stress. Sunflower seeds and pumpkin seeds are high in zinc. But dosage should not exceed 100 mg daily, since high doses can raise cholesterol levels.

"Pyridoxine $B_6$ promotes antibody production and reduces lymphatic and thymic tissue shrinkage. It also reduces PMS and fluid retention for many women. A very high-protein diet, alcohol, and birth control pills create unnatural deficiencies. $B_6$ increases zinc and $B_{12}$ absorption, and promotes HCL (hydrochloric acid) production. Some beneficial foods are parsley, beef, bananas, wheat germ, whole grains, and many vegetables. $B_6$ holds magnesium in solution to normalize calcium delivery to the bones. The coenzyme, or converted formulation of $B_6$, is pyridoxal 5 phosphate, or P5P. It is a biologically available nutrient the liver does not have to convert. A daily dose of 20 mg is the equivalent of 100 mg of B$_6$, a safe dosage for adult daily usage.

## Herbs that Reduce Stress

"A few herbs to help the body adapt to stress over a period of time, and increase longevity, include *Eleutherococcus senticosus,* or Siberian ginseng. The Orientals call it *Wuchaseng* and prepare a *pian* (pill) of a cooked extract to increase immunity and stamina and to balance blood sugar during an immune response. It is beneficial for diabetics, and even reduces jet lag and arthritic symptoms when used for several months. Wuchaseng is more subtle than Korean and American ginseng and usually does not cause headaches and tight shoulders. Hypertensive fairies should check with a healthcare practitioner before using herbs.

"Another powerful, yet lesser known, herb in the west is *Polygonum multiflorum,* also called *Ho Shou Wu* or *foti.* Its action is most remarkable in cleaning the blood through the liver and kidneys and building tremendous stamina without being a stimulant. It is a great cardiovascular tonic with the ability to rejuvenate and preserve hair color and bone strength. The adaptagenic herbs strengthen the body over one to three years with daily or frequent doses. *Polygonum multiflorum* has hypotensive qualities, reducing high blood pressure over one to three years."

## Essential Oils that Reduce Stress

"Essential oil blends are the quickest, easiest way to reduce stress with aromatic herbs. The body also responds well to aromatic sedative herbs, such as lavender, sage, and sandalwood. Rosemary is refreshing and uplifting. Thyme and sage can be effective to combat colds, flu, and sinus congestion. Eucalyptus and peppermint are stimulants useful to abate pain and asthma. Dilute essential oils in hot water as a steam, in oil or lotion and apply them directly to the body."

When Flora finished lecturing, only Lao Poo gave her a standing ovation. All the fairies had fallen fast asleep, another way to rejuvenate the body from a stressful day.

As Flora stepped down from her mushroom, she looked defeated and slightly frustrated. Lao Poo moved toward her very cautiously. When Lao caught her attention, he encouraged her with a smile.

"Why isn't anyone interested in nutrition and better health like me?" she sighed.

"Well, I'm sure the fairy community is interested, replied Lao Poo. "They just don't have the passionate conviction you carry in your heart."

"Why don't they realize they'll be pushing up stars if they don't continuously work on their health?" Flora cried.

"Fairies are born with a desire for pleasure. That's why they are so compatible with flowers. Fairies create beauty from their desires and share it with all of us. Nature blesses those who share their wealth of experiences and expertise." Lao Poo gently stroked Flora's shoulders as she wept softly into the palms of her hands.

"So, do you think there's a way to make nutrition pleasurable and exciting?" asked Flora, wiping the tears from her cheeks.

"Sure! You can create some recipes with exciting names and claims to fame!" replied Lao Poo.

Flora's eyes brightened as ideas began to formulate in her mind. She looked around her for a pen and notebook to jot down some recipes, completely absorbed in her thoughts.

Lao Poo chuckled as he quietly walked back to his room. Combining Flora's knowledge with a little sensationalism should have some interesting results, he mused as he disappeared into the forest.

## FLORA'S STRESS REDUCERS

Meanwhile, Flora stayed awake all night tapping out sensational recipes on her laptop, to be distributed amongst the fairies the following day.

### HIGH-ENERGY DRINK

Try this before a workout.

**Ingredients**
> 1 teaspoon each of fresh parsley, dandelion, and salad burnet leaves
> 1 tablespoon of fresh spearmint leaves or another mint
> 2 cups boiled water

Add ingredients to the water. Cover and remove from the heat and steep for ten minutes. Strain and serve over ice with a twist of lime. Serves one.

## SUPER-CHARGED SNACK

Nibble a tablespoon for a high-energy snack during the day.

**Ingredients**
- ½ cup raw sunflower seeds
- ½ cup pumpkin seeds
- 1 tablespoon raw wheat germ
- ⅛ teaspoon ground cayenne pepper
- ¼ teaspoon cinnamon
- 1 tablespoon sesame seed oil

Preheat oven to 300°. Mix ingredients thoroughly until the seeds are coated. Roast in the oven on an un-greased cookie sheet for thirty minutes. Serves eight.

## DR. POO'S SEXUAL TONIC

Dilute a tablespoon daily in warm water or cold juice and enjoy a youthful, virile body.

**Ingredients**
- 2 ounces Ho shou wu (*Polygonum multiflorum*)
- 1 ounce prepared Ti huang (*Rehmannia glutinosa*)
- 1 ounce Schizandrae fructus (*Schizandra chinensis*)
- 1 ounce Lycie fructus (*Lycium chinensis*)
- ½ ounce Fu ling (*Poria cocos*)
- ½ ounce Suk Gok (*Dendrobium hancockii*)
- 1 quart brandy

Steep the herbs in the brandy for three to four weeks in a glass jar. Strain and begin with one teaspoon daily and increase the dosage to one tablespoon daily over the next three weeks. (Add brandy as necessary to cover the herbs during steeping.)

## Preserving Youth Vitality Tonic

Dilute one teaspoon daily in warm water or juice to add light-years to your body!

## Ingredients

  2 ounces Wuchaseng (*Eleutherococcos senticosus*)
  1 ounce Chinese yam (*Dioscorea batatas*)
  1 ounce astragalus (*Astragalus membranaceus*)
  ½ ounce Fengwang, a Royal Jelly bee secretion (available at health food stores)
  ½ ounce Jujube red date (*Zizyphus jujube*)
  1 quart of brandy or rice wine

Steep the herbs for three weeks in the brandy or rice wine. Strain and dilute one teaspoon daily.

## Fairy Pleasurable Aromablend

Wear two drops of this blend on the neck and behind the ears and experience the best time of your life!

  6 drops rosemary essential oil
  3 drops lemon grass or lemon verbena essential oil
  1 drop thyme essential oil
  1 ounce vegetable oil

Combine the essential oils in the vegetable oil. Cap in a dark brown glass bottle or heavy plastic lotion container.

## Unending Energy Blend

Wear two drops on the neck or hair and feel the energy rising!

  6 drops peppermint essential oil
  4 drops eucalyptus essential oil
  2 drops spearmint essential oil
  1 ounce vegetable oil

Combine the essential oils with the vegetable oil. Cap in a dark brown, glass bottle.

CHAPTER 7

# Preparation Time
## Teas, Tonics, and Fairy Food

*Flowers Bloom When Fairies Sing*

The fairies spent the winter brewing Flora's energy teas and tonics. Their vitality and stamina increased as each week passed. The tonics also built their resistance to cold weather. Instead of feeling lethargic, the fairies were bustling with energy.

There was every good reason to stay busy. The most exciting occasion would be taking place in the forest of the oaks very soon. A real fairy wedding would commence and everyone in the Land of Thyme was invited!

The fairy world was busy gathering all the materials necessary to celebrate the upcoming wedding of Nimbus and Sweet Tooth. The fairies were electrified with anticipation. This would be no ordinary wedding. The whole clan of Mother Nature's garden would participate: herbs, flowers, vegetables, shrubs, and trees. Why, even the grass was getting a manicure for this occasion!

Special invitations were being etched on pressed wood violets and mailed in handsome silver maple leaves. Everyone looked forward to receiving an invitation with a R.V.S.F. (reserved for a very special fairy) for a fairy reception afterwards:

*Mother Nature is proud to announce*
*the dimpled hand of*
*Sweet Tooth Petal to Nimbus Cloud*
*in Holy Matrimony*
*on this fairy day of February 14*
*since the beginning of Thyme in the Forest of the Oaks.*
*Reception following.*
*Please reserve a place on the Fairy Float for the procession to the garden altar.*

## Weight Loss Behavior Modification

The big day was approaching and everyone was hurrying. The fairies were busy baking the cakes for the bride and groom and Flora was busy removing all the fat. The bees and wasps were designing a gorgeous wedding gown of wisteria flowers fit for a queen. This was a first: Other fairies had gowns sewn from silver lace vine flowers, but Sweet Tooth wanted to be different. Besides, the tiny white flowers were a wee bit too small for her generous hips. So, the lavender-pink colored wisteria was gathered from vines where they hung in clusters like grapes.

Nimbus stayed far away from the wisteria vines. He had a few run-ins with the bees and wasps that hung out around the flowers. Nimbus didn't want to be stung again and need to wear a bandage at the wedding. It would show through his tight leotards and he knew that Vinnie would notice, and blurt something out at the most inappropriate moment.

Of course, Nimbus had trimmed down quite a bit since meeting Sweet Tooth. His workouts were paying off. He had reduced to a smaller size since the fall. His tuxedo was being designed from the oldest flower: the great, white blossom of the southern magnolia. The waxy outer coating would give his tuxedo the appearance of being shiny.

"How do I look?" squeaked Nimbus.

"A little pink. You look more like the blushing bride than Sweet Tooth," exclaimed Butterfly, the tailor.

"Whew! I can't tell you've lost any weight today, Nimbus," panted the butterflies in attendance. "Hold your breath and we'll try this again. One, two, three, stretch!"

"Where did you say you lost that weight, Nimbus?"

"My feet! I lost the weight in my feet; they're a whole leaf size smaller," joked Nimbus. "Do you think you could loosen the belt a little, fellas?"

"Uh, we didn't make one. You won't be needing a belt to hold up these petals!" exclaimed the butterfly as he fluttered gracefully around the groom-to-be. Nimbus was amazed at the elegant butterfly that danced with its wings.

"Could you give me a few ideas on how to stay light on my wings like a butterfly?" pleaded Nimbus. "I don't want to break out of my petals when I reach over to kiss the bride."

"Sure. How about a fast on fruit nectar?" suggested one of the butterflies.

"No," Nimbus replied. "It's not good for my blood sugar. I have to eat often or I faint. The last time I fainted, I fell in the wood violets."

"Is that where all those pressed violets for the invitations came from?" whispered the butterfly to another attendant.

Nimbus ignored the whispering. "Actually, I don't like to diet," he confided. "It depresses me. I like to eat and look forward to mealtime. Do you have any other ideas that will work for me? This magnolia-petal tuxedo is getting tighter as we talk."

"How about practicing a little behavior modification?" suggested a passing glowworm. "There's nothing wrong with carrying a little extra weight. You just need to do some shape shifting with some sound dietary practices. There's a visitor who specializes in helping dieters make constructive changes in their eating habits without really changing a lot of what they eat."

"I like that idea. How do I start?" Nimbus asked.

"Let's see what knowledge June Bug has brought from the earth this year." Glowworm slid through the garden to find June Bug. "He studied behavior modification during the grub worm stage of his development. It's amazing what knowledge is available from the earth."

"I hope we find him before he hangs on the screen door. It's hard for me to climb that high," remarked Nimbus.

"Nimbus, what would the fairy world do without you?" laughed the glowworm. "Here's June Bug, now, fresh out of the mud!"

June Bug looked a little dazed as he adjusted to daylight.

"Hey, June Bug. Nimbus wants to know how to lose weight effortlessly," joked Glowworm.

June Bug nodded his head slowly and faced Nimbus.

"The easiest way is to give up one high-calorie food," he instructed. "You can lose at least two pounds in one month. For example, if you eat ice cream every night, or even once a week, you can eat a piece of fruit instead and still drop some weight by the end of the month," June Bug explained patiently.

Nimbus paled at the thought of giving up his favorite pleasure food, lavender ice cream. It reminded him of the first time he saw Sweet Tooth.

"What's the next easiest way?" he asked.

"Choose to eat less of your favorite high-fat food, like chocolate-covered donuts," said June Bug, unaware that he was picking another favorite food of Nimbus.

"Could I substitute with the kind that has powdered sugar all over it?" asked Nimbus. "It would save a lot of calories to have chocolate-free donuts," Nimbus smiled hopefully.

June Bug did not agree and chose to continue.

"Let's go on, Nimbus. Always eat sitting down at the table and put all your food on one plate," advised June Bug.

"The plate's not big enough, June bug!" Nimbus said with much consternation. He was feeling a little defensive.

June Bug continued. "Weigh and measure specific food portions . . ."

"How big of a scale can I use?" asked Nimbus. He had never heard of a food scale.

June Bug droned on like a broken record. "Never allow second helpings to be served."

Nimbus brightened at this idea.

"Oh, I can eat it all in one helping. That's easy!" Nimbus said as he laughed and uncomfortably crossed his legs.

June Bug cleared his throat to demonstrate his displeasure.

"A-hem! Always leave uneaten food on your plate to affirm willpower, Nimbus."

"Isn't that a sin?" asked a horrified Nimbus.

"No, no, and no, Nimbus. Now, thirty minutes before eating, sip eight ounces of water or herbal tea."

Nimbus looked terrified as he interrupted June Bug.

"Herbal tea? Do you mean like Ginseng Elixir?" Nimbus paled at the memory of the fateful flight of the Phoenix. He flapped his fairy wings and ran away into the forest.

"Nimbus, come back! Be sure to brush your teeth so you won't be tempted to eat between meals!" yelled June Bug as Nimbus disappeared in a cloud of dust.

Nimbus was not heard from again that day, but here are a few tips June Bug left him on the way to the screen door.

- Never allow yourself to become very hungry before mealtime. This will encourage overeating. Schedule small snacks or nibble on some raw vegetables before lunch and dinner.
- Do not drink large amounts of liquid during meals. It will inhibit protein digestion by diluting hydrochloric acid. Sip one glass of water or tea during a meal. Drink more fluids in between meals.
- Eat crunchy raw vegetables or rice cakes if you are a nervous eater. Chewing reduces anxiety.
- Do not eat in front of the TV. Sip a non-calorie drink to help transition your previous eating habits.
- Do not eat on the run. Eat in a designated dining area at home and at work.
- Concentrate on what you are eating. Take time to notice the taste, texture, and feeling the food gives you.
- Exercise thirty minutes every other day. Choose an enjoyable exercise or sport.
- Weigh yourself only once a week.
- Reward weight loss with a non-food-related gift to yourself, like an aromatherapy lamp.
- Keep a daily journal of the foods and beverages you ingest. Include the amount consumed and how you feel after eating.
- Never dine at an "all you can eat" restaurant!

# FAIRY FOOD

Meanwhile, the fairies were creating recipes for the fairy feast and reception. For some reason, there was an abundance of pressed violets available from the garden, so the fairy decorator decided to candy them. She found a tiny paintbrush and tweezers to create the following edible decoration.

## PRESSED CANDIED VIOLETS

Gather one cup of fresh violets in the morning after the dew evaporates. Remove the stems. Place them flat, without touching, on waxed paper (or allow Nimbus to flatten them). Using a tiny paintbrush, coat each violet thoroughly with one large beaten egg white. Turn the violets over with tweezers to coat each side. Sprinkle superfine sugar on both sides of the violets. Allow the violets to dry on the wax paper for six hours. Use a spatula to remove them one at a time.

**Note:** Although the violets found for this recipe did not intend to volunteer for this service before Nimbus fell on them, it is very likely they will recuperate quickly by moving to a more remote area of the garden.

## ELDERBERRY FRUIT PUNCH: THE RED FRUIT PUNCH

This drink is a delicious and attractive punch for an elegant occasion such as a wedding. Substitute apple or white grape juice for the fruit punch if Vinnie, or any other hyper-fairies, are attending. They are often sensitive to red and yellow food coloring.

**Ingredients**
    2 thinly sliced lemons
    2 thinly sliced limes
    1/2 cup fresh spearmint leaves
    1 cup fresh elderberry flowers
    2 cups sparkling mineral water
    1 quart frozen fruit punch
    fresh spearmint leaves for garnish

Layer fresh spearmint between the citrus slices. Allow them to stand while preparing an elderflower concentrate. Steep freshly picked flowers from an abundant source in two cups of mineral water for thirty minutes. Strain and add one quart of fruit punch prepared with sparkling mineral water or distilled water. Add the lemon and lime slices. Serve over ice garnished with fresh spearmint leaves.

**Note:** Elder bushes bloom in abundance and won't mind having a few blossoms trimmed off for this recipe. Dried flowers can be substituted for fresh. Use one cup dried flowers.

## ROSEMARY AND THYME COOKIES

After a bit of experimenting, the baker took out the parsley and sage and left the rosemary and thyme in this recipe.

**Ingredients**

    1½ cups all-purpose or whole-wheat graham flour or wheat-free flour**
    1 teaspoon baking soda
    1 teaspoon minced fresh or dried rosemary leaves
    1 teaspoon fresh minced lemon thyme
    1 cup unsalted butter or ghee***
    ¾ cup sugar or date sugar (available at health food stores)
    1 tablespoon fresh lemon zest
    1 small egg or egg replacer*
    1½ tablespoons fresh lemon juice
    1½ teaspoons grated and peeled ginger root

Begin by preheating the oven to 350° and prepare this basic sugar cookie recipe: Sift flour and baking soda. Stir in herbs. In another bowl, cream butter and sugar and add lemon zest. Beat in egg, lemon juice, and ginger root. Add flour to the mixture and form into dough. Roll into a log. Refrigerate for thirty minutes on wax paper. Cut into one-quarter-inch slices. Place cookies one inch apart on an un-greased cookie sheet. Bake until golden, about ten to twelve minutes. Remove with a spatula and cool on racks. Dust with fairy dust: one-half teaspoon powdered ginger in one-half cup powdered sugar. Sprinkle lightly on top of the cookies.

### *EGG REPLACER

**Ingredients**

    1 teaspoon egg-free baking powder
    1½ tablespoons water
    1½ tablespoons cold-pressed vegetable oil

Combine well and add to a recipe to replace one egg. This recipe may be doubled for two-egg recipes.

### **WHEAT-FREE FLOUR

**Ingredients**
- 1 cup cornstarch
- 2 cups rice flour
- 3 cups potato starch
- 2 cups barley or soy flour (barley is best for cakes)

Combine and sift three times. Bake at 325° for ten to twenty minutes. Store any leftovers in a closed container.

### ***GHEE (CLARIFIED BUTTER)

**Ingredients**
- 1 pound unsalted butter

Melt unsalted butter in a skillet until it bubbles. Scrape off the bubbles. Pour into a wide-mouth container and refrigerate. When the milk fat separates and hardens, scrape it off. Use only the yellow ghee.

## HEAVEN SCENT WEDDING CAKE

**Modified for egg-free and milk-free diets.**

The wedding cake had to be chocolate to please Sweet Tooth. It also had to be low-fat to please Flora, who went to work creating this recipe for the wedding reception.

**Ingredients**
- 1½ cups cake flour
- 1½ teaspoons baking soda
- 1 teaspoon baking powder (non-aluminum)
- 1½ cups skim milk or 1% cocoa/soy milk (milk substitute*)
- 1 tablespoon vinegar added to the milk of your choice
- 2 tablespoons softened butter or ghee
- ¼ cup date sugar
- 1 egg or egg replacer
- 1 teaspoon vanilla
- 2 teaspoons chocolate extract (or chocolate syrup if Flora is not watching)
- 3 tablespoons cocoa powder
- 1 tablespoon chocolate mint leaves pureed in a blender
  with ½ cup milk of choice

Sift flour, baking soda, powder, and cocoa. Cream the butter, extracts, sugar, and egg (or egg replacer). Alternately beat in butter, milk, and dry ingredients. Pour into a nine-inch greased round cake pan. Bake for twenty minutes in a preheated 350° oven until the top of the cake does not stick to your finger. Cool for fifteen minutes before removing from pan. Loosen with a knife.

*Calcium-rich milk substitutes:

SESAME MILK
**Ingredients**
> ½ cup sesame seeds
> ½ cup water

Combine sesame seeds and water. Blend at high speed for forty-five seconds. Strain the liquid through double cheesecloth. Sweeten to taste.

ALMOND MILK
**Ingredients**
> ¾ cup almonds
> 1⅔ cups water
> 1 teaspoon vanilla extract

Combine almonds and water. Blend at high speed for one minute. Strain the liquid through double cheesecloth. Add one teaspoon of pure vanilla extract.

COCONUT MILK **(Recommended only for slender fairies)**
**Ingredients**
> ½ cup grated fresh coconut
> 1 cup fresh coconut juice

Combine fresh coconut and fresh coconut juice. Blend at high speed for one minute. Strain if desired, or fold into the cake batter.

# FAIRY SNACKS

Here are some tasty dips Flora prepared for the wedding reception. Flora served them with dry Melba toast. However, the Melba toast was still there after the feast. Jason crushed it and served it to the birds, who left it for the ants.

## HUMMUS

Serve with whole grain crackers

**Ingredients**
- 2 tablespoons olive oil
- Juice of 1 medium lemon
- 1 clove garlic
- ¼ cup Tahini (ground sesame butter)*
- 17-ounce can of garbanzo beans, drained
- ½ teaspoon dried winter savory or sage leaves, crushed

Blend at high speed for one minute.

### *TAHINI (GROUND SESAME BUTTER)

Tahini is calcium-rich seed butter, high in protein and vitamin T-increasing blood platelets.

**Ingredients**
- 3½ cups hulled white sesame seeds (about 1 pound)
- 2 teaspoons sesame oil

Spread sesame seeds onto an un-greased cookie sheet. Toast at 325° for eight to ten minutes, stirring occasionally. Remove the seeds when they turn a pale straw color. Browning seeds will cause them to taste bitter. Blend at high speed until it makes butter. Add two teaspoons sesame oil (if necessary), for smoothness.

**Note:** Tahini and rice make an excellent complementary and easy complete protein. Tahini can be used as a peanut butter substitute or in any nut butter recipe.

# LENTIL MOCK GUACAMOLE

Serve as a side dish or with fresh vegetables as a dip.

## Ingredients

10 ounces frozen petite peas (cooked and strained)
1 tablespoon safflower or canola oil
1 tablespoon mayonnaise or potato flour mayo substitute**
2 teaspoons ground cumin
1 teaspoon minced fresh spearmint
½ teaspoon lemon juice
½ garlic clove or 2 tablespoons onion

Blend at high speed for one minute. Add garnish such as olives, pimento, and cilantro.

## **POTATO FLOUR MAYONNAISE SUBSTITUTE

Wheat-free, egg-free, milk-free, gluten-free, yet it tastes good!

## Ingredients

1½ tablespoons potato flour
¼ teaspoon dry mustard
1 teaspoon fructose
½ teaspoon salt-substitute seasoning
¼ cup cold water
¾ cup boiling water
2 tablespoons lemon juice
1 tablespoon vinegar (preferably apple cider vinegar)
½ cup vegetable oil

Combine dry ingredients in a saucepan. Add cold water and mix well. Add hot water and cook until mixture clears. Cool until lukewarm, then beat in remaining ingredients. Refrigerate any leftovers.

# Cashew Paté

Serve with cocktail bread or whole grain crackers.

## Ingredients

    2 cups cashews
    1 cup cucumber
    2 stalks celery (pureed)
    1 medium carrot (peeled)
    1 tablespoon powdered vegetable broth
    dash of cumin
    2 tablespoons Tahini
    1 tablespoon fresh basil leaves
    dash of cayenne, chili powder, or paprika

Blend cashews and cucumber until pasty. Add remaining ingredients. Blend well.

# The Wedding Punch Nectar

Nimbus and Sweet Tooth would toast to their nuptials with elegant Tiffin Palais Versailles crystal. The fairies chose the dainty cordial for Sweet Tooth and the much-larger seafood cocktail glass for Nimbus. Chocolate kisses surrounded Sweet Tooth's cordial as she drank this wedding punch nectar.

## Ingredients

    2 cups grape juice
    12 ice cubes
    2 teaspoons honey or flavored honey
    1 tablespoon lemon zest

Blend at high speed. Yields four cups.

**Note:** To flavor honey, set a two-cup jar of honey in boiled water. Remove the water from the burner. Add two tablespoons of herbs and flowers. Combine thoroughly; cover and allow to steep for thirty minutes before straining into a clean glass jar. If desired, thin with one tablespoon of orange juice.

Fresh lemon verbena leaves
Rose petals, jasmine, honeysuckle, or gardenia flowers
Orange mint or spearmint leaves
Lemon thyme and rosemary leaves

# VIOLET TEA

For those who favor tea over punch, a delicious recipe for violet flower tea was tested until the following tea was brewed.

## Ingredients

1 cup boiled water
1 heaping teaspoon fresh violets
1 candied violet flower
Twist of fresh lime

For each cup of boiled water, steep one heaping teaspoon of fresh violets, covered in a teapot, for five minutes before serving. Serve with a candied violet and a twist of fresh lime.

# CHAPTER 8

# A Fairy Wedding
## A Celebration of Love

*All the love you share with others is really meant for you.*

### The Nervous Bridegroom

As the fairies baked and created new recipes, the decorating committee met to plan the reception. A fairy feast would follow the cake-cutting ceremony with colorful treats to experience before enjoying their favorite sport, a baseball game to end the evening. The fairies sure knew how to have fun! The party would extend into the evening, as fairy parties generally do.

This wedding was a very special one. There was no holding back on decorations, especially since Sweet Tooth was a renowned teacher in the community. It was rumored that even Mother Nature would be attending. Therefore, the decorating committee wanted the most elegant reception and fairy feast in the Land of Thyme. Everyone had ideas about which decorations would look best. The only thing on which they all agreed was using fine glass settings instead of plain papery leaves. And they wanted to find crystal bowls, plates and cups of every color in the rainbow in the smallest sizes available.

One of the fairies had heard of a crystal shop nearby with a wide variety of patterns and unique colors. The committee voted unanimously to visit the shop and choose the patterns and colors fit for a fairy feast. The display they created was striking, a dazzling work of fairy art, complementing the happiest day of Nimbus and Sweet Tooth's life.

During the day, Collie found Nimbus working furiously in the garden, tilling the same soil over and over again. Collie first looked surprised and then angry.

"Nimbus! What are you doing? You're going to re-injure your shoulders tilling the garden! Why, it's not even time to till! The fall gardens are planted and spring is yet to come," he chided.

"It's either work or eat, Collie. I just have to stay busy!" Nimbus groaned.

"Are your feet getting cold before the wedding?" asked Collie.

"Oh, no! It's not that! I just feel overwhelmed about what June Bug told me earlier today, that's all," sighed Nimbus, as he sat down next to Collie and wiped his brow.

"I didn't even know June bugs could talk, much less have anything important to say," Collie said.

"Well, this one did! He taught some guidelines for behavior modification for people who love to eat like me. He must have absorbed all that wisdom from stored knowledge deep within the earth while he was in the larvae and grub stage," explained Nimbus.

"Ugh! You'll never convince me there's any wisdom in being a grub, or even a June bug, but that's okay. Just explain to me why a bug's great wisdom overwhelmed you, Nimbus. You have all the innate wisdom of a gardener combined with the surrealistic magic of a fairy. How could a bug living out his last hours intimidate you?"

"Well, he gave me all these reasons not to eat! What will I do if I give up the comfort of eating until my whole body hums?" asked Nimbus with a frightened look on his face.

"There are a lot of things you can do if you don't numb your senses eating, Nimbus! What are you afraid of?" asked Collie, intently looking into Nimbus's eyes.

"Well, life, I guess," answered Nimbus, keeping his gaze to the garden floor.

"How about responsibility?" Collie fired back. "That's what self-actualization is all about — taking responsibility for making your life better everyday in a way that benefits others."

"Ouch! You got me there. I guess better doesn't mean a better meal, does it?" Nimbus said, feeling slightly self-conscious. "I just don't have enough self-confidence to do anything but eat and garden," Nimbus replied, thinking out loud.

"Well, that's where most everybody starts, Nimbus. You just have to go about this slowly so you make gradual changes over a period of time. That's what behavior modification really means."

"It's great to have a friend like you, Collie. With your support, maybe I can take some effective steps toward a leaner diet."

"Oh, I'm sure," nodded Collie. "Why, even Flora would approve of your efforts."

"That reminds me!" exclaimed Nimbus as he flew into the air. "Next spring Flora is sending Sweet Tooth and me to a garden so we can learn how flower essences and essential oils support conscious growth."

"Good idea! Let me know if I can give you a ride," replied Collie as he stood up to leave. "I have to go now, I hear my owner calling. We're going to the groomer. I want to look sharp for your wedding, buddy!"

Nimbus blushed and left the garden, thinking maybe he really could make some behavior modification changes in his diet.

## The Wedding

The big day finally arrived, and everyone was hurrying with last-minute preparations. Nimbus was nervous. He had to eat constantly to keep from fainting. Collie ran back and forth from the kitchen to bring him some low-calorie snacks.

"Whew! I wish someone would invent a decent fairy deodorant for times like this," complained the carnation in Nimbus's lapel. Nimbus looked helpless as he mopped his brow. His best man suddenly appeared with a solution.

"Here's some fresh parsley to chew on, Nimbus. With any luck, it will quickly filter through your sweat glands," offered St. Francis, patron of the gardens, making a rare appearance as the best man.

"Why does it taste like the grass people eat so frequently?" Nimbus asked as he chewed on the parsley.

"It's low-fat, low-sodium, low-calorie, high-fiber, and much lower maintenance," St. Francis patiently explained. "Better yet, it's a natural deodorant and breath freshener."

"I knew something that tastes this bad had to be good for me," Nimbus said while looking at this watch.

Suddenly, an enthusiastic cupid appeared. "It's time to escort you to the altar, you lucky guy! Would you like a ride too, St. Francis?"

"No, I'd rather walk," he replied. "I enjoy the simple life. What happened to the Phoenix? I thought he always accompanies the bridegroom!"

"The Phoenix declined," replied the cupid. "Something about a bad back from a previous flight. He's on disability for a while yet."

"What are you going to do after the wedding?" asked St. Francis.

"I thought I'd stick around and hold a candle for the fairy feast," the cupid replied.

"Good idea," said St. Francis. "I'll gather my birds and forest friends and be right there."

## The Ceremony

Fairies, flowers, and friends gathered from every corner of the Land of Thyme to witness the big event. The forest floor was carpeted with freshly fallen leaves. The sun rose for this special occasion and blanketed the altar with a pink glow of warmth. The wind gently flowed through the trees calling all the little forest animals. A silver mist lotus and lute welcomed Lao Tzu and Kuan Yin to bless the rings. Pink carnations decorated the altar.

A Justice of the Garden stepped forward to lead the ceremony. It turned out to be none other than the chief Fairy SEAL of Operation Fairy Storm. Nimbus winced, then blushed. The ceremony commenced. Nimbus was ready to go on with his life. His past foibles were no longer part of him. As his thoughts drifted, he heard the Justice of the Garden asking, "Nimbus, do you take Sweet Tooth Petal for your lawful, wedded wife?"

"I think so. What's an awful wedding wife?" Nimbus queried, puzzled, and turned to his beloved.

Sweet Tooth whispered something in Nimbus's ear. He blushed bright red, started sweating again, and blurted, "Oh, yes, I do! I really do!" Everyone clapped.

The chief went on. "Sweet Tooth . . ."

All of a sudden, a familiar voice rang out of the audience. "Hey, Nimbus! What's that poking out of the back of your petal tux? It looks like the outline of a toothbrush."

It was Vinnie, the hyper-fairy, always available to blurt out an embarrassing question. A ripple of laughter moved through the audience. Nimbus laughed nervously. He never went anywhere without his toothbrush, especially if he was going to be alone with Sweet Tooth. With his head in the clouds thinking of spending a honeymoon alone with her, Nimbus turned and smiled at Sweet Tooth.

"Sweet Tooth, do you take Nimbus Cloud for your lawful, wedded husband?"

Everyone's eyes turned to gaze at the beautiful bride. Sweet Tooth looked ravishing. Nimbus couldn't take his dreamy eyes off her. Apollo himself made an appearance to give the bride away. Naturally, he couldn't resist flirting with Mother Nature during the ceremony, who overtly winked back. As they flirted, Sweet Tooth's life flashed before her.

Sweet Tooth had tears in her eyes. This was the moment she had waited for her whole life. Her dream lover and a chocolate wedding cake! And now she was remembering the cherry blossom tea ceremony before the wedding.

She turned to Nimbus, put her arms around him, and planted a kiss right on his lips. "I do!" exclaimed Sweet Tooth. "I sure do."

The audience cheered as the Justice of the Garden pronounced Sweet Tooth and Nimbus man and wife. Nimbus felt numb and had the silliest grin on his face as he exchanged gold rings with his new wife.

The fairies threw their hats in the air, cheering and clapping loudly. They gathered around the altar with the intention of carrying the bride and groom to the cake ceremony, but quickly changed their minds. They decided to carry the Justice of the Garden instead. He was embarrassed at first, but soon began to enjoy the festive moment with the crowd. Soon he was flexing his biceps and showing off, hoping Flora would notice him, but she was too busy counting fat grams and calories in the wedding cake. Everyone gathered behind the newly-weds to continue the celebration with a cake ceremony.

## An Intimate Fairy Dinner

They all marched to the cake ceremony in the most festive mood. Everyone was dressed in the finest floral designs. The flowers put forward their prettiest petals, aromas, and foliage for the feast. The pine trees shook with joy, spilling showers of cones and scattering the crowd.

They came together again in the banquet hall at the forest clearing. Talk continued of how lovely the bride looks and how attractive the outline of the toothbrush looks in Nimbus's leotard. "How can he sit down with a toothbrush in his pants?" asked Vinnie.

"How can he brush his teeth afterwards?" remarked St. Francis quietly.

The idle talk was interrupted when the wedding cake was unveiled.

"Oh, look!" the crowd exhaled. "The wedding cake is beautiful! Is that a chocolate-covered bride and groom on top of the cake?" asked one of the smaller fairies.

"I think so," yawned Jason, as he stretched up and up above the crowd. "Sweet Tooth just ate them!"

"Oh, and a chocolate-covered cherry for the groom's cake," sighed Mother Nature, still drying the tears from her eyes.

"Yes, Sweet Tooth thought she'd order Nimbus a cake she would enjoy just in case he didn't like it," said St. Francis with a chuckle.

"I've never known Nimbus to dislike anything gooey, fattening, and sticky-sweet," recalled Mother Nature. "He does look a little firmer and thinner since he's been on an exercise kick and behavior modification program, and his pant seams aren't quite as pronounced!"

The crowd became silent as the bride and groom walked to the front of the banquet hall.

Finally, it was time to cut the cake. All the condiments were chocolate, much to Flora's chagrin. There were chocolate roses, chocolate leaves, chocolate ribbons, and chocolate maple leaf wafers for dishes. Sweet Tooth ate them all and she loved every morsel. She promised herself she would make up for all those extra calories much later. Her petals grew tighter as she ate, while Nimbus watched in admiration. He lovingly wiped the chocolate smudges from the corners of her mouth before the photographer took the next photograph. No one noticed her teeth were dark chocolate as she smiled. She was the happiest bride the fairies ever remembered seeing. Her eyes filled with tears of joy as she handed Nimbus a cup of wedding punch.

The couple tipped their Tiffin cordials filled with wedding punch as they vowed to share every meal together for the remainder of fairy time. Everyone clapped and agreed they made a wonderful couple, a great boon to the fairy society where love is always welcome.

## The Dance

As the crowd quickly ate their cake and sipped wedding punch, music floated through the forest as the band began to play. The Garden Friends Band was playing their theme song, as the wind cleared the forest floor. There was Snail playing bass and Preying Mantis on lead guitar. Cricket took his seat at the drums next to a pill bug, Roly-Poly, playing the piano. A chorus of ants knew every tune and sang as the bumblebees hummed in the background! This was the party the fairies waited for: good food, good music, and a happy couple to lead the first dance.

The crowd called out to Nimbus and Sweet Tooth for the first dance. Bagworm requested "Twist and Shout," and the music echoed through the forest. Everyone was singing and dancing to the music. Nimbus was shuffling his feet, a little embarrassed by his awkwardness. He had never made it to his dance lessons during adolescence. They were held after lunch, the moment when Nimbus always felt the need to curl up for a nap. Now he wished he knew how to dance. He didn't want to let down Sweet Tooth on their wedding day.

Sweet Tooth was surprisingly light on her feet. All that chocolate didn't slow her down a bit. She was jiggling and twirling all around Nimbus, spinning closer and closer. She was so close he could smell her rose perfume. He thought he would faint until Sweet Tooth wrapped herself around him and helped Nimbus move to the music. The friction warmed up the forest in a hurry. Sweet Tooth leaned closer and they disappeared in a cloud of steam. From that moment on, Nimbus was never the same. He whirled Sweet Tooth around and as the steam rose, Nimbus realized he, too, could dance!

The crowd roared, stomping and clapping to the rhythm. The band played on, and on, and on as Nimbus led his graceful sweetheart in dance after dance. The chocolate kiss marks left on his face from the steamy encounter with Sweet Tooth were melting down his neck. All he felt was rhythm and feet that thundered. He became the music and the music became him. They danced until the band took a break and everyone migrated to the fairy feast for refreshments. Everyone congratulated Nimbus as they walked by.

Sweet Tooth went into the kitchen to find the recipe for those delicious chocolate condiments and, hopefully, several more of them to eat. However, all that remained on the counter was an open *Betty Cricket Cookbook* with several pages ripped out. The following recipe appeared inside.

## How to Make Melba Toast

Cut bread into diagonal slices. Remove crusts. Place on un-greased cookie sheets and bake at 200° for four to five hours, or "until the bread tastes like cardboard," said Sweet Tooth with a yawn.

Variations: Before baking, brush lightly with your favorite herbal ghee (basic recipe on page 117).

Rosemary ghee: Simmer one teaspoon fresh or dried rosemary in one cup of ghee or olive oil for ten minutes. Cool and strain. Refrigerate leftovers in a covered container.

Herbal substitutes: Instead of rosemary, use one-half teaspoon of freshly grated ginger; one-half a clove of mashed garlic; two teaspoons of fresh lemon thyme; one-half teaspoon of dried oregano; or one-half teaspoon of fresh winter savory.

## The Fairy Feast

Meanwhile, the fairies and visiting forest animals, insects, and devas began the feast. They ate, played games, drank punch, and demonstrated their floral skills on the nearby flowers. Everyone was happy to see Nimbus really let go of his insecurities and dance! Dancing is an act of abundance to fairies, and Nimbus certainly demonstrated that. Of course, Mother Nature was concerned that Nimbus might overexert himself, but Apollo assured her it was good for his waistline!

As the guests stood around and talked, ladybugs flew around them and filled their empty demitasse cups with iced drinks or red fruit punch. Apollo was leaning closer and closer to Mother Nature, making small talk about the garden industry, when Vinnie, the hyper-fairy, bounced by. He was trying to make conversation with Flora, who managed to ignore him, so he decided to talk to the shell of a deceased snail. Vinnie didn't mind a one-way conversation at all.

Apollo heard him jabbering and called out to him, "Hey, son, how's the organic gardening work going?" Mother Nature looked uncomfortable, expressing sudden interest in her toes. Flora looked puzzled, turning slowly toward her parents.

"Son? I thought I was an only child! Dad, did anything happen between you and Aphrodite?"

"No," he said with a chuckle. "I got turned into an anemone first. I spent years waiting for a frog to kiss me so I could get back into a body. You just don't know how tough it is being a wildflower. When it rains, fairies curl up in your petals. One time Nimbus tried it and I thought I would die before the storm was over." Apollo winked at Mother Nature, who knew he was kidding Flora, and trying to change the subject.

"Then why did you refer to Vinnie as a son?"

Vinnie loved the attention and reached over to have some refreshments, grinning from pixie ear to pixie ear.

"Well, Flora, didn't your mother ever tell you about your brother?"

"Ah!" Flora screamed. "My brother! He can't be related to me. He must be a reject from the compost pile!"

"Actually, he's your twin, Flora," Apollo gently replied. Mother Nature was very uncomfortable now, watching Flora from the corner of her eye.

"But he's hyper and he drools!" screamed Flora as she wildly flew out of the forest towards the lake. Apollo and Mother Nature looked at each other as they began to follow Flora.

Just then Vinnie picked up the wrong glass and drank the red elderberry flower fruit punch. His eyes bulged as his hyperactivity kicked in. He couldn't stop bothering everyone with teasing, touching, and interrupting. His wings crossed, his feet left the ground, and his eyes gleamed as he squealed, "Flora! Wait for me!"

Flora screamed louder and beat her wings wildly to get away from Vinnie.

The forest became quiet except for the flap of wings and Mother Nature screaming, horrified, "No, Vinnie! Not the red fruit punch!" But it was too late. The red color of the fruit punch put Vinnie into orbit. He followed Flora as she ran away. Mother Nature searched for her lavender essential oil, in vain, to calm him. Vinnie was flying high, skimming the tops of the trees in the forest.

Suddenly, there was a loud splash. Everyone moved forward in unison towards the lake. Apollo looked alarmed as he grabbed Mother Nature by the arm.

"Oh, it's all right, darling. Flora always falls into water, even for no reason, especially when she has her best wings on. She must have some latent water nymph genes in her DNA." Mother Nature patted Apollo's arm as they flew towards the lake. No one was worried about Vinnie hurting himself. He inherited a hard head.

As everyone gathered near the water, a gasp went up from the crowd. Flora was nowhere to be found. A few bubbles came up to the top of the water, then nothing!

"My baby!" cried Mother Nature. Apollo ran to catch Vinnie, who was flying upside down in circles nearby, and poured the rest of the red fruit punch down his throat. Vinnie flapped wildly.

## The Rescue

"Go rescue your sister!" shouted Apollo, pointing Vinnie toward the lake and giving him a nudge.

There was no time to waste. Vinnie flew to the lake, bursting with energy. Instead of diving in and saving Flora, he grabbed a demitasse cup and scooped out all the water in the lake cup by cup! Water flew out of the lake as Vinnie's arms twisted relentlessly. In moments, Flora's feet were seen wiggling outside of the water.

"Oh, my baby's alive! She loves to play with her feet!" cried Mother Nature happily.

Vinnie flew towards Flora with fire in his eyes, almost as wet as she was. Flora gurgled, then screamed, "Help! He drools!" She fainted momentarily, clutching what seemed to be some Betty Cricket recipes in her hand. The crowd cheered Vinnie as he carried Flora to safety. She ran away as soon as she came to her senses with Vinnie happily bouncing after her.

"Want to be my friend? Huh, Flora? I'll show you my pet snake collection!" Vinnie wanted to be friends with Flora more than ever now, but Flora was not amenable.

"Ah!" screamed Flora, as she flew away into the forest, dripping as she flapped. She just wasn't prepared to face her kinship with Vinnie. Flora felt out of control and very vulnerable inside. She quickly disappeared into some nearby verbena flowers to find solace and a sense of peace.

## The Grand Finale

After everyone dried off from Vinnie's demitasse frenzy, a baseball game began. The flowers all shook their pollen to mold it into a ball. Vines were stripped for bats, and bases were drawn with diatomaceous earth. Of course, since Apollo was a great athlete, everyone wanted to be on his team, while Mother Nature got all the runts. Vinnie was assigned to her team. She smiled graciously, but her mind was already racing.

Mother Nature had a plan. Every time Apollo's homerun hitters slammed a run, Vinnie was given red fruit punch to drink. He came out of left field spinning like a top. He would leap into the air catching every hit before the batter made it to first base. The score was 0 to 0 in the last inning, and now Mother Nature's team, the Short Stops, was up to bat.

"Batter up!" yelled the wise old umpire owl.

The pitcher threw a wild curve ball. It curved at least three times before it got to home plate. Mother Nature's team was so used to running all over the garden to hit one of her wild pitches that the batter had no problem hitting this ball.

Whack! The ball sped into left field with an outfielder moving in on the grounder. The little runts had such short legs no one thought they had a chance until Mother Nature pulled out her famous Red Hot Pepper Sauce! She quickly poured a few drops down the throat of the panting little fairy.

Zoom! The fairy took off like a bolt of lightning. He passed first base and headed for second. The outfielder threw the ball to second base. The hot pepper sauce activated the runt's sinuses into a great big sneeze. The resulting wind blew over the second baseman before he could catch the ball. The fairy landed on second, wings down!

"You're safe!" cried the owl.

By the time Vinnie came to bat, the bases were loaded with two outs. The crowd was restless and noisy. Vinnie was bouncing up and down. He missed the first ball. "Strike one!" Then he missed the next. "Strike two!" The crowd booed. Vinnie bit his lip, scared but determined not to let down his teammates.

Mother Nature had another plan. She called a timeout and motioned Vinnie to join her at the sideline. From deep within her pockets, she pulled out home-made Melba toast and stuffed them into his mouth. The starch in the crumbs slowed him down. Vinnie relaxed, stopped drooling, and stepped up to the plate. Everyone held their breath as Mother Nature sprayed Vinnie with an Alert Aroma blend. "Pay attention!" she called out to him.

Wham! Vinnie smacked the ball clear out of the garden. The fairy crowd threw their hats into the air. The flowers repeatedly opened and closed their petals to share in the joy. Everyone was cheering on Vinnie as he ran the bases as fast as his little legs could travel.

Apollo yelled, "Run! Show 'em what you're worth, son!" Both teams threw their hats into the air as Vinnie spun into home base. The crowd moved toward home base as both teams ran to congratulate Vinnie. Mother Nature stood at the sideline, smiling in approval.

The game was over. Vinnie had become a hero twice in one day. His tiny teammates hosed him down with a sedation aroma blend so they could carry him off the field.

Spider, top reporter for the *Fairy Morning News,* took down all the recipes, typed them, telephoned the paper, and waited in line for Vinnie's autograph using all eight busy hands.

## ENERGY RED HOT PEPPER SAUCE

Serve with caution. To sedate, heat and serve on homemade Melba toast. Mmmm.

**Ingredients**
  2 poblano chilies
  6 tablespoons onion
  ¼ teaspoon garlic
  1 tablespoon fresh lemon or lime juice

Chop and seed the poblano chilies and grate the onion. With a garlic press, juice the garlic. Add the lemon or lime juice and stir and cover at room temperature for two hours.

## WINNING COMBINATION ALERT AROMA BLEND

This blend allows the wearer to focus on winning.
  10 drops lemon grass essential oil
  2 drops Indian paintbrush flower essence
  3 drops spearmint essential oil
  1 ounce jojoba oil

Combine the ingredients and wear on temples or forehead.

## HEAVY SEDATION AROMA BLEND

To release tension and reduce over-activity, apply this blend on the face and neck or on the soles of the feet.
  3 drops sage essential oil
  3 drops verbena flower essence
  2 drops sandalwood essential oil
  1 tablespoon sesame oil

Combine the ingredients and relax.

## The Honeymooners

After Sweet Tooth and Nimbus finally finished packing several suitcases, they were ready to leave and enjoy their honeymoon! They first tried to make reservations on the TransButterfly Airlines, but the fairy pilots found out and immediately went on strike. They rightfully complained that their fairy pilot wings just weren't equipped for carrying such a heavy load!

Instead, they decided to take a long romantic honeymoon cruise on a beautiful velvet swan. Besides, the food is better, and more desserts are served on a cruise! Their days would be filled with a variety of activities and their nights would be filled with music and dance.

Sweet Tooth looked stunning in a suit made with passion vine and hand-embroidered roses. Nimbus wore petal-pushers made with amaryllis blossoms and his favorite tennis shoes tied with bindweed, his usual attire. His shoes never came untied! As the swan began to move gracefully out of the port, the couple smiled and waved to the crowd. They were ready to go.

Everyone gathered to throw pollen as the happy couple danced gracefully to elevator music. Nimbus now referred to Sweet Tooth as his "honky-tonk woman." She turned to throw her wedding bouquet of gardenias to a crowd of single, giggly female fairies. Candy wrappers flew everywhere as Sweet Tooth released the gardenia bouquet into the air. The fairy girls were jumping and screaming in unison, knocking into each other's wings. Petite climbed atop Jason's shoulder to get a better view. As the bouquet flew into the air, everyone scattered as his friend, the German shepherd, jumped into the air. The bouquet landed on Jason's shoulder with Petite popping up in the middle of it, balancing a gardenia on her head. The crowd clapped, Petite blushed, and Jason gave the German shepherd a big hug!

The happy couple sailed away with thunderous applause. Sweet Tooth waved and Nimbus danced a few fancy steps for the crowd until his bindweed shoelaces wrapped around each other. He sat down rather abruptly to avoid falling. The crowd held their breath until the velvet swan recovered from the shock waves. Then, the fairies waved and called out to the honeymooners until they disappeared into the sunset!

## The Gift

As the crowd dispersed, Flora appeared with a neatly wrapped box. "A little late for a wedding present," said a fairy passing by.

"This is for Vinnie. Have you seen him?" asked Flora sweetly.

Nearby, Mother Nature and Apollo had to hold onto each other to contain their joy. "How sweet of you, darling! Have you prepared Vinnie a thank-you gift for rescuing you?"

"Yes. I've been in the kitchen all afternoon. Can you call him, Daddy?"

Apollo complied with a whistle that shook the leaves off the trees. "Hey, Vinnie! Flora has a present for you!" Then he whispered under his breath, "I hope it's not red."

Vinnie bounced over the treetops to join them. He smiled with genuine appreciation and friendship, then wildly tore into the package. He uncovered homemade checkerboard cookies and wolfed them down in a few slobbery bites. He turned to thank Flora, but she had already left.

"Oh well," he thought. "I'll thank Flora later when I share my pet snake collection with her." He was delighted that he had a new friend and a twin sister who could bake yummy cookies. But what was this underneath the crumbs? Why, it looked like a T-shirt! Vinnie unfolded the white shirt to read the stenciled lettering. It said EVIL TWIN.

"An 'evil twin' T-shirt! Now, that's really interesting," a crow remarked. Vinnie's eyes grew big, but he had nothing to say. He wasn't sure what Flora meant, but he felt a little anxious and scared. "Maybe she didn't want to be friends after all," he sighed sadly.

Apollo and Mother Nature quickly walked over to Vinnie. Mother Nature and Apollo encircled Vinnie as he started to walk away. Apollo put his hand on Vinnie's shoulder. "That T-shirt is really going to be a hit with all your friends, Vinnie. Nobody has one like it!" Vinnie brightened a little when Mother Nature suggested they take his picture. Apollo went to find Flora, determined to settle the sibling rivalry.

The next day, Spider had a front-page news story about Vinnie's valiant rescue of Flora and winning hit in the baseball game. And there on the front page in full color was a large photo of Vinnie proudly wearing his T-shirt and holding a box of homemade Melba toast. The stencil had a horizontal arrow pointing to none other than Flora, holding Vinnie's pet snake! What a happy photo for all of fairydom to see! And on the second page was Flora's delicious and soon-to-be-famous high-fat, high-cholesterol, and loaded with sugar Evil Twin Cookies.

# EVIL TWIN COOKIES

## Ingredients

2½ cups bleached flour (unless you like your twin, then use unbleached flour)

⅓ cup chopped pecans or hazelnuts

2½ tablespoons cocoa powder

2 sticks softened unsalted butter (use salted butter for an "old" taste)

¾ cup sugar

1 egg

1 teaspoon pure vanilla extract

1½ tablespoon freshly grated lemon zest

½ teaspoon instant coffee dissolved in 1½ teaspoons hot water

Combine nuts and cocoa powder and pulverize in a blender. In a medium bowl, blend butter and sugar until fluffy; then, add the egg, vanilla, and lemon zest. Beat until smooth. On low speed, blend half of the flour and then stir in the remaining flour with a wooden spoon. Divide dough in half and return half to the mixing bowl, adding the cocoa and nut mixture. Knead thoroughly. Mix in dough. Divide the dough in half.

Roll out the white and chocolate dough on sheets of wax paper into a six-by-ten-inch rectangle. Place on an un-greased cookie sheet and freeze for twenty minutes. The dough must be very cold to be assembled into checkerboards.

Peel wax paper off and lay one portion of dough on a cutting board. Peel the second dough from the wax paper and place on top of the first dough. Trim uneven edges. Cut into thirds lengthwise, making three two-by-ten-inch strips. Stack on wax paper, alternating colors like a checkerboard. Press to form an even two-by-ten-inch block. Wrap in wax paper and freeze for twenty minutes.

Cut combined layers lengthwise into quarter-inch-by-ten-inch strips. Stack in checkerboard fashion, alternating colors. Wrap in wax paper and freeze for twenty minutes.

Knead the extra discarded chocolate pieces and roll into a nine-by-ten-inch rectangle. Place on an un-greased cookie sheet and refrigerate for five minutes. Remove top wax paper. Place checkerboard dough in the center and enclose it with chocolate dough. Trim any excess dough. Wrap in plastic wrap and freeze for twenty minutes.

Preheat oven to 350°. Grease baking sheets. Carefully cut frozen block crosswise into one-eighth-inch slices, using a sharp knife and cutting board. Transfer the slices to the greased baking sheet and space one inch apart.

Bake on center rack for five to eight minutes, or until the edges begin to brown. Remove from oven and allow cookies to cool for one minute. With a spatula, remove cookies to wire racks. They will become brittle when thoroughly cooled. Store in an airtight container or freeze until an evil twin appears in your life. Yields sixty cookies.

# CHAPTER 9

# Flora's Dream
## Empowering the Chakras

*Flower essences transform our inner world.*

### Heart to Heart

After the wedding party, Apollo had a heart-to-heart talk with Flora. She now had a new perspective of Vinnie and the fairies who lived under her guidance. She realized that maybe life wasn't as easy for them as it was for her. Flora knew how to achieve and maintain a healthy lifestyle. Vinnie and some of the fairies had to really work at achieving their disciplines. Apollo counseled Flora about opening her heart and accepting people as they are to enhance their creative change. This wasn't easy for a young goddess like Flora. She always wanted to fix everyone and make him or her better. She immediately noticed what was wrong instead of what was right.

Flora really wanted to please her father, but she couldn't let go of her desire to lead the fairies into optimal health. And yet, she never dreamed it would be so hard and take so long to convert them to a healthy lifestyle. For every calorie or fat gram she saved, a hundred more would find their way into the fairies' diets. As for Vinnie, well, she wasn't sure how to help him. He was a good gardener and liked her Melba toast, but he got on everyone's nerves. Suddenly she remembered a poem Vinnie wrote for her.

*"Look Before You Speak"*
*My brain has a mouth*
*That precedes good taste*
*Sometimes it strikes*
*Always with haste*
*Can it be silenced*
*Will it be tamed*
*The answer may surprise you*
*But the problem remains unchanged.*

These thoughts traveled through Flora's mind as she wearily climbed into bed. Maybe they all needed her help, the fairies and Vinnie. Then, they would be more likely to want to do everything right like her, rather than just have fun.

As she drifted off to sleep, Flora felt the presence of her guardian angel hovering over her. She often felt this presence before she received guidance during her sleep. She smiled in anticipation of helping the fairy world become more like her.

Her guardian angel smiled at Flora's modesty! Little did she realize that teaching the fairies would also help her to open her heart.

As Flora slept, she dreamed of the many inner challenges that affect the external world of fairies, pets, and even their human owners. Feelings of self-esteem and self-worth, rejection, and feeling unloved took form and marched before her. She felt these feelings like she never had before, to the very depth of her goddess-soul. Suddenly, Flora felt compassion for others, as well as a sense of responsibility to help them. She noticed that as feelings such as guilt and loneliness would take form, a flower would appear growing beside it. Flora then dreamed of growing a garden with a flower to heal the broken hearts and lonely souls of every fairy. Why there must be a flower for every feeling! She had understood flowers to be only an aromatic healing agent for the body. Now, she realized they could soothe the soul and the many feelings contained within the psyche, hidden within the darkness of the subconscious.

As she dreamed, Flora was suddenly transported to gardens all over the world, each with flowers blooming to support the feelings of the population. This opened a whole new world for her to explore. She understood flowers as sources of pleasure rather than for healing old hurts. Everyone could use flowers to heal their feelings!

Just then, Flora envisioned Nimbus standing in his garden, looking sad and forlorn. "Help! Get me out of this body!" he cried out to Flora.

"Oh, yes, Nimbus, I can help you now!" cried Flora, as she awakened and flew out of her bed.

"There's something to all this emotional pain I never realized before! It must be the next step to a healthy fairy community. My dreams never lie!"

"Where are my notes on flower essences? I never gave them much thought before," mumbled Flora, as she scrambled through her old school books. "Ancient healers brewed flowers to heal mental and emotional anguish.

"Ah, heck, this one's on Star War rules, I'll just throw that one out! Fortunately, that part of my life is over!"

As the book tumbled to the floor, a small, folded piece of paper fell from the opened page. "Hey! I don't remember taking notes in Star War class. It was too boring. What's this piece of paper?" Flora pondered.

As she opened the handwritten note to its full size, an address appeared in Flora's handwriting.

"Oh, yes! I've been looking for this! It was right here in my room the whole time! Flora chuckled. "It's not like me to make a mistake!

"This is the garden I've been wanting to send Nimbus and Sweet Tooth to visit. Sweet Tooth does seem to keep Nimbus happy. His whole life has turned around since he fell in love with Sweet Tooth. He's even somewhat interested in nutrition now," Flora mumbled happily to herself as she dressed hurriedly.

Suddenly, she stopped, her eyes opening very wide as she made a connection. "Apollo was right, as dads often are! Nimbus opened his heart first, and then his life began changing. Maybe other fairies will heal like that too! This could be the key to filling my nutritional classes. Surely everyone would want to reduce their salt, fat, and sugar intake once they open their hearts and eliminate all those uncomfortable, judgmental feelings."

The thought of fulfilling her nutritional dreams throughout the Land of Thyme made Flora sing joyfully. She hadn't noticed it was the middle of the night when everyone else was fast asleep.

The moon snored peacefully until Flora's singing rudely awakened him. He frowned and disappeared behind a cloud to withdraw the moonlight.

As Flora's room returned to darkness, she panicked. "Where's my paper? I can't see in the dark. I have to find the address for Nimbus."

"Go back to sleep, Flora," hooted a barn owl.

"Who do you think I am, you old owl? You're as blind as a bat! I'm Flora, goddess by day and dreamer by night," replied Flora, very curtly, as she climbed back into bed.

She threw the covers over her head to shut out the Land of Thyme and quickly fell asleep. As she slept, she dreamed she was taken by the hand by an unknown yet compassionate spirit into an immense library. She was then seated at a table in the presence of a gnome who opened a very large book written in an ancient language. The writing resembled hieroglyphics, which Flora didn't understand.

The gnome perched at the top of each page. As he moved his finger across each symbol, Flora understood its meaning. It all seemed so natural, yet she was not really reading at all. She was learning from this little gnome whose gaze mesmerized her.

When she awoke, Flora attempted to write what she learned in her dream.

## The Enchanted World of Mother Nature

The hidden structure of nature works on a level unknown to the intellect, yet this seemingly magical world will enchant and protect you. Like the creative mind, the enchanted world of Mother Nature knows no age or order of difficulty in healing. The body's cells work on this level. As long as they have the electromagnetic energy and necessary nutrients, they can heal and regenerate like a newborn child. The consciousness of the cells does not understand the concept of incurable disease or illness. It knows how to create and regenerate from the pure enthusiasm inherent throughout all life forms.

The centers of this consciousness align from the coccyx to the crown of the head. Ancient healers called them *chakras*, describing whirling vortexes of energy with color, sound, and vibrational frequency. Chakras are large, integrated circuits of the central nervous system directing energy to every organ and muscle via neurochemical coded messages to the brain. These sensory centers create the image of an open flower, whirling in a clockwise motion like a fan.

Chakras are very sensitive and integrate with the inner world of our emotions, feelings, and desires. Emotional stress can create an imbalance immobilizing the free flow of light, color, and sound resonating from the chakras. Each chakra resonates to a unique frequency, affecting neurochemical changes in cells of a similar vibratory pattern. Tension and stress can block this smooth flow of energy, depleting vitality and altering the emotional response of an individual. An imbalance or inactivation of this vital life force can create an atmosphere that may lead to disease. Neurochemically, it can alter mental and emotional perception as well.

Flowers are very beneficial instruments for reducing emotional stress. The energy fields they radiate are similar to the frequencies vibrating from the chakras and reduce toxic and nutritionally deficient systems caused by stress.

Ancient healers made essences from flowers to balance the chakras and re-establish a harmonious pattern of health. Essences were extracted from fresh blooms, added to a medium of alcohol, water, or oil and applied topically to each chakra.

Essential oils were then applied externally to enhance the immune response. The recipient would also be encouraged to wear a corresponding color and listen to music associated with a chakra to enhance mental acuity, emotional well-being, and endocrine function.

Chakra balance was essential to spiritual growth and self-actualization. Flower essences and essential oils were worn on a daily basis to encourage an open mind and body in tune with nature. This is known as subtle body healing when the heart and the mind act as one.

Before Flora put down her pen, she decided to explain each chakra and chart what she knew about each.

"I'll add nutritional and dietary suggestions, as well as essences and essential oils," Flora said out loud as she tapped her pen to the table. "I'll explain subtle body health so the fairies understand how stress indirectly causes disease by increasing dietary and nutritional demands. Surely then the fairies will want to eat like I do! My recipes will be in demand and my lectures will have standing-room only!"

Then Flora bounced up and down in her chair like Vinnie as she proceeded to write about chakras.

## The Empowerment Center

At the very tail of the spine, the base chakra resonates from the coccyx. This chakra relates to the self-identity of the ego. Sexual identity and self-acceptance begin to structure the personality as a sense of enthusiasm and vitality increases regeneration throughout the body. The will to live and reproduce resides in this chakra, as memories of survival are stored here.

The challenge experienced by the personality is trust. All memories of abandonment, abuse, and fear of others block the vitality and free flow of energy from the legs, knees, ankles, and feet to the coccyx. Pain or degeneration in these areas is an indication that the chakra is blocked.

The base chakra is ruled by the kidneys, which filter metabolic waste from fluids passing through them. Optimal function of this chakra enhances the quality of blood and ability to have children.

An imbalance or immature function of the basal chakra may be expressed as self-doubt, hyperactivity, selfishness, fear, and anxiety. A tendency for depressed thoughts, crying, and feelings of loss may occur.

The following chart details the color, flower essence, and essential oil that supports the blossoming of the chakra.

| | |
|---|---|
| **Location:** | Coccyx |
| **Color:** | Red, the color of enthusiasm |
| **Jewel to be worn:** | Ruby |
| **Musical note:** | Key of C, marching music |
| **Dietary guidelines:** | Increase cooked greens, soy products, animal protein, blackstrap molasses |
| **Nutritional support:** | Folic acid, B$^{12}$, vitamin E, iron and zinc |
| **Flower essence:** | Fimbriata antique rose increases a passion for life |
| | Salvia enhances self-esteem |
| | Amaryllis sedates anxiety of the unknown |
| | Red rose reduces depressive thoughts |
| | Marigold clarifies sexual identity and acceptance |
| | Viridflora enhances personal power |
| **Essential oil:** | Vanilla enhances a feeling of protection |

**Herbal compress:**   Comfrey

Steep two ounces of fresh comfrey leaves in two cups of boiled water, covered, for fifteen minutes. Strain and apply topically with a clean cloth. Flower essences and essential oils may be added to the compress after straining the leaves. Recommended dosage is two to five drops of each. Apply topically to the lower spine or add to bathwater. See the listing above for specific essences.

## The Friendship Center

The second chakra is cradled by the sacrum, located in the pelvis, below the navel. This chakra relates to the development of inner guidance, self-protection, and emotional balance. The personality develops a sense of knowing what to do and how to take care of needs, leading to a success consciousness. The basal chakra establishes identity as the sacrum realizes, "I can take care of myself and share this with others."

A sense of inner peace enhances immune function by lowering the fight-or-flight stress response. As the endocrine organs harmonize, the roller coaster of emotions subsides into a sense of security. An imbalance would result in oversensitivity, addictions, low blood sugar, food cravings, premenstrual mood swings, and pleasure seeking.

The personality learns social skills during the flowering of the sacral chakra. The ego perceives the world through a window rather than a mirror, reflecting at the base chakra. Male and female sexuality and preferences, skills and differences are developed. Social inhibitions and socially unacceptable behavior block the sacral chakra. The personality will revert to behavior developed from the fight-or-flight stress pattern, displaying a variety of emotions such as anger, fear, hiding, or running away, and seeking pleasure through recreational drugs, alcohol, or sex.

The adrenal cortex and medulla rule the sacral chakra. They are located on top of the kidneys. The cortex is an endocrine gland wrapped around the inner medulla. It generates energy to the brain and body like a car battery, demanding sugar from the liver. The cortical also controls electrolyte balance for the kidneys, allowing nutrients to be taken into the cells. The medulla balances membranes in nerve fibers and other cells using chlorides as a catalyst.

A balanced, functioning sacral chakra enhances neuromuscular tone, stamina, and a sense of joy in living. Sexual function is often enhanced and experienced as a truly beautiful expression of love.

The following chart outlines support for this chakra:

| | |
|---|---|
| **Location:** | Four inches above the coccyx, in the pelvis |
| **Color:** | Orange, the color of joyful renewal |
| **Jewel to be worn:** | Gold or yellow sapphire |
| **Musical note:** | Key of D; songs that evoke deep feelings |
| **Dietary guidelines:** | Wheat germ, whole grains, bananas, peaches, oranges, sesame seeds and sesame seed butter |
| **Nutritional support:** | Magnesium, chlorophyll, niacin, pyridoxal 5 phosphate, the coenzyme of $B_6$ |
| **Flower essences:** | Indian paintbrush enhances a success consciousness for better health, prosperity and beauty |
| | Old Blush antique rose enhances stamina and neuromuscular tone |
| | Lily reduces anxiety about specific future events, such as passing an exam |
| | Bamboo aids those searching for a new direction in life |
| | Snapdragon encourages discernment and judgmental skills |
| | Cecil Brünner antique rose aids in creating realistic boundaries and goals in relationships |
| | Grüss an Aachen antique rose reduces food cravings and settling for less in relationships |
| | Country Marilou helps release uncomfortable feelings about the physical body |
| **Essential oils:** | Jasmine enhances sexuality |
| | Siberian ginseng increases social interest |
| **Herbal tonic:** | Dilute eight to fifteen drops of Siberian ginseng extract (*Eleutherococcos sinticosus*) in four ounces of warm water daily and drink as a tea to promote longevity. Start with two to four drops daily, and then add a few more drops daily until maximum dose is achieved. Fairies and pets under fifty pounds should not exceed eight drops daily. |
| | Raspberry tea is also soothing to this center. Steep one teaspoon of dried leaves in one cup of boiled water, covered, for ten minutes. Strain and sip. |
| | Chocolate mint tea reduces chocolate cravings. Add one teaspoon of fresh leaves in one cup of boiled water or warm milk. Cover and steep for ten minutes. Strain and enjoy. |

## The Vital Energy Center

The third chakra enhances the digestive organs, providing nutrients, heat, and energy for a long productive life. Muscle strength is a sign of a strong, functioning vital energy center. The assimilation of nutrients, minerals, and their coenzymes is absorbed throughout the blood and circulating fluids.

The challenge of the personality is to develop self-appreciation and overcome the fear of loss. As an "I can do it" attitude prevails, a belief in loss and failure subsides. Success is measured in the rebound as the tough gets going. A sense of community spirit invites the individual to create a healthy environment, as well as a healthy body.

Poor digestion and incomplete assimilation reduce the efficiency of the vital center, creating poor concentration and eventual memory loss. The personality may display angry outbursts or experience a feeling of uncomfortable fullness in the intestines and chest, acid reflux, or even an inconsiderate attitude toward others. Self-importance may be exaggerated or deflated as financial stability is adversely affected.

The stomach, pancreas, liver, and gallbladder rule the vital energy center. These organs break down proteins, fats, carbohydrates and sugars. Their metabolic processes direct a smooth flow of energy to the muscles, preventing spasms and shaking. Complete breakdown of protein and nutrients enhances neurochemical messages to the brain and blood flow to the heart. This center is most affected by stress-related diseases, such as ulcers, colitis, hyperacidity, and acid reflux. The following chart outlines support for this chakra:

| | |
|---|---|
| **Location:** | Navel |
| **Color:** | Yellow for vitality and mental stimulation |
| **Jewel to be worn:** | Topaz |
| **Musical note:** | Key of E, stimulating music with a beat |
| **Dietary guidelines:** | Papaya, if ulcers and inflammatory bowel are not present; oatmeal is beneficial for many that suffer from hyperacidity; reduce caffeine and carbonated beverages or avoid them. Eat four smaller meals daily and reduce fatty and fried foods. |
| **Nutritional support:** | Water-soluble chlorophyll, bioflavonoids, vitamin C, choline, deglycyrrhized licorice |
| **Flower essences:** | Peppermint reduces fear of loss |
| | Pink geranium dissipates pent-up feelings and suppressed anger |
| | Crossandra reduces the fear of making major changes in life. Fortune's double yellow reduces excessive desires and the feeling that the individual won't get what they want from life |
| **Essential oils:** | Peppermint increases digestive processes |
| | Ginger to disperse excess energy and nausea |
| | Marigold mint (*Tagetes lucida*) reduces colic and cramping |
| | Lemon grass enhances liver and digestive functions |

| Herbal teas: | Combine peppermint (one teaspoon fresh or one-half teaspoon dried leaves), chamomile (one-half teaspoon fresh or dried flowers), and lemon grass (one teaspoon fresh or dried leaves). Steep in ten ounces of boiled water for ten minutes; strain and sip with meals. |
| --- | --- |
| | For an upset stomach, steep one teaspoon of chamomile flowers in one cup of boiled water for ten minutes. Strain; add one-half teaspoon of honey. Stir and sip. |
| | For gastrointestinal distress and signs of inflammation, ulcers or colic, simmer one teaspoon of whole fennel seeds, crushed with a mortar and pestle, in ten ounces of water for five minutes. Remove from heat; add one teaspoon of fresh or dried spearmint leaves, one teaspoon of fresh lemon verbena leaves (optional), and one-quarter teaspoon of hops. Cover and steep for ten minutes before straining. Serve with one teaspoon of honey, if desired. |

## The Heart Center

The heart chakra is centered in the mid chest and radiates throughout the upper torso. It provides energy for the cardiovascular system, lungs, thymus immune organ, wings, shoulders, arms, and hands. The heart center holds the key to compassion, forgiveness, and the seed of faith and surrender. It is believed to be the instrument of the soul and nourishment of the psyche. When the emotional nature of an individual becomes restless, it is a sign of a troubled spirit. Surrender to the heart's desire allows faith to express itself through compassion. As the heart center opens, the breath flows freely and the diaphragm expands. The wings release to flap freely as the spirit soars.

The heart center increases sensitivity to touch and encourages intimacy with all of Nature. The attitude of forgiveness allows the mind to remain impartial and non-judgmental. Others are treated with respect. Kindness is a child of the heart.

An imbalance in this center leads to arrogance, pride, degrading others, and self-deception. Feelings of guilt, responsibility for others' actions, and not releasing feelings of hurt can cause stress hormones to injure this center and reduce the efficiency of the cardiovascular system. Closing off the heart to the needs of others injures the soul and dims the eternal light within all nature.

Healing from the heart is the challenge of every heart to beat as one. Success is first measured in intimacy patterns allowing the individual to be free of the stresses that inhibit a loving heart. Love structures the family, the community, the nation, and the world for the benefit of all.

The following chart supports opening the heart center:

| Location: | Mid chest |
| --- | --- |
| Color: | Green for growth |
| Jewel to be worn: | Emerald or jade |

| | |
|---|---|
| **Musical note:** | Key of F, romantic and environmental tunes |
| **Dietary guidelines:** | Add spices appropriate for taste and tolerance: cinnamon, cayenne, ginger, tumeric |
| **Nutritional support:** | Niacin, copper, chromium, magnesium, potassium, taurine |
| **Flower essences:** | Wisteria opens the heart chakra |
| | Lilac enhances forgiveness |
| | Daffodil aids in overcoming shyness |
| | Louis Phillipe antique rose encourages surrender |
| | Dancing Lady Orchid makes peace with the past |
| | Penta aids those who withhold love |
| | Bougainvillea releases guilt |
| | Archduke Charles antique rose aids in feeling safe when touched, for those who pull away in close relationships |
| **Essential oils:** | Geranium encourages intimacy, reduces depression |
| | Eucalyptus opens the lungs for easier breathing |
| | Sweet Annie encourages a graceful unfolding of self-actualization |
| | Lavender encourages feelings of romance and love |
| | Sage reduces congestion in the breasts and lymphatics |
| **Herbal tonics:** | To calm the heart center and release blocked emotions: |
| | Simmer five lotus seeds (*Nelumbo nuciferae*) in ten ounces of water, covered for fifteen minutes. Strain; add one fresh gardenia or five honeysuckle flowers, when available, and steep, covered, for five more minutes. Strain and sip. |
| | To increase cardiovascular strength: Simmer ten hawthorn berries in two cups of water, covered, for twenty minutes. Remove from heat and add one tablespoon of dried or fresh motherwort (*Leonnorus cardiaca*). Steep for ten minutes and strain. |
| | For clogged arteries: The Chinese ingest one teaspoon of raw, powdered tienchi ginseng daily or as a food. (Available through Chinese herbalists.) |

## The Communications Center

The throat chakra is a channel of the mind co-creating through the power of the spoken word. As it opens, artistic and latent creative talents may emerge. It is the key to encouragement and the power to heal or hurt.

Suppression leads to depression, loneliness, fatigue, and autoimmune reactions. The body processes may become sluggish or hyperactive in an attempt to regulate metabolism. Headaches may occur from tension held in the neck and cervical spine. Stress may occur for those who feel they have no purpose, such as an "empty nest" syndrome.

The development of the personality is to keep promises and speak only what is desired to manifest and speak the truth. Cooperation is finely tuned during this level of development and compromise will surely advance communicative skills. It is very important to have supportive friends and associates during this time.

The following chart will detail support for this center:

| | |
|---|---|
| **Location:** | Anterior of the neck |
| **Color:** | Royal blue |
| **Jewel to be worn:** | Amethyst |
| **Musical note:** | Key of G, soothing, flowing music |
| **Nutritional support:** | Thiamin ($B_1$), vitamin A |
| **Flower essences:** | Red crepe myrtle enhances the spoken word |
| | Azalea enhances creativity |
| | Pansy releases grief |
| | Meadow sage aids in the expression of strong emotions without blaming others |
| | Chamomile helps those who swallow hurt feelings and disappointment |
| **Essential oils:** | Lemon balm calms the heart to express deep feelings |
| | Thyme guards against viral invasion |
| **Herbal tonic:** | Astragalus tea strengthens immunity and regulates weight: Boil six three-inch slices of astragalus in two cups of water for twenty minutes. Strain and drink two cups daily. |
| | **Note:** High-quality astragalus yields yellow slices. |

## The Imagination Center

The imagination center is located in the center of the forehead, a third eye seeking inner wisdom. It is best utilized to visualize what is desired, a new set of wings, a healthy lithe body, a happy ending. As the mind sees, feels, and experiences the visualization, it accepts this reality. Our outer world results from our inner thoughts and beliefs. Introspection of the outer world allows an individual to take a closer look at motives and actions. At any time one can begin anew.

The masterminds of the visual center are the pineal, pituitary, and hypothalamus glands, guiding the endocrine and stress responses through chemical and hormonal messages. They unite to become the decision maker qualifying emotions and attitudes.

As the third eye opens, creativity is activated from the love that inspired it. The result is fulfillment.

The following chart details support for the visual chakra:

| | |
|---|---|
| **Location:** | Center of the forehead |
| **Color:** | Indigo, the color of knowledge |
| **Jewel to be worn:** | Lapis lazuli or pearl |
| **Musical note:** | Key of A, soft melody |
| **Dietary guidelines:** | Sunlight or full spectrum lighting (available at light stores) |
| **Nutritional support:** | Manganese, melatonin, phosphatydlcholine, vitamin D |
| **Flower essences:** | Iris enhances creative expression |
| | Sunflower makes peace with our Creator |
| | Red carnation enhances self worth |
| | Madame Alfred Carrier antique rose enhances prophetic dreams |
| | Kalanchoe corrects the illusion of opposites, the black-or-white perception |
| **Essential oil:** | Basil increases oxygen to the brain |
| | Rosemary lifts the spirits and releases fond memories to share with others |
| | Sandalwood calms the mind and opens the heart |
| **Herbal tea:** | Lemon grass tea is an herbal source of vitamin D. It is especially soothing on a cold, dreary day. Steep one tablespoon of fresh or dried lemon grass in one cup of boiled water. Add one-half teaspoon of wintergreen tea leaves, if desired. Cover and allow to set for ten minutes. Strain and enjoy. |

## The Crown Center

The crown center is a fountain of light flowing over the top of the head. Here the gift of intuition and knowledge allows the spiritual and physical ideals to receive guidance from the higher self. Answers are often realized by an inner voice, evidence that the crown chakra is following nature. There are also times of deep inner silence and peacefulness as the present moment unfolds under grace.

Signs of imbalance may include disorientation, confusion, or incessant weeping. Living in the past or unreality in the present time indicates resistance to inner guidance, blocking the flow of endorphins from this center.

The personality learns that decisions and actions must be for the good of all. The energy flow will then form a figure-eight pattern with the empowerment center bringing in a similar resonance from the earth. The result is illumination.

The following chart supports the opening of the crown center:

| | |
|---|---|
| **Location:** | Above the top of the head |
| **Color:** | White, the color of illumination |
| **Jewel to be worn:** | Sapphire or diamond |
| **Musical note:** | Key of B, sacred music |
| **Dietary guidelines:** | Lipoic acid available in flowering plants |
| **Nutritional support:** | Phosphatydl serine, pyridoxal 5 phosphate, the coenzyme of $B_6$ |
| **Flower essences:** | Sunflower enhances a feeling of peace with creation |
| | Verbena enhances inner peace |
| | Silver moon enhances a contemplation, reducing obsessive thoughts |
| | Cherokee rose opens the crown center to increase creativity in daily activities |
| **Essential oils:** | Rose balances the crown and heart centers to increase compassion and enhance union with the soul |
| **Application:** | To affect the crown chakra and promote union with the soul, the ancients applied flower essences to the right ear, where five cranial nerves converge into the ganglia. It is called *shen wen* and is located in the right ear just above the ear opening. |

# CHAPTER 10

# The Visit

## Discovering the Subtle Body

*"The journey may seem rough, but it always takes you*
*where you need to be."*
Vincent Ermis, "An Easter Poem," 1999

### The Missing Piece of the Puzzle

As Flora finished writing, she put down her pen and read through her chakra charts. She felt that this was very valuable information. However, she wasn't quite sure how to use it. She did admit to herself that healing from the heart held the key to helping the fairy community evolve. Certainly flower essences must be the missing piece of this puzzle!

She began to daydream and reminiscence about her childhood days when she gardened alongside her grandma. As Grandma tended the flowers, she would converse with them like they were real fairies. But Flora was busy playing and didn't pay attention to what the flowers told Grandma. Now it was too late to ask.

Yet Flora was not a goddess who accepted no for an answer! She was determined to learn more about flower essences, healing from the heart, and what to do with her chakra charts!

Flora became very excited about all the possibilities before her. She loved learning adventures. It brought out the pioneer in her, a side too often contained in the environment of the classroom. Surely, there was someone who would help her. As Flora's mind raced, she spontaneously grabbed the chakra charts and ran out the door. She planned to consult with Sweet Tooth, the most knowledgeable fairy on the subject of aromatherapy.

### Flora and Sweet Tooth Chat

When Flora arrived at Sweet Tooth's place of business, she found Nimbus leaving for the gardens with his lunch box and her perfumed hankie to wipe off the delicious kisses she left on his cheeks and forehead.

Today was Nimbus's first day at work after his honeymoon. He was wearing his favorite T-shirt that he bought on the cruise with his name monogrammed above this slogan:

*Save your wings*
*and fly with me*
TransButterfly Airlines

"Good morning, Flora! What brings you here so bright and early in the morning?" Nimbus said graciously.

"Oh! I'm glad you're leaving, Nimbus. I want all of Sweet Tooth's attention," began Flora. "By the way, how was your vacation?" Flora looked around nervously. She was surprised at how quickly the past few weeks had passed.

"Thanks for asking, Flora. We had a great time and now look forward to visiting the garden you told us about last winter." Nimbus squeezed Sweet Tooth's hand and smiled at Flora.

Flora looked down, hedging a bit and shuffling her feet before answering. "Well, I've had a dream that makes me want to go to the garden and learn about flower essences, too."

"Wow! That would be great!" exclaimed Nimbus. "Wouldn't you love to have Flora join us, honey?" Nimbus smiled at Sweet Tooth, who showed her displeasure.

"Honey?" Nimbus tried to look into his loved one's eyes, but Sweet Tooth looked away. Flora finally broke an uncomfortable silence.

"Well, I guess that answers that! Maybe I could visit another time." Flora's enthusiasm faded. Obviously disappointed, she shuffled the papers she had brought to show Sweet Tooth.

Sweet Tooth sighed, unable to turn down Flora. "Look, Flora, it would be great to have you with us as long as you have a friend travel with you."

Flora brightened as she thought about Sweet Tooth's suggestion. "Well, I'm sure everybody will want to be my partner! I'll have a contest so the best fairy can win!"

"Excellent idea," yawned Sweet Tooth, as she nibbled on a chocolate mint leaf. "Here's the chocolate mint you gave us as a wedding gift, Flora. This is my opportunity to thank you in person," smiled Sweet Tooth politely.

"Why, you're quite welcome. I was hoping to keep you away from the other kinds of chocolate," replied Flora curtly.

Suddenly, Sweet Tooth turned to Flora, looking her straight in the eye, and replied, "Flora, not even a goddess can keep me away from chocolate!"

"Oh, my!" Flora stepped back, surprised by Sweet Tooth's adamant reply. Nimbus gulped and giggled nervously.

"Now, now, girls, let's change the subject!" Nimbus said while smiling and patting them both on a shoulder.

"Of course," replied Flora, clearly shaken. "I came to show Sweet Tooth some information I gathered on essential oils and flower essences. We'll discuss chocolate another time."

"Oh! Let me see," Sweet Tooth replied as she reached for the papers. "This looks very thorough," she said as her eyes searched through each page.

Flora grinned widely, as she nodded her head in agreement. Nimbus took the opportunity to fly to work, with wings beating furiously to keep him in the air.

Sweet Tooth turned and waved goodbye. She was so very proud that Nimbus was lighter and could fly again.

"This is clearly inspired," murmured Sweet Tooth, purposely sucking on a chocolate chosen from the depths of her pocket.

Flora's pixie feet lifted right off the floor in excitement. "I had a dream! I had a dream and woke up clearly inspired!

"Why, Flora, you really did some great work on this heart chakra," mused Sweet Tooth, shaking her head in amazement. "Here, have a chocolate." Sweet Tooth chose a variety of individually wrapped chocolates from her pocket.

"Oh! I don't eat chocolate, Sweet Tooth. As a goddess, I'm expected to remain perfect at all times," Flora nodded.

Sweet Tooth held the chocolates right under Flora's nose. "Well, if you're already perfect, then you can try one."

As Flora sniffed the chocolates, her mouth began to water. She steadied herself. Before she realized what she was doing, Flora grabbed a chocolate and munched it down in a few sloppy bites.

"Mmm!" Flora's eyes grew as big as saucers, as she licked her lips.

"Try another one," Sweet Tooth offered, "but this time remove the wrapper first."

Flora didn't waste any time finishing off every one of the chocolates in Sweet Tooth's hand. She beamed a chocolate-covered smile to Sweet Tooth, agreeing that they did taste better without the wrappers.

Suddenly, guilt overcame Flora, as she realized what she'd done.

"Oh, my!" she cried. "I've lost control of myself, haven't I? Now I can't be an example of perfection to all the little fairies under my care!"

Sweet Tooth chuckled as she invited Flora into the house.

"You'll be perfect with a little roundness to those hips, darling."

"Oh!" cried Flora in surprise, as she turned to examine her backside. "I didn't know chocolate was good for the hips," exclaimed Flora, as she followed Sweet Tooth through the door.

"It's good for a lot of things," replied Sweet Tooth, as her hands smoothed her full figure. "Now, have a seat on this buttercup and let's go over your paper." Sweet Tooth smiled as she patted the couch made of fresh buttercups.

Flora sat down and giggled as pollen flew around her and dusted her nose. She sneezed and then began.

"Sweet Tooth, my main concern is the difference in the essential oils listed under the heart center. For example, you always listed lavender as an essential oil that opens the highest center of the brain and I list it for the heart center."

"I see what you mean," pondered Sweet Tooth, as she compared her lecture notes with Flora's. "There is an explanation for this, Flora. Lavender affects the highest cortical function of the brain because the scent directly opens the crown chakra. As the body lets down and relaxes, blood flow to the heart increases, literally warming the heart. A warm heart, of course, attracts a love and then the heart chakra bursts into full bloom! For some fairies, lavender is an aphrodisiac."

"Oh, my! What have I done to Nimbus, assigning him to the lavender gardens from new moon to full moon. I'd better give him some relief!" sighed Flora, as she lay back onto the buttercup couch.

"Don't you *dare*!" chided Sweet Tooth. "I'll take care of Nimbus! You should announce the contest for the best fairy to accompany you to the garden we plan to visit in March."

"Oh! The contest!" cried Flora. "Of course! But can I ask you just a few more questions before I leave?" Flora asked with the innocence of a child.

"Okay, but I don't have any more chocolates," laughed Sweet Tooth.

Flora blushed until her ears burned. She self-consciously wiped her mouth with her hand before continuing in a whisper.

"I'd appreciate it if you kept the chocolate binge between us, Sweet Tooth. Now I understand what makes a fairy prefer it to my Melba toast."

Sweet Tooth nodded, suppressing an urge to burst into laughter.

Suddenly, Flora changed the subject, opening her heart and sharing her deepest feelings with Sweet Tooth.

"It's hard being a goddess sometimes. And it's lonely. Fairies don't understand what it's like being on top of creation's chain of evolution. I have to be everything to everybody, but who can I lean on and depend on to make my day?" Flora flapped her wings anxiously as she talked, waving her hands in the air as she tried to explain her feelings.

"Every fairy sometimes feels alone. That emptiness can only be filled from an inner strength, the kind that builds character, and, ultimately, your destiny."

"Well, I already know my destiny, Sweet Tooth. I'm a goddess here to enlighten the fairies living in the Land of Thyme. They would become obese and unhealthy without me."

"Oh, dear," sighed Sweet Tooth. "You *are* young. Father Time will add wisdom and understanding to your beautiful presence in a few light-years when you learn the difference between a goddess and a heroine."

"Well, actually, I was wondering if flower essences would help me," Flora murmured a little shyly.

"Flower essences reduce stress, and essential oils do too, but there's a difference. Flower essences are meant to catalyze the innate wisdom and goodness inherent within. They are more delicate and cooling than essential oils. The chemistry of flower essences is also more stable, while essential oils are volatile and evaporate quickly. Flower essences are taken into the body in ten to fifteen seconds, like an essential oil, but are not detected in the urine two to three hours later as are essential oils. Flower essences are broken down by enzymes in the skin with little, if any, to be detoxified by the kidneys. Topically, they are considered nontoxic."

Sweet Tooth sipped some chocolate mint tea and poured a cup for Flora, who listened intently. Then, she folded her dimpled hands and continued.

"When flower essences are applied topically, they have a cooling effect on the nerves under the skin, which relays this message throughout the nervous system immediately."

"How does this happen?" asked Flora, sipping her tea.

"Remember, the brain is a hologram. What happens in one part of the body is relayed immediately through the nervous system and subtle body," nodded Sweet Tooth.

"I've been around flower essences and essential oils since I entered the Land of Thyme, but I *really* don't know what a subtle body is!" exclaimed Flora.

## The Subtle Body

"The subtle body is a cloak of electromagnetic energy draping the body. It looks like clothes we don't normally see and clings like static electricity. The subtle body is often referred to as the *aura*. It projects varying shades of color, magnitude, and thermal energy," Sweet Tooth answered.

"What does it do?" inquired Flora politely.

Sweet Tooth moved toward the kitchen to brew another pot of tea. "The subtle body is a body of light which is considered to be very protective to the denser body we can easily perceive. It works like an external immune system complete with a neurological system known as the sixth sense," Sweet Tooth answered as she re-entered the room with a tray of freshly brewed tea and tiny teacakes.

Flora's eyes lit up as her nose picked up the fresh aroma of spearmint and lemon verbena tea. Then she spotted the teacakes and pulled her hand back before she spontaneously grabbed one.

"Are these teacakes fattening?" she asked Sweet Tooth.

"Oh, no," she answered the curious goddess. "They're too little to be fattening," she said while smiling as she offering Flora a teacake.

"I wondered if you'll be staying for lunch." Sweet Tooth asked softly.

"Oh, no!" Flora laughed. "This will do for awhile," as she reached for a handful of teacakes. "These are really good; you must share the recipe with me," she smiled happily as she popped a few teacakes into her mouth.

"Oh, dear," mumbled Sweet Tooth under her breath. "I'll have to look around for the recipe," she hedged. "Now, where were we?"

"Mmm, oh, yes," Flora thought out loud as she sipped some tea. "Where does the subtle body originate? It seems to be outside the body."

"To my knowledge, it originates from the chakras," Sweet Tooth replied. "So that means it begins at the base of the spine." Sweet Tooth smiled as she dabbed a pretty folded napkin to her perfect lips.

"So, if the chakras are not functioning and interacting properly, then the body could lose energy or become ill," Flora added.

"Yes," agreed Sweet Tooth, "but the first sign of imbalance is often an emotional response, especially when it's out of character, like rage from Nimbus."

"Or, calmness from Vinnie!" laughed Flora. Sweet Tooth soon joined in the laughter. Her whole body laughed as she threw back her head, enjoying a good joke.

"Okay, okay." giggled Flora. "What is the second sign of imbalance?"

"Well," Sweet Tooth cleared her throat. "An imbalance in the chakras can lead to an improper mental attitude, like prejudice, or a separation from nature."

"That ought to include just about everybody," Flora popped off.

"What do you mean, Flora? Do you know fairies like that?" queried Sweet Tooth in a surprised voice.

"Well," answered Flora, hesitantly.

"I see," said Sweet Tooth. "Well, I won't ask any more leading questions. What about fairies that think they're fat?"

"Like Nimbus? Yes, flower essences, chakra balancing, and you will help him," replied Flora, smiling. "Nimbus is one of the nicest fairies I ever met, but he's hard on himself. He seems to find things wrong with himself, but he's not that way with others. He's very complimentary and helpful. I don't understand why he doesn't lose weight."

"Yes," Sweet Tooth agreed. "He is a good fairy. It's just taking him awhile to realize he can achieve what he wants. Deep down inside his kind heart he doesn't believe he can do it."

"Did he have a bad childhood?" asked Flora, wrinkling her brow in concern.

"Not that I know of," replied Sweet Tooth. "He has developed a pattern of eating under stress and has a body type that gains weight easily."

"Would it help if I made him a large order of Melba toast?" asked Flora.

"Well, probably not, Flora. Fairies like to eat comfort food to sedate or soothe feelings, not Melba toast."

"I could sprinkle cinnamon on the Melba toast!" interrupted Flora.

"Drizzle some gooey chocolate on it and it's a deal," Sweet Tooth answered while laughing.

"Oh! I never thought of that!" Flora answered with surprise.

"That's because you don't think and feel like we do, Flora. But flower essences will help all of us. They will help us understand each other and catalyze our ability to change for the better."

"I like that, Sweet Tooth. I am eager to visit the flower essence garden with you and Nimbus," Flora said as she flapped her wings and grinned.

"Oh, well, then, you need to announce the contest so you have a travel pal," Sweet Tooth suggested.

"Oh, yes!" Flora flapped with even more excitement. "I must hurry! I'll have *so* many applicants to weed through! I only want the most intelligent, witty, and accomplished fairy!"

"Well, if you're looking for perfection again, Flora, you might want the captain of the Fairy SEALs. He sure has a crush on you! From what I've heard from the grapevine, he drives by your kitchen flexing his muscles most every day."

"Ugh!" Flora's wings lost their lift, as she flopped down on the buttercup couch. "I'd rather bring Vinnie's pet snake!"

Sweet Tooth fell back in her stuffed tulip chair laughing. "Stop! You'll make me split my petals!" she giggled.

"Well, on that happy note, I'll make my exit," Flora announced. She hesitated just inside the door and turned to Sweet Tooth.

"I just want to thank you," she stopped as her eyes met Sweet Tooth's.

Simultaneously, they fell into each other's arms, wrapping their wings around one another in the grandest hug.

"I'll let you know how the contest goes," Flora said, as she squeezed Sweet Tooth's hand. "Wish me luck!" She left, turning several times to wave goodbye, exhilarated from the visit and feeling energized from the chocolates.

## The Contest

After the visit, Flora flew around town posting announcements about the contest on every large magnolia tree. The announcement created more work for Flora. She wrote equal opportunity entry forms and made a placement box. Then, she flew around posting entry forms on every contest poster.

She spent the week working every waking moment to take great care of every detail. Her excitement grew as the time drew near to choose her perfect travel companion. Every night she fell asleep dreaming of her new-found friend.

The day finally arrived! Flora hardly slept a wink the night before. She had asked Owl to accompany her to select a winner, but her curiosity got the best of her. Owl could only see at night and Flora thought it would be fair to shake the box and maybe even take a quick peek inside.

She soon talked herself into visiting the contest box. By sunrise, Flora was flying as fast as her wings could carry her to a hollow in an oak tree. There Flora would find the applications of each contestant.

"Wow!" she thought. "I hope I can make a decision! Maybe Owl will be able to help me, but maybe I should look through the applications and weed out some of the hopeful contestants."

Flora continued to talk herself into going through the applications before Owl would join her at night. She felt sadness for all the fairies that would be disappointed they were not chosen. Then, she felt guilt, then remorse, then more sadness, until she arrived at the hollow oak.

Excitement roared inside Flora, as she neared the contestant box in the hollow oak. She tiptoed softly toward the tree, just in case a hopeful fairy was leaving an application.

As she neared the tree, Flora closed her eyes and reached into the hollow box to shuffle the applications.

"Gee! They must have fallen to the bottom," she thought. "I wonder where all the applications are?" she asked herself, as she felt all around the hollow. "Maybe I'm at the wrong tree," she mumbled.

"No, you're not" the oak answered. "Keep looking." Oak then went back to sleep.

With Oak's encouragement, Flora shoved her arm deep into the Oak's hollow, searching for a leaf, or any sign of an application. She produced two folded oak leaves and one scroll and that's all.

"That's all!" Flora exclaimed out loud, as her eyes looked at the applications in disbelief.

"Yup," answered Oak momentarily, before closing his sleepy eyes once more.

"Why, this is unbelievable!" complained Flora, as she shoved her head and then her whole body into the hollow for a closer look.

"Ouch! Nothing here but the ants. Ouch! Okay, I'm leaving!" Flora huffed, as she crawled out of the hollow.

"Well!" she sighed as she sat down in the nearby grass. "This scroll must be a long list of hopeful fairies. I'll just take a peek and scratch through the names of those I don't want as a travel pal."

Flora quickly opened the scroll and began to glance through the information. Her eyes grew larger by the line as her mouth opened wide.

"Oh, no! This whole scroll is an application from Chief, captain of the Fairy SEALs and Justice of the Garden!" As she flipped through the pages, she frowned with obvious displeasure.

"All these pages are lists of his qualifications and achievements! Who cares? I don't want a conceited flapper flying next to me!" Flora stormed. "He's not the only fairy in the Land of Thyme," she fumed as she lifted the two folded oak leaves in her hand.

The oak tree suddenly opened its sleepy eyes and added, "Those two oak leaves represent the only two applicants brave enough to sneak past the captain to enter an application."

"What do you mean, Oak?" cried Flora.

"I mean, the captain of the Fairy SEALs stood in front of me for the past week blocking any applicants from entering their forms. Then he would clear the hollow once a day to ensure no fairies escaped him."

"How did these two escape?" asked Flora as she stared at the two oak leaves in her hand.

"They wrote their application on one of my small leaves, crumpled the leaves, then dropped them in my hollow from my highest limb at daybreak this morning."

"Brave fairies!" exclaimed Flora. "I will certainly reward such diligent and intelligent efforts," she sighed dreamily.

"Well, one of them," began Oak.

"No, no!" Flora interrupted. "Both of these braves fairies will be rewarded by accompanying me as travel pals." Flora smiled as she opened the first leaf and read aloud.

"'Qualifications: flexible.' That's good," Flora nodded her approval.

"'Achievements: sleeps using only a rock as a pillow.' I hope that won't be necessary." She continued to read. "'Eats only one time a week.' My wings! What a role model for Nimbus!"

Flora turned over the leaf to find the identity of this brave fairy.

"*SNAKE!* Oh, no! It's Vinnie's pet snake! I can't take a pet snake as a travel pal!"

"Vinnie does," answered Oak. "And, besides, it was Snake who climbed to the top of me and threw the applications in my hollow. Then, he slithered down my trunk and scared Chief away!"

"A Fairy SEAL afraid of a little grass snake! Ha!" cried Flora. "I've even had my picture taken holding that disgusting creature and I wasn't scared," Flora replied as she tossed her head into the air.

"Well, he sure knows how to keep Chief away," Oak suggested. "And, he only eats once a week! Sounds like a cheap date to me, Flora."

"Oh, Oak!" Flora shouted. "You've been around too long." Oak's limbs shook with laughter as Flora opened the second leaf. She began to read out loud.

"A gardener, yes, that's good. A loyal and honest friend! Well, this sounds interesting. Enjoys large servings of Melba toast!"

Flora thought about the last statement for a moment before tossing the second leaf into the air.

"It's Vinnie! Oh, no! This can't happen to me!" she cried. "I can't show up at the Garden of Beauty with a pampered pet snake and a fairy that drools!"

"But, you will," replied Oak fondly. "And, you will be well cared for by those two brave, ahem, fairies."

"Oh, what a cruel world," cried Flora. "I deserve better than this for all the good I do!"

"I'm sure Chief will be saying the same thing when he finds out you chose a snake," chuckled Oak. "Life seems to serve us exactly what we need to grow."

But Flora didn't hear Oak's wise words. She had already dried her tears and flown away.

As Flora flew away, Snake crawled from under a nearby rock, his head particularly more flat than usual.

"Hey, Oak! How did it go? Are we in?" Snake asked as he slithered toward the large oak tree.

"Yes," replied Oak as he closed his sleepy eyes.

"Yeah, well, it was nothing. Vinnie painted stripes on my back and fitted me with some fake fangs so I looked dangerous. Then, he put a rattle on my tail. Whew! That was a lot of work, hissing, slithering, and rattling all at once. I have more respect for other snakes now."

"Gee, thanks for that observation, Snake. Why don't you slither along and tell Vinnie the good news. The two of you should be packing," suggested Oak, as his sleepy eyes closed one more time.

Snake took the hint and made his way back to Vinnie, the only other creature in the Land of Thyme that could talk as much as Snake.

CHAPTER 11

# The Journey
## Into the Garden of Beauty

*In the subtle body, health relates to spiritual growth*
Judy Griffin, *The Healing Flowers*

## Time Traveling

Snake wasted no time getting ready for his journey. He wiggled right into his nest and packed everything he owned, including his toy mouse. Then, he quickly returned to Vinnie's abode, dressed in his best tie and dark sunglasses.

"How do I look?" he asked Vinnie.

For the first time in his life, Vinnie had nothing to say. His eyes grew big with disbelief.

"I can tell you don't approve of the tie, when your eyes grow into saucers," complained Snake. "I just want to make a good impression with Flora."

"Oh!" replied Vinnie, suppressing his laughter. "She'll remember you!"

"Good! Now tell me why we're going to this garden," demanded Snake.

"Flora wants to learn how to heal from the heart," replied Vinnie as he neatly packed his belongings.

"Great, but I can't get any lower to the ground than this," answered Snake as he adjusted his tie in front of a mirror.

"Snake! I mean, like how to feel good about yourself under any condition and how to get past your fears," corrected Vinnie.

"I have a fear of heights since I had to climb up to the top of Oak dragging a rattle," hissed Snake.

"I'm sure Flora will be interested, Snake, but remember, we're going to help and protect her."

"I hope I get the opportunity to wrap myself around her," Snake thought out loud.

"Hey! That's my sister, you know. It's more likely you'll get stepped on. Those sunglasses are reflecting the light into my eyes. I can't see where I'm going!"

The two friends were soon on the ground wrestling and kicking up dust until they simultaneously noticed someone standing over them.

"Ahem." Flora cleared her throat from all the dust. "Are you boys ready?"

The boys danced to an upright position, smiling sheepishly and brushing the dust from each other.

"Gee, Flora, you look nice," smiled Vinnie as he nudged Snake.

"Oh, yes, very nice," hissed Snake. "Say, since I didn't come equipped with a nice set of wings like you, how about I crawl on your shoulder as we travel?" winked Snake.

"Oh, that won't be necessary, Mr. Snake," replied Flora. "We're going to time travel to another dimension. We'll have to cross several time zones to float into the earth plane."

"I can't wait till we're safe in the garden," Vinnie said nervously. "There's lots of pure air around the plants. Even on ground level, Snake."

"It's Mr. Snake now, Vinnie. She must really respect me," whispered Snake.

"I thought you were going to say she really looks up to you, Mr. Snake," laughed Vinnie.

Just then Nimbus and Sweet Tooth joined them, escorted by Collie.

"Thanks for the ride!" they waved to Collie as he wiped away his tears, smiling weakly.

As everyone gathered together, they formed a fairy ring for safe travel. Flora broke the silence by announcing her plan.

"We'll be time traveling to another dimension by light years. Each of us will be assigned a color of the rainbow to travel from the Land of Thyme to the Garden of Beauty, which seems far away. Actually, the Land of Thyme and the Garden of Beauty exist like two sides of a coin. So, the distance is merely our perception."

"So, how do we hop this rainbow and go back to the future?" joked Snake.

Flora was quick to answer. "We close our eyes, take three deep breaths, and think of our assigned color until we totally identify with it. If it's pink, just think pink, then experience what pink feels like until you become pink. In a flash, you will travel through the time barrier to the opposite dimension."

Everyone clapped and cheered as if they had already accomplished their task.

Then Snake slithered forward. "Flora, I've never seen the colors in a rainbow. What can I do?"

Flora's jaw dropped in silence. The fairies caught their breath until Vinnie stepped forward.

"Rainbows have green in them, and you've seen lots of grass."

"So you'll get green!" everyone said at once.

"Yes," answered Flora. "And the girls will go with pink, the boys blue."

Then everyone walked to the end of the rainbow, always present and glistening in the sky. Their excitement mounted as the time grew near to time travel. Even Snake thought it would be much more exciting than shedding his skin each year.

Flora called a practice session. Each fairy imagined his or her time travel color. Deep breaths were sighed as each counted to three.

However, Vinnie was having a hard time focusing and concentrating, as hyper fairies often do. Somehow, he kept seeing brown instead of blue. As he reached for a calming aroma blend, Spider, the journalist, jumped out of his pocket and into his hand.

"Pssst!" Spider called out to a startled Vinnie.

"What are you doing here?" asked Vinnie, staring at Spider in disbelief.

"I wanna log onto this trip. Can you help me?" inquired Spider. "This will make a great story for the *Fairy Morning News*."

"Oh! Uh, what colors can you see, blue, pink, or green?" offered Vinnie.

"Brown," answered Spider dryly.

Vinnie looked stumped as his brow wrinkled. His eyes lit up as a new idea popped into his head.

"Do you have your laptop computer?" he asked.

"Always," answered Spider, abruptly.

"Then, we'll set the screen on blue, set you on the screen and beam you up," Vinnie answered quickly.

Spider agreed and climbed onto the computer screen after it was programmed on blue. To Spider's surprise, Vinnie abruptly shut the case, locking Spider screaming inside.

"Hey! Give me some space! I can't move in here! I may never walk again!" Spider cried.

"But your voice still sounds strong," laughed Vinnie. "Shhh! Here comes Flora. Don't make a noise!" ordered Vinnie sternly.

Flora walked quickly from fairy to fairy with her "take charge" attitude. She wished each fairy, and then Snake, a safe journey. As she patted each fairy's shoulder, one by one, they joined Snake on the ground, face down. Nimbus winked at Sweet Tooth as she nuzzled the earth. It was time to launch!

"Four, three, two, one," they chanted together. "TAKE OFF!" Flora cried as each color of the rainbow resonated throughout every cell in their bodies. As each one mentally joined with pink, blue or green, they launched into the rainbow, as if in a chute, disappearing before the rainbow's end.

Every cell in their tiny bodies vibrated to the speed of light. The noise was deafening as flares of bright lights flashed past them. As they traveled, they lost all sense of time and space. Soon, their self-identities were stripped away. Only the sound of their breaths remained.

## The Landing

Within seconds, the fairies began landing on the other side of the rainbow. Each floated from the sky as if supported by a parachute. Snake hung in the sky like a twisted tube of toothpaste, his head perfectly flattened by the experience.

At first, the fairies looked stunned as they gently drifted to the ground. Their legs felt weak and their little bodies shook all over until they acclimated to the new environment.

Vinnie immediately reached into his pocket to free Spider. He searched deeper and deeper without success.

"Where's Spider?" asked Vinnie as he looked around.

Everyone was too preoccupied with acclimating to their new environment to pay attention to what Vinnie was saying. Vinnie began to panic as he thought about what might have happened to a defenseless little spider without wings to support his flight.

Vinnie began to fly around aimlessly, a normal reaction for him during stress. He flew up and down, unable to decide what to do. Visions of Spider suspended in the rainbow, unable to weave his way out, raced through Vinnie's anxious mind. While Vinnie obsessed, a small object passed before his eyes on the way to the garden ground. A muffled, familiar voice echoed in the air before it hit the ground. "Help! I hit the delete button!"

"Delete button?" Vinnie's brow wrinkled as he thought out loud. "That must be Spider!" Vinnie sped toward the area of the garden, where he thought Spider had landed abruptly. He flew around searching and calling his name to no avail. Vinnie knew Spider was nearby. Frustration mounted as he fluttered in and out of a clump of fragrant herbs and sprawling rose bushes looking for Spider.

Suddenly, Vinnie's sharp eyes spotted Spider's laptop stuck in the heavily mulched garden. He dove for the ground as fast as his wings could flutter, determined to save a friend in need. Then, he felt a sharp jerk from behind, tugging at the back of his neck. No matter how fast he fluttered, Vinnie stayed right where he was, suspended in mid air, caught on a very long thorn belonging to a nearby rose bush.

To make matters even worse, a large black dog ran to where Spider lay, silently waiting to be rescued, and began to bark. Vinnie tried in vain to quiet the dog before its owner was alerted to the situation, but it was too late. First he heard footsteps, then he saw a pair of tan legs walk in front of him as he wiggled helplessly in the air.

"What are you barking at?" the gardener reprimanded the black dog, as she carefully prodded the garden floor with a spade. "It's not going to hurt you!" The gardener patted the dog as she reached over to pick up the box.

Just then, Vinnie's tireless efforts set him free as the thorn sprung him into the air. He flew right in front of the gardener's eyes, dazzling her with every acrobatic trick he could perform.

The gardener stepped back, shaking what appeared to be the stars out of her eyes. She looked around a little dazed, as Vinnie valiantly continued to buzz around her head.

"Oh, my gosh!" she exclaimed. "I think I really am seeing fairies this time!" the gardener cried aloud as Vinnie buzzed in front of her face. Her eyes crossed as Vinnie landed on the tip of her nose.

"Why, you're a wet little fairy," the gardener laughed, as Vinnie wiped his chin.

"I'm here to defend my friend from the clutches of this vicious canine!" Vinnie announced proudly.

"Mom!" the gardener laughed in surprise. "Mom's a pushover if you pet her," explained the gardener, as the dog instinctively rolled on her back for attention.

Vinnie took the opportunity to fly over to the laptop enclosing his friend.

"Spider! Spider, are you in there?" Vinnie called out to his friend. But the box lay silent on the ground, as Vinnie fluttered around feeling like his heart would explode inside him.

The gardener reached over and opened the tiny box as Vinnie's tears spilled inside it. Spider lay flattened inside the box, his little heart weak but still pumping. As the gardener turned to Vinnie with a puzzled look, he answered the question she never asked, the words spilling out faster and faster.

"It's my friend, Spider, from the Land of Thyme. He time traveled with us to do a story for the *Fairy Morning News*."

Seeing Vinnie's distress, the gardener interrupted him and ran off to find help for Spider. She quickly returned with a tiny bottle she sprayed on Spider to revive him. Vinnie wrung his little hands as he flew around, repeating over and over, "He pushed the delete button with one of his legs."

Just then, Spider began to move ever so slowly. As the gardener sprayed, Spider groaned. Finally, his head popped up and his legs began to bend and take form.

"Spider's alive!" screamed Vinnie as he flew off to find his fellow fairies. Soon, he returned with the entire entourage of travelers, cheering Spider on as he gathered strength to walk out of his laptop. At that moment, the other fairies did not understand what happened to Spider and how he arrived in the garden.

Vinnie flew around in circles, relating the whole story, as the gardener stood back watching the scenario in amazement. Before her dazzled eyes stood a wide variety of what appeared to be fairies of every size and proportion.

Suddenly, they turned toward her and asked in unison, "What did you spray on Spider?"

"Oh!" she cried, as she was startled into "reality." "It's a blend of flower essences and essential oils I make from my gardens," the gardener proudly explained, as she held up the bottle.

"Wow! We must be in the right place," Nimbus exclaimed, turning to Flora.

For the next several minutes, the fairies flew past the gardener and introduced themselves, with one exception. Nimbus couldn't stay up long enough and landed in the gardener's lap, giggling nervously. Flora took the opportunity to explain their mission.

"So," answered the gardener, "you want to learn how flower essences catalyze healing from the heart. Well, you certainly came to the right place. These plants have traveled and naturalized here from all over the world for just that reason. They seem to have a group consciousness to open our hearts."

"Where did you learn about flower essences?" inquired Flora.

"Oh, it's a tradition handed down to the women in my family for at least four generations," explained the gardener. "The knowledge seems innate, just like organic gardening."

"Have you always made flower essences?" asked Sweet Tooth.

"Well, no although I always knew how. I began seeking answers through nature after I had children. My eldest are twins. They had a physical condition beyond what our modern science and technology could help. I returned to my roots in nature to find the answers that always exist in some form of plant life. I used both herbal tonics and flower essences. A few years later, my youngest child displayed allergies that greatly reduced his hearing. I added essential oil aromatherapy to decongest his sinuses and restore his hearing."

"When did you have time to make flower essences?" queried Sweet Tooth.

"I began to open my heart to Mother Nature's flower essences while suffering from a serious disease. I felt overwhelmed, not to mention scared and in pain. I was even more afraid of surgery, since I watched my parents have at least twenty major surgeries during my childhood. It just didn't seem right for me at that time in my life. However, I remained open to all my options during a very long recovery."

The fairies gathered around the gardener as she continued.

"My answer came as an inner message to work with flowers, as well as other forms of complementary healing. It's not exactly the answer I expected from prayer," the gardener chuckled. "All I really wanted was to get out of pain."

"How did you get through all those problems?" asked Flora. "I feel overwhelmed just listening to you."

"These flowers gave me the strength to transform my perception of life, leaving behind fears, disappointments, and all the old hurts and beliefs that were dragging me down," the gardener replied, as she pointed to her gardens. "I was a prisoner to my mind, enslaved to belief systems that didn't work. I was blocking any real healing, because on a very deep level I had given up on life."

"I feel the same way about being fat," Nimbus replied, as he stomped the ground. "I just feel trapped inside these fat cells, ruled by an ego that makes me eat too much. When I get under stress, I eat comfort foods."

"How does that make you feel, Nimbus?" asked the gardener.

"It makes me feel vulnerable," he replied, "because I've never even seen my ego."

"Well, it makes all of us vulnerable," agreed the gardener. "Our ego literally rules how we see reality and what we believe to be true."

"Slow down, *slow down*!" interrupted Spider. "I'm not yet up to speed on my typing," he explained, as he typed with all eight legs.

"Did you and your children ever shake all these problems?" he inquired as his legs slowed to a halt.

"Why, yes, but it wasn't overnight," the gardener replied. "It took years for my health to transform, although the progression was steady. The children blossomed into better health in a very short time."

"Would you say the flower essences made you well?" Spider asked as he typed.

"The flower essences catalyzed my will and ability to heal. Not even drugs really heal. The body has innate healing abilities that can be catalyzed by flower essences. The body doesn't know how to get sick, it only understands how to get well. When emotions, stress, and perceptions upset the balance of homeostasis, this innate healing ability is locked out. That's when flower essences help. They can reconnect with our biological source of health. We not only get healthier but we also tap and utilize our talents and potential gifts with a hearty zest."

"I'd like a flower essence to make me bloom!" Vinnie chimed innocently. As the gardener turned to acknowledge him, Vinnie added, "Did you know Flora and I are twins?"

"Why, no!" exclaimed the gardener in surprise, as Flora frowned.

"I was born first!" Vinnie continued, his spirits soaring, quite enamored with the gardener.

"That's because I kicked him out," added Flora, wryly.

"Well, life gives us just what we need to grow and bloom," answered the gardener, laughing. "Flower essences not only heal the wounds and expectations of the personality, but also encourage a sense of unity with others," she offered. Then she turned to the gardens and asked, "Would you like to tour the gardens?"

"Yes!" The fairies fluttered about gathering around the gardener.

"Wait! Wait one minute!" called Spider, as he finished typing.

"Do you believe that your flower essences healed your body from all those problems?" he inquired, still looking for a sensational story.

"I believe my body healed itself and flower essences catalyzed a transformation of my personality, as well as my reason to be here. To me, they were as much a part of healing as any herbs or treatments I used during my recovery. They gave me faith that my body can heal itself."

As the gardener turned to enter the gardens, Spider could be heard talking to himself. "Faith! That's it! We'll call her Faith."

## Into the Garden

Faith transformed as she entered the garden. Her voice became lighter and she seemed to float as she walked down the garden paths. The fairies fluttered all around her like butterflies dressed as tiny pixies. Spider stepped over Snake, who was fast asleep on a rock.

"When I work in my gardens, I enter a world where flowers talk and nature sings. Flowering plants are such wonderful teachers. They see the sadness in our eyes, yet catalyze the potential of what we can be. Flowers speak to us from the heart of creation, and heal wounds from the deepest part of the psyche. Their fragrance, shape, color, and beauty remind us that all true healing comes from the heart." The fairies nodded in agreement.

"Each flower has a unique message and healing potential that can be captured in an essence at the peak time of its bloom," Faith continued. "I choose flowers that bloom under stress from an inner joy that expresses the wonders of nature."

"Why do you pick flowers that bloom under stress?" asked Nimbus innocently.

"Because they help us bloom under stress," Faith answered, smiling at Nimbus.

Nimbus blushed as red as a rose, but felt confident in continuing his inquiry.

"That would make every stressful situation an opportunity to bring out the best in me, wouldn't it?" he raised his voice, as he looked around for approval.

"Yes, but not everyone I know would see it that way," sighed Faith. "I understand what you're saying is true, but I still find myself complaining sometimes," she chuckled under her breath.

"As ethereal beings, we understand there are ups and downs in life. Nature supports both the good and unwelcome bugs as equals. We don't see the bigger picture to understand why," explained Flora. "We exist on the ethereal plane and actually see the aura of flowers and plants. Although we understand flowers are soothing and healing to the psyche, we have a lot to learn about healing from the heart. That's why we're here. We want you to teach us what you know and have experienced so we can also teach the fairies in the Land of Thyme." Flora sat down on a nearby flower as she finished talking, as if out of wind.

Vinnie seized the opportunity to gain Faith's attention and add something important to the conversation.

"Flora wants the fairies to open their hearts so they'll eat her Melba toast," Vinnie explained. "I'm the only fairy that eats it willingly."

Flora slapped her forehead then hid her eyes with her hand.

Faith laughed aloud as Nimbus and Sweet Tooth burst into uncontrollable giggles.

"That's quite a job you've taken on, Flora," Faith replied, looking directly at Flora, as she smiled sweetly.

"I'm teaching the earth fairies dietary and lifestyle changes to improve their health and reduce the extra weight their wings have been carrying around." Flora answered matter-of-factly, as she turned to look at Nimbus and Sweet Tooth.

"We believe opening the heart is the key to our growth," explained Sweet Tooth, as she looked past Flora and squeezed Nimbus's hand.

"But not the kind of growth that makes our petals stretch," added Nimbus.

Faith laughed, then explained, "What I can teach you is how to balance the personality and the subtle body with flower essences. They unlock the deepest layer of creative potential to catalyze and soften the process of conscious growth." She glanced at her audience to make sure they understood before she continued.

"In the subtle body, health relates to spiritual growth. The roles that no longer serve us fade away and we leave behind all that is not true to our nature. An inner atmosphere of peace overcomes the ego's illusion of separation. For what is divine cannot be separated from its source."

"How will these essences affect us when used?" Spider queried.

"Most people, or I mean, fairies too," Faith stumbled, "feel lighter because the subtle body is less dense. But these essences also reduce stress, anxiety, and compulsive, unconscious actions."

"What do stress and unconscious actions have to do with the subtle body?" asked Spider, as he continued to type.

"The subtle body has an electromagnetic charge like static electricity," Faith answered. "Flower essences reduce the charge. The let-down response reduces stress like an exhalation of a deep breath," Flora replied.

"That's it!" Spider answered excitedly. "I'll title my story 'Gardener Unlocks Miraculous Cure for Stress.'"

The fairies broke their stunned silence with a noisy applause. Faith laughed, shaking her head.

"Experience has taught me that for every impossible situation or incurable illness, Mother Nature has provided a flower to support us," Faith answered, looking down humbly.

"Can you give me any examples?" Spider asked.

"I can teach you how over a hundred flower essences support health and emotional balance," answered Faith. "Over the past twenty years, I have used these essences with thousands of folks who often came to me in serious health and stressful situations. At a deep level, the essences catalyzed attitude changes and emotional balance, which allowed a process of renewal to regenerate the body and spirit. The body, like a garden, continuously transforms and recreates itself from the subtle body to the dense physical form."

"So you're saying an inner harmony leads to a healthy lifestyle," added Spider. "And disharmony can lead to stress that ultimately initiates or even causes disease."

"Right," answered Faith. "The physical body expresses disharmony in three ways: endocrine imbalance, expressed by emotional distress; immune depression, expressed by nutritional deficiencies and leading to many physical and mental disorders and illnesses; and neurological dysfunction, often displayed in intimacy patterns and auto-immune reactions."

"So, when can we learn more about all of them?" queried Flora. "This sounds like what we need to know to help the fairies in the Land of Thyme."

"Yeah! We're ready to learn," agreed the fairies.

"Wait, wait!" laughed Sweet Tooth. "Maybe we should treat Faith to some of our floral cordials and have a break before the lecture."

"Excellent idea," agreed Flora. "I'd like you to brew some lemon verbena and spearmint tea for starters."

"Yea!" The fairies flew to the kitchen with equal enthusiasm. A party of any variety excited the fairies and this was close enough to a celebration for them! They joined together and whipped up the following recipes to dazzle Faith with their wit and charm.

## Lemon Verbena and Spearmint Tea

Sweet Tooth named this her "beat the heat" recipe for weary gardeners.

**Ingredients:**

2 tablespoons fresh lemon verbena leaves
2 tablespoons fresh spearmint leaves
1 cup of boiled water

Blend all ingredients for one minute. Strain. Add two cups of cold water and serve over ice. Serves three.

While Sweet Tooth brewed tea, Nimbus went to work making a garden preserve and butter to serve with teacakes.

## Rose Petal Jam

**Ingredients:**

2 cups scented rose petals, torn into small pieces
2 cups brown sugar (or date sugar)
2 cups sugar
4 cups cored and peeled cooking apples
1 cup water
2 tablespoons freshly squeezed lemon juice
vanilla essential oil (optional)

Pound rose petals with brown sugar in a mortar and pestle until well mixed. Simmer apples in one cup of water and two cups of sugar over low heat for twenty minutes, covered. Add rose sugar and lemon juice and boil twenty minutes longer. Pour into sterilized jars. Refrigerate leftovers.

## Scented Geranium Butter

**Ingredients:**

1 stick unsalted butter
1 tablespoon finely minced scented geranium leaves, such as rose, lemon, lime, cinnamon, ginger, or coconut.

Simmer butter until it begins to bubble. Reduce heat and skim off the bubbly milk fat. Add the scented geranium leaves. Cover and remove from heat for ten minutes. Strain and refrigerate before serving. Serves eight.

Meanwhile, Snake slithered in, complaining there was nothing edible in the kitchen. "Where's the food?" he asked. "All I see are flowers, creams, and lotions! How am I going to survive on all this pretty stuff?" Snake pouted.

Faith became quite uneasy with Snake in the kitchen. She sent Vinnie and Snake into the garden to pick lemon thyme to flavor teacakes. Snake could be heard complaining to Vinnie from the kitchen.

"I'm your pet! You're supposed to take care of me, Vinnie. Look at me! I'm starving! I'm so weak I can hardly drag myself around!"

Vinnie carefully lifted Snake into his arms and affectionately wrapped him around his neck while he pinched lemon thyme for the following teacakes.

## LEMON THYME TEA CAKES

**Ingredients:**
   2 tablespoons unsalted butter
   1 teaspoon finely minced lemon thyme
   1/3 cup boiling water
   3 cups oat flakes
   1/2 teaspoon baking soda
   pinch of salt (optional)

Melt unsalted butter and lemon thyme. Add the boiling water and allow to cool. Preheat oven to 350°.

Combine remaining ingredients. Stir in melted lemon thyme butter to make a soft dough. Place the dough in an eight-inch un-greased baking pan. Pat the dough into place. Bake for forty minutes, until golden brown. Cut into bite-size slices and serve with rose jam and scented geranium butter. Serves six to eight.

**Variations:** Substitute one of the following for lemon thyme: one teaspoon minced fresh rosemary, sage leaves, curry leaves, lavender leaves, or lemon verbena leaves.

# CHAPTER 12

# Freeing The Personality

## Herbs and Flowers for Different Personality Types

*"As we return to the source, we express a passion for life."*
Judy Griffin, *The Healing Flowers*

## How Flowers Perceive Us

As the fairies wiped their plates and cleaned the kitchen, Faith prepared her lecture. First, she opened her cabinet to prepare a blend of dry potpourri to scent the room.

She gathered and mixed:

1 cup fragrant rose petals

1 cup lavender flowers

½ cup rosemary leaves

½ cup lemon thyme leaves

½ cup sweet annie flowers

Faith crushed the leaves with a mortar and pestle to release their natural fragrance. She placed them in a glass container over a pan of simmering water, adding a few drops of rose essential oil.

The fairies gathered around Faith as she began to lecture, sniffing the sweet aroma.

"The souls of flowers perceive the human personality as an emotional legacy including upbringing, present environment, inherent strengths, and weaknesses. The personality can be defined by understanding underlying fears and pain; specific flower essences will encourage healing and growth. During stress, the personality will act out characteristically to a dominant personality trait. First, I will outline how the personality perceives the world on a daily basis according to past experiences. Then, I'll answer questions to help determine your personality's strengths and weaknesses according to emotional stress, immune response, and intimacy patterns. I will describe flower essences that aid in balancing each response, without making claims for healing disease. They catalyze potentials and encourage the personality to express its greatest good.

"All true healing comes from opening the Heart."

The fairies applauded and moved to the edge of their cushions in anticipation of the lecture. They weren't sure they understood everything yet, but they were eager to learn more.

"The personality develops dependent, controlling, and competitive traits by the age of seven. These traits have negative and positive qualities. During stress, we are likely to act out some of the negative qualities. These actions developed from the needs and fears of our early childhood experiences. They become part of the behavior of the ego that drives us from an unconscious level. We refer to any constructive changes stemming from ego fears as *conscious growth*."

"Is that what drives me to eat under stress?" asked Nimbus innocently.

"Yes, and as we discuss in depth how the personality develops, you will understand how you can change these habits," Faith replied. "First, let me briefly describe the dependent, controlling, and competitive parts of the personality. Then, we'll go into details."

## The Dependent Personality

"Those with the Dependent Personality are humanitarians concerned with the plight of others — their needs, desires, and problems — and are always willing to share. They put faith in others and divine intervention. They are concerned with family, friends, and the community. This is the worker, the one to put a plan into action while being compassionate and present for others. They represent the mass of humanity.

"Dependents become imbalanced when they believe someone else knows better, can do a better job, or is necessary in their life to feel complete. This leads to a tendency to cling to and smother the people they love or need to love. They give away their power to avoid abandonment, rejection, or being alone. Their worst fear is being unlovable. They often mimic the behavior of their parents or a dominant personality, unable to be their own person. Their commitment is to security and they may use manipulating, pleading, and helplessness to have their way. The result is often being the victim. Circumstances control their lives.

"In a relationship, co-dependency can occur. A dependent person will do almost anything to avoid abandonment, the ego's greatest fear."

"When does a person learn to fear abandonment?" asked Flora, wrinkling her brow.

"Good question," smiled Faith. "Abandonment is a child's first and greatest fear. As a baby, we are all helpless and afraid, even goddesses."

"Flora's a goddess," offered Vinnie.

"Then, you are a god," replied Faith, "because she is your twin sister."

Vinnie was so shocked he stood up and looked all around himself, like he expected to grow a tail.

Spider stopped tapping his laptop as the room grew very quiet. Everyone was looking at Vinnie.

"Well! I guess that's why I'm such a good gardener," Vinnie grinned broadly. Just then Snake woke up and crawled out from beneath a chair.

"Just remember, Vinnie, you're made of the same stuff as the compost you're spreading in the gardens."

Everyone laughed and began clapping, as Vinnie proudly bowed, loving the attention.

"Oh, great," complained Snake, as he slithered under a chair. "Now I have to deal with a hyper *and* conceited owner."

"Don't worry, Snake. I'll see to your needs," chided Vinnie, as he returned to his seat with a huge grin. "Remember, we came here to take care of Flora."

However, Vinnie had received the gift of a new self-image from the journey. He returned to the lecture with renewed interest and a sense of well-being he had never felt before. He seemed much calmer as Faith continued her lecture.

"We can think of the dependent stage of the personality as developing from birth to two years of age. The next stage is the controlling part of the personality. It develops as a child realizes he or she can get his or her way by certain actions: smiling, pouting, crying crocodile tears, or even blaming others. In society, balanced controllers are leaders. So, let's just put the controlling personality type in a nutshell and then we'll discuss it."

## The Controlling Personality

"The Controlling Personality is a great organizer, manager or researcher, concerned with being exact and correct. They often work behind the scenes, taking charge of getting the job done right and on time. They are responsible members of society. These people take control of their environment as lawmakers, researchers, scholars, financial analysts, and group leaders.

"Controllers become imbalanced when they have to be right. Their greatest fear is failure or losing control. These people feel powerless when they are not in charge, even to the point of being critical, vindictive, and holding grudges. They can be resentful of those who do not take them seriously and blame others rather than accept fault. In relationships, they can accept respect more easily than affection and may appear to be cold, aloof, and demanding. In life situations, their biggest challenge may stem from denial."

When Faith finished her outline, Sweet Tooth was the first to speak up.

"Gee, I wonder who we know that is a controller?" she asked in a soft voice.

"I know," replied Flora in a firm voice. "The captain of the Fairy SEALs. He tried to control who won the contest to be my travel partner."

Sweet Tooth turned toward Faith to direct her next question. "Do controllers feel like they're perfect, or have to be perfect, by any chance?"

"Oh, they're definitely perfectionists," replied Faith, not catching the underlying meaning of Sweet Tooth's question.

"Flora's perfect," Vinnie offered, smiling.

"Yeah, she's certainly a ten," added Snake, as his head poked out from under a chair.

"Oh!" laughed Flora shyly. "I don't relate to either of the personality types so far. What's the last one?"

"It's the competitive personality," Faith answered quickly, a little uncomfortable with the conversation.

## The Competitive Personality

"The Competitive Personality is an extrovert in search of praise. Their thrust is to please others and have many talents to support them. They not only want to be praised—they also want to be remembered. As their achievements exceed the height of human capability, they excel as leaders as well as great achievers. They may be entertainers, athletes, politicians, artists, or corporate celebrities. These are the superstars one would call on to slay the dragons in society.

"When appreciation of their talents is lacking, the competitive personality may resort to questionable ethics, showing a very insensitive action. Their concern is to be number one. There's only one place to be and that's on top of the world.

"Appearance is a useful commodity that helps them achieve recognition. They notice every flaw in their physical appearance and consider aging to be an enemy.

"In relationships, their needs evolve from gaining attention and praise and being the only one. They may need to be reminded of the individual needs of their loved ones."

As Faith finished, she looked around the group and asked, "Did you find yourself in all three personality types? The psyche is a complicated combination of checks and balances, and sometimes denials. You should find familiar strengths and weaknesses in each trait. If any particular trait limits your expression, it will put you into a psychological reversal that stunts your growth and creativity."

## How the Subtle Body Affects the Personality

"How would these traits relate to the chakras and the subtle body?" asked Flora.

Faith looked quite surprised at Flora's question. "Why, that's an excellent question, Flora. Let's outline the chakras on the board."

In the subtle body, the chakras most affected by the dominant personality traits are:

| Identity and self-worth | Coccyx | Competitive |
|---|---|---|
| Security issues, social and sexual expression | Sacral | Dependent |
| Personal power and influencing others | Navel | Controlling |
| Forgiveness and compassion | Heart | Controlling |
| Co-creating though the spoken word | Throat | Competitive |
| Imagining what you want to manifest | Third Eye | Controlling |
| Expressing spiritual ideals into actions, as a humanitarian | Crown | Dependent |

"So, if we want to work on any imbalances, can we use your flower essences?" asked Nimbus.

"Of course, we can build what I call 'shield of health' by utilizing the support of nature: flower essences, herbal tonics, proper nutrition, chakra balancing, and essential oil aromatherapy. The goal is to create a harmonious expression for each personality trait," replied Faith.

"Now, let me get this straight," Spider spoke out from a long silence. "When we get under stress, we display a dominant personality trait. Will it always be the same?"

"Not necessarily," answered Faith. "You might be whiny or a victim in an intimate relationship. At the office, you could be demanding and with siblings you could be competitive."

"Yeah, you could have a dominant personality trait for each leg, Spider," sneered Snake.

But Snake was lost in his notes and too preoccupied with his laptop to hear Snake's smart remark. The fairies giggled as Vinnie carefully lifted Snake and carried him outside to a nice warm rock for his nap.

"Tell us more about the shield of health, Faith," requested Sweet Tooth.

"Well," began Faith, "I believe balancing the personality ultimately leads to optimal health because the energy is free flowing throughout the chakras in a figure-eight pattern. This forms a shield that nurtures and protects the body and helps to keep the head and the heart in the right place. For every potential imbalance, Mother Nature has provided a flower to catalyze optimal creativity and personal growth."

"Can you outline the flowers and nutrients for each dominant personality?"

asked Nimbus.

"Yeah, you said you'd tell us more about each trait also," flapped Vinnie, as he twirled around the room.

"Okay, okay," Faith smiled warmly. "I do appreciate your interest and enthusiasm. This is going to be a lot of new information, so be sure to take notes."

Spider spun around in his chair with all eight legs typing. The fairies cheered and Faith began to explain.

## Dependent Shield

"The dependent personality is governed by the need to be loved. An imbalance is created by the underlying anxiety of the unknown: Am I lovable? Will my emotional needs be met by others? Am I saying and doing the right things to receive love? The dependent ego's greatest fear is anxiety separation, the ultimate fear of abandonment and death. Subsequently, every sign of loss, rejection, or disappointment, real or unreal, is perceived as abandonment. Dependency fears originate from feeling rejected by the parents. The fear of rejection creates a pattern of holding on in subsequent intimate relationships. Control is only attempted through manipulation or being the victim.

"As a child, the dependent is sweet and loving, but takes it personally if love and rewards are not returned. At this stage of development, a child does not understand that parents are teachers. They have their own needs, some of which have not been met since childhood. Therefore, they are incapable of noticing and providing all the love and attention a child desires. Neither can parents control external conditions such as moving, illness, divorce, and sibling rivalry. The child becomes predominantly dependent as he matures without developing the ability to go within and determine how to resolve his emotional needs, love, and attention.

"Dependents enter into adult relationships with the same emotional needs of a child. Often they are excellent nurturers; they just don't know how to get their needs met. The fact that they are needy ensures defeat. Every frustrated attempt brings out fear from the past. Doubt opens the historical questions: Am I lovable? Will I be abandoned? Dependents often act and look as helpless as a kitten to receive care. They will stay in a relationship and settle for less rather than risk being alone.

"They will repress angry feelings and confrontation for the same reason. Dependents may subject themselves to abusive relationships, sometimes attracting a partner that expresses the anger they cannot feel. Dependents are not very critical of others because their efforts go into being irresistible. They will take anger out on themselves through chronic pain, depression, and feelings of guilt.

"Feeling unloved or unfulfilled in love relationships can lead to food cravings, anorexic behavior, excessive spending, bingeing, and compulsive behavior. Emotional unfulfillment creates an endocrine imbalance. Blood sugar levels and cellular insulin response can create a host of symptoms, the most severe being hyperglycemia and hypoglycemia. The most severe emotional response is suicide, for death can be kinder than abandonment.

"To build a shield of the dependent personality, it is necessary to release past hurts. Focusing on what is right and good about life and remembering pleasant memories will help release endorphins and facilitate new neuronal pathways. This will build a perception of life that does not see everything as loss. Depression may lead to frequent viral and secondary bacterial infections, such as sinusitis, bronchitis, and middle ear infections (otitis media). Repressed anger can be linked to allergic rhinitis. The dependent personality is oversensitive until the dependent's emotional response is balanced.

"Oversensitivity can also result from nutritionally deficient food and poor eating habits. Dependents prefer sweets and sometimes use them as a substitute for affection. Tenderness and touch will sedate the oversensitive nervous system and concentrate neurotransmitters to abate suppressed anger and depression.

"The feeling of separation from love and Nature stems from abandonment. The ultimate separation is from the Self, the consciousness of true identity, and a sense of destiny as an individual. In order to empower the individual, autonomy must be achieved. This develops by dropping the roles others have chosen for the dependent, such as, 'He looks like his father' or 'She is just like her mother.' When dependents give their power away, someone else steps in to make their decisions. The career, schooling, and even life partner are influenced by a parent's decision and desires. The dependent personality matures to be like the dominant parent, including having similar diseases, opinions, and intimacy patterns. Becoming aware of one's true nature is a process that will resume development of a unique personality with a balanced emotional response and competent immune pattern.

"To remain balanced, the individual will have to practice decision-making and feel a purpose in life with guidance and nurturing from the soul. Insight into the depth of the feeling nature will enlighten the unconscious fears and empower the personality with the ability to be self-sufficient. For what is divine cannot be separated from the source."

After she finished lecturing, Faith looked at each fairy, open for questions and comments.

"Gee, it seems as if we all relate to some part of the dependent personality," Sweet Tooth commented.

"If I work on the part of me that's dependent upon eating under stress, will I become self-actualized?" asked Nimbus.

"You'll certainly be on the right path," answered Faith.

"Which essences help empower the dependent part of the personality?" Nimbus asked, sensing the need to learn more very quickly.

"Let's make a list of some of the most important ones," Faith replied, turning to the chalkboard.

## Nature's Support for Dependent Personality Traits

Wear two drops twice daily on the navel chakra. A combination of four or five synergistic essences may be used simultaneously.

| | |
|---|---|
| Abandonment: | Dill |
| Afraid to release the past: | Bachelor button |
| Anxiety of the unknown, feelings of dread: | Amaryllis |
| Separation: | Dill |
| Being a victim: | Japanese magnolia |
| Separation from the body's wisdom: | Dill |
| Disappointment, swallowing hurt: | Chamomile |
| Fear of death: | Dill |
| Feeling insecure: | Begonia |
| Feeling of lack, unsatisfied: | Moss rose |
| Fear of loss: | Peppermint |
| Lack of direction in life: | Bamboo |
| Rejection or loss of a loved one: | Pansy |
| "Love hurts": | Lemon grass |
| Learn from past intimate relationships: | Autumn damask |
| "Fat" complex: | Pink rose |
| Food cravings: | Primrose |
| Obsessive behavior, bingeing, overeating, overspending: | Knotted marjoram |
| Unproductive relationships: | Fimbriata |
| Uncomfortable feelings about the body: | Country Marilou |
| Settling for less in relationships: | Grüss an Aachen |
| Withdrawn, apathetic: | Dianthus |
| Oversensitive: | Lantana |
| Lack of assertion: | Ligustrum |
| Living in the past: | Morning glory |
| Desire to withdraw: | Vanilla |
| Guilt: | Bougainvillea |
| Learning to say no: | Lobelia |

## Flower Essences for Weight Reduction

"Wait! Wait, just a minute!" Nimbus pleaded. "I'm starting to feel overwhelmed! I think I need all of them!" he sighed.

Faith laughed, as she answered, "I know what you mean. The flower essences seem to hit the spot. Let's start with the most important ones. What is most important to you right now?"

"Being fat," he answered bluntly.

"Then start with Pink rose for the pound you lose and gain time and again," Faith answered.

"How did you know that?" Nimbus asked, amazed.

"Because I have educated and counseled people with many complaints and problems for twenty years," Faith replied.

"Wow! What other essences do you have to help me?" Nimbus asked.

"Well, you probably eat when your feelings are hurt, and that's chamomile."

"That's right!" exclaimed Nimbus. "Keep going!"

"Bingeing and overeating calls for knotted marjoram; food cravings indicates primrose. If you eat to satisfy an emptiness inside, moss rose helps."

"Gee, can I mix these together or try them one at a time?" queried Nimbus.

"Either way," Faith answered. "Most people receive the most benefits from a mixture."

Faith walked to the kitchen and mixed the essences and handed them to Nimbus. "Try these," she offered. "Just rub a few drops on your tummy."

Nimbus was quick to apply the essences, giggling as he rubbed them onto his tummy. "Am I cured?" he asked.

"The essence or soul of a flower already sees you as complete. So, in a way, you are cured. Using them daily will reinforce the lifestyle change, as well as your daily habits," Faith answered.

"How do you feel?" asked Spider, as he looked up from his laptop.

"Well," Nimbus thought a moment, "I feel lighter, like a burden's been lifted."

"Is there anything else he can do to establish healthy daily habits?" Sweet Tooth asked with greater interest than she'd shown before.

"Why, yes," answered Faith. "Dependent personalities need to balance their blood sugar and subsequent endocrine response by eating small meals with an in-between snack."

"What foods should we accent?" asked Sweet Tooth.

"Proteins of animal or vegetable origin, such as soy, and complex carbohydrates, such as oatmeal and whole grains," replied Faith.

"What foods should they avoid?" asked Spider.

"Caffeine and lots of raw foods and sugars. They digest very quickly and often leave them hungry in an hour," replied Faith.

"I thought lots of raw foods were good for us," commented Vinnie in a surprised voice.

"Dependents need balance, so it's best to eat salad with a protein, such as beans or a slice of turkey. It keeps them from craving sweets and getting hungry between meals," continued Faith.

"I get hyper when I eat a lot of sweets or raw food," added Vinnie.

"You might do well on lantana for oversensitivity," Faith answered quickly, as she offered him a few drops.

"I guess chocolate's not on the list of foods to accent," Sweet Tooth interrupted in a meek voice.

"A small amount is okay," answered Faith. "But, dependent personalities are very sensitive. Stimulants make them oversensitive. Not only chocolate, but highly spiced foods or bitter herbs, like aloe and goldenseal."

## Flower Essences for a Chocoholic

"So, let's get back to the subject of chocolate," moaned Sweet Tooth. "What if we eat just a little bit more chocolate than the average person?"

"People who crave chocolate are often temporarily depressed or overtired. With women, it can also indicate a hormone imbalance due to insufficient fatty acid production. They crave chocolate for the high fat content, as well as essential nutrients, such as magnesium and copper," Faith lectured. "Some people use the caffeine in chocolate for an energy boost."

"Not me," replied Sweet Tooth, "I love it because it makes me feel good about myself. When life lets me down, chocolate lifts me up!"

"Do we have an essence for that?" asked Nimbus, squeezing Sweet Tooth's chubby hand.

"Probably evening primrose because chocolate is a substitute for love. Often, children feel rejected by a parent's actions and never really feel good about themselves on a deep level. When that feeling tries to surface, they eat chocolate," Faith replied.

"Well, I was ignored by my father," Sweet Tooth answered. "He was ashamed of me because I've always been heavy."

"How do *you* feel about yourself?" asked Spider, typing nonstop at his computer.

"I *like* myself the way I am! I feel powerful as a large woman," Sweet Tooth answered adamantly.

"How do you feel about the way your dad treated you?" asked Faith in a soft voice.

"Well, I feel rejected," answered Sweet Tooth with tears in her eyes.

"Oh, Honey!" cried Nimbus, as he wrapped his arms around her.

"That's lemon grass!" replied Faith. "Lemon grass helps release the feeling of rejection by a parent. Often, the individual goes through subsequent love relationships where the one they love hurts them. I call it a manifestation of love hurts. In the subtle body, a belief that loving someone is going to hurt them attracts exactly that. Until the underlying pain is removed, the fear is always there."

"That's true!" agreed Sweet Tooth. "I went through many relationships feeling rejected, until I met Nimbus! However, sometimes I still feel nervous or insecure and start eating chocolate for no apparent reason."

"The flower essences will help you feel more grounded and secure under stress, even if the stressor is unidentified," suggested Faith. "At least eating chocolate will be a choice, then," she laughed.

"I wish I could hold you until all those uncomfortable feelings go away," sighed Nimbus.

## Aromatherapy and Flower Essences

"The whole consciousness of the flower essences is that we have to help ourselves by changing our inner image," Faith commented. "As Sweet Tooth lets go of the memories of rejection stored throughout her body, her world will change for the best."

"How do these images get stored in the body?" asked Flora, intently leaning over a table.

"The brain is a hologram," Faith continued. "What we see, believe, and experience is relayed from the brain to every part of the body through the communications system we call the subtle body."

"So we're back to the chakras," Flora nodded. "Do you think the aromatherapy Sweet Tooth practices also helps to heal wounds from the past?"

"Of course!" exclaimed Faith. "Essential oils distilled from fresh, organically grown blooms directly affect brain chemistry so we can reprogram how we feel about ourselves. As the inner world changes, what we attract in life changes, too. And, if we feel good about ourselves, so will others," she smiled.

"Why do you use both flower essences *and* essential oils?" asked Vinnie, as he flew around the room.

"There are so many feelings and stressors we experience in life," replied Faith, "and there's a flower essence to support us through all of them. Many do not have fragrances that we can detect, which helps sensitive noses. However, fragrant flowers do not all have essential oils. I think of essential oils as immune enhancers because they contain immune properties of the plant. Essential oils can be derived from many parts of plants in a variety of ways. Leaves, flowers, citrus rinds, and tree bark can contain essential oils. Some are steam distilled, some are separated by alcohol, or even chemicals. They can affect healing in many ways or be enjoyed as fragrances. Flower essences are used specifically for personality growth with or without fragrance. Even if we like fragrances, there are times we don't need or want to use aromas in subtle-body balancing."

"So, can we use essential oils and flower essences together?" asked Sweet Tooth, as she rubbed lemon grass onto her navel power center.

"Definitely," replied Faith. But, before she could continue, Sweet Tooth turned toward the group and munched a chocolate.

"Sweet Tooth!" cried Faith and Flora simultaneously.

Sweet Tooth laughed as she licked her fingertips. "I thought I'd experiment to see if chocolate still tastes good after applying lemon grass for rejection of my father," Sweet Tooth teased, as she looked at Flora from the corner of her eye.

Everyone looked at Faith and Flora to see their response.

"Well, how does it taste?" asked Flora.

"Like chocolate without the wrapper," she replied, as the two girls fell into each other's arms laughing.

"This is a good time to take a break," Faith suggested.

## How Non-Fragrant Flower Essences Work

Vinnie followed Faith down the hall, flapping as fast as he could fly.

"Hey! Faith, how do the non-fragrant flower essences work?"

"Well, Vinnie, I extract a catalyst that makes flowers bloom under stress. It's called lipoic acid," Faith explained, as she continued walking. "In the body, lipoic acid is very protective and encourages natural detoxification through the liver. It seems to have antiviral properties also."

"Oh, kind of like beneficial insects in the garden, huh?" Vinnie did his best to sound like he knew what Faith was talking about.

"Well, it is beneficial, Vinnie," Faith replied. "Lipoic acid is an antioxidant that protects the body from free-radical damage and certain environmental and heavy metal toxicity. Wearing it as a flower essence is likely to affect the subtle body."

"And, then what happens?" asked Vinnie, as he slowed to turn a corner.

"The subtle body affects our mental and emotional balance. This reduces stress on a physical level," she replied. "There can be various physical benefits from reducing stress with flower essences. Each flower essence seems to help with different types of conditions. I will give Spider a copy of that research if it will help the fairies in the Land of Thyme."

"I'll go ask Flora," Vinnie suggested, as he flew down the hall.

Faith stood alone wondering when Vinnie would be able to make a decision by himself. She turned toward the kitchen as she heard the fairies gathering nearby. Sweet Tooth approached her as she entered the door.

"Can you recommend a tea or tonic to build a healthy body and promote longevity?" asked Sweet Tooth. "I want to live as long as the old timers in the gardens," she chuckled.

"Oh! Then we'll brew some herbal tonics that enhance health," replied Faith, as she reached for her pots and pans.

Faith brewed the following tonics for tea tasting.

## Tonic to Support Endocrine Health

This is an excellent tonic to balance blood sugar fluctuations.

**Ingredients:**
> 2 cups water
> 2 tablespoons *Rehmannia glutinosa* (prepared)
> 2 tablespoons *Astragalus membranaceus*
> 2 tablespoons *Zizyphus jujube* dates, fresh or dried

Simmer each herb in two cups of water in a covered pot for thirty minutes. Strain and sip one-half to one cup of the slightly sweet-tasting tea daily. Serves two.

## Tea for Immune Support

This is a relaxing tea, especially beneficial for the onset of a cold or flu.

**Ingredients:**
> 1 cup water
> 1 teaspoon chamomile flowers
> 1 teaspoon lemon thyme or thyme leaves
> 1 teaspoon catnip leaves or blossoms

Boil one cup of water. Remove from heat. Steep one teaspoon of each herb, fresh or dried, for ten minutes. Strain, sweeten if desired, and sip one or two cups daily. Serves one.

## Controller Shield

After the fairies enjoyed tea tasting and experienced the effect of flower essences, they were ready to learn more about healing from the heart. They gathered around Faith as she began to teach.

"By the time children are two years old," Faith explained, "they realize that they have some control over their environment. For example, crying may get a parent's attention or smiling may make grandma to want to hold them. They grow up perceiving the world to be safe only if they can control their environment. Under stress, the controlling part of the personality will experience anxiety, anger, and a diminished sense of importance and power.

"To the controlling personality, emotional pain, loss, and abandonment are often expressed through anger and rebellion. Anger is the only easily expressed feeling when the emotional nature is threatened. It is expressed with justification and blame, often by pointing a finger at the other person. It has to be somebody else's fault because the controller has to be right. Expressing hurt is not possible because it reveals weakness. The hormones released with anger help the controller feel strong. Their strong intellectual skills support their need to be right.

"Control is not meant to be a weapon. It is a learned response meant to secure love and meet the dependent's needs. An infant learns very quickly that every smile and syllable secures attentive love. They learn to point when they want something, a skill they will often use as adults.

"During childhood, the controller often had to grow up before his time, abruptly, or had to avoid dependence on an unreliable or absent parent. The child will learn to control the environment to combat the fear of losing control.

"The underlying anxiety is fear of change or control of the environment. When confronted with unfamiliar or fearful situations, this person will regress to unusually childish and needy behavior. Overwhelming stress instigates excuses, denial, and hiding to temporarily block pain or avoid explanation. Feeling helpless, powerless, alone, and unloved increases the desire to control the environment, for power minimizes the fear of being rejected. By the age of two, the child realizes the power of saying no as a form of defense.

"However, the fear of being wrong kept the child from speaking his mind, releasing past pain and visualizing a future. Being in control actually makes the personality powerless to make changes for the better. Major lifestyle changes are avoided. Any change is unwelcome. As the controller interacts with any of society's rules, rebellion becomes an expression of anger. Creativity may be blocked by the need to be in control.

"Letting go of past pain and mistakes to make peace with the past is a real breakthrough for spiritual growth. Letting go includes letting down defenses, being wrong or stupid, and being vulnerable. It could even mean accepting change as part of life. Changing workaholic habits and being available for social interactions will give the personality a chance to relax and slow down the intellectual dominance. Seeking answers in dreamtime is another way to let go and let life flow through with ease.

"When letting go is threatening, denial will occur and block progress. The inner world and physical reality will separate into two different realities. Alcoholism, disorientation, confusion, and schizophrenia can occur. A more common feeling of separation is from God and Nature. The person questions God. When feeling separated from Nature, the personality may experience several ways to insult the environment without realizing the longterm consequences.

"In the body, neuromuscular response may become imbalanced. Spasms, such as irritable bowel, temporomandibular jaw discomfort, and migraines can result. Adrenal exhaustion can occur from the increased state of tension, as well as increase in bacterial infections, aching, and malaise from chronic viral infection. Opening the heart chakra will help overall by encouraging cardiovascular flow and harmonizing neuromuscular response, as well as a warm smile.

"A controlling personality can be difficult to get along with in intimate relationships. A controller may become jealous and possessive, spoiling the spontaneity of passion. Differences in opinion may become threatening, leading to outbursts of anger or cold indifference. If divorce or separation occurs, it is very difficult for the controller to let go and adapt to change.

"In new relationships, controllers are cautious. They are likely to hold back from entering new relationships and resist being persuaded. To feel secure in a relationship, controllers must learn to accept others as they are, as well as themselves. They will realize they are in control when they are peaceful within.

"In spiritual matters, the personality is at peace when guided by a compassionate heart. Denial is overcome when this person follows his heart.

"From stillness of a quiet mind, pure awareness emerges."

After Faith finished her lecture, Spider broke the silence.

"Wow!" Spider exclaimed. "I'm ready for some pure awareness. "Will flower essences help the controlling part of the personality?"

"Yes! Let's make a list of flower essences for letting go of the pain that causes anger and rebellion," Nimbus called out in anticipation.

"Okay," Faith replied, as she turned to the chalkboard and began to write.

## Nature's Support for Controlling Personality Trait

Wear two drops on the heart chakra.

| | |
|---|---|
| Demanding needs: | Texas tulip poppy |
| Letting go: | Lilac |
| Rebellion | Jasmine |
| Workaholic; making peace with the past: | Dancing lady orchid |
| Suppressed anger: | Pink geranium |
| Willfulness (stubbornness): | White carnation |
| Denial: | Alfredo de Damas |
| Uprooting old patterns: | Rose campion |
| Surrender: | Madame Louis Levique |
| Avoiding change: | Morning glory |
| Holding onto the past: | Bachelor button |
| Fear of speaking out: | Crepe myrtle |
| Jealousy; hard to get along with others: | Double yellow |
| Inconsiderate: | Penta |
| Making peace with your Creator: | Sunflower |
| Holding back from a relationship: | Cecil Brunner |
| Encourage relaxation: | Verbena |
| Critical thoughts: | Garden mum |
| Enhancing willpower: | Old blush |
| Visualizing the future: | Bronze fennel |
| Creative change: | Azalea |
| Answers from dreams: | Madame Alfred Carrier |
| Opening the heart (chakra): | Wisteria |
| Cooperation with others: | Indian hawthorne |
| Need to escape or control environment: | Kalanchoe |
| Encouraging others: | Blue Danube aster |
| Follow the heart's yearning: | Marie Pavie |
| Guidance from a peaceful heart: | Maggie |
| Quiet the mind: | Silver moon |

## Healing the Heart

Faith paused as she turned to face the fairies. A solitary tear fell from the corner of Flora's eye as she spoke.

"Now I know what healing from the heart means."

Spider placed all eight hands on his heart and sighed. "Where do we go from here?"

"Let's define dietary and personal habits to build an immune shield of health," responded Faith.

"Overall, we want to promote personal warmth and cardiovascular flow," she began. "Green vegetables, whole grains, and legumes are especially helpful."

"What foods should controllers avoid?" asked Sweet Tooth.

"Alcohol, fermented foods, beverages in large amounts, and fatty foods, like coconut and palm oil," replied Faith.

"They should probably avoid fatty meats, pastries, and lots of whole milk products, too," added Flora.

"Wait! Before you continue, if there are dependent and controlling parts to heal, where do I start?" asked Spider.

"Go with the dominant symptoms," explained Faith. "If you're feeling alone and abandoned, take dill for dependency. A controlling personality fears the same experiences, but this person will display anger or rebellion and may need pink geranium or jasmine."

"What about foods?" asked Nimbus sheepishly.

"The dependent part of the personality is more likely to have food cravings and endocrine imbalance, like low blood sugar. The controller is more likely to drink too much alcohol or sedate feelings with heavy fatty foods. Their weakness is immune related and, later, problems like hypertension may occur," answered Faith.

"How does that happen?" asked Flora, wrinkling her brow.

"At first, the person feels out of control in some area of their life. That's when a flower essence really helps. Over time, the system breaks down and an illness occurs," Faith explained.

"Then can we say that flower essences prevent all diseases?" prodded Spider.

"We can say that flower essences certainly promote healthy attitudes, creativity, and gifts from the heart," replied Faith, as she walked toward the kitchen.

The fairies followed single file. As Flora passed by Spider, she poured a whole bottle of white carnation essence onto his heart chakra. "Don't worry so much about the cures," she warned him. "Sensationalism is for untalented journalists. We're looking for quality in our lives."

Spider quietly followed the group into the kitchen where Faith was brewing a tonic to enhance a controlling personality's health. He sat down at the table and started to type.

## TONIC TO SUPPORT CARDIOVASCULAR FLOW

Drink this tea to relax and tone the heart muscle.

### Ingredients:
2 cups water

5 lotus seeds (*Nelumbo nucifera*) available packaged at specialty grocery stores

10 hawthorn berries (*Crataegus* species)

1 teaspoon gotu kola leaves, fresh or dried

1 tablespoon red raspberry leaves, dried

1/8 teaspoon fresh or dried ginger

In two cups of water, simmer lotus seeds and hawthorn berries for twenty minutes, covered. Remove from the heat. Add gotu kola, raspberry leaves, and ginger. Cover and steep for ten minutes. Strain. Enjoy one cup daily. Serves two.

## TEA TO ENHANCE IMMUNITY

At the onset of a flu or cold, make a tea of the following herbs.

### Ingredients:
1 cup water

1 teaspoon hyssop, fresh or dried

1/2 teaspoon sage leaves (fresh is best)

1 teaspoon thyme, fresh or dried

1/2 teaspoon of fresh or dried orange peel

Steep for ten minutes in one cup of boiled water. Strain and drink one cup up to three times daily to relieve symptoms. Serves one.

Suggested supplements to correct imbalances and promote longevity include copper; vitamin C; L glutamine taken thirty minutes before breakfast; bioflavonoids, especially quercetin; procanthanins from grape seed or berries; magnesium; taurine; and glutathione.

## Competitive Shield

To finish a long day of lectures, the fairies decided to sip their tea as Faith explained the competitor's shield for longevity.

"The competitive personality is driven by a need to win to affirm self-worth.

They have a win-or-lose attitude that makes life a constant struggle to succeed. Although they are hard workers, they hide failures and humble beginnings that might invite criticism. Competitors believe they have to be the best at all times and value praise and flattery over love and friendship. They enjoy giving their best performance and need to be center-stage in order to feel worthy. Discouragement devastates them and judgment is avoided. They are often self-learners and self-starters. Competitors can develop a great imagination to live in a fantasy world of success. They may feel too vulnerable to admit shortcomings and disappointments, pretending they don't care. They are often leaders in their career who learned to emulate and imitate others since childhood to achieve higher goals.

"In childhood, competitors are often pressured to perform and achieve to please their parent. Competitors feel they have to be successful to 'make up for' their parents' lack and unfulfillment. Their greatest childhood disappointment is realizing their parents' limitations and failures. They are driven to great achievements by an underlying fear of growing up to be like them.

"There is another gnawing anxiety inside. Competitors fear if they are not successful, they will not be loved. This results in a feeling of emptiness, even when success is achieved, and a propensity to feel frustrated and resentful. How can a competitor ever win when he looks to others to fulfill his need to gain attention? All the competitor's efforts are focused outside himself.

"The competitor may seem calm and confident, but may be nervous and vacillating inside. Indecision and shyness dampen natural spontaneity until self-love is attained. Only then are they able to focus on priorities, quickly respond to opportunities, and learn from setbacks.

"Inner conflict may manifest as autoimmune and inflammatory disease. This may include allergies, Crohn's disease, cardiovascular disease, fevers, migraines, and acute illnesses. Nutritional deficiencies caused by overwork and stress may result in burnout with depression, neuronal degeneration with motor weakness and lack of coordination. They can experience dizzy spells from stress. When a competitor does take time to visit a doctor, the diagnosis is 'it's only nerves.' But grounding and balancing the chakras can recharge energy and heighten a sense of well-being. However, the most profound healing comes from touch. Developing and experiencing a sense of touch will relax and strengthen the nervous system and enhance intimate relationships.

"Developing intimacy will require patience. Competitors seem aloof, remaining detached and guarded to prevent the insecure feeling of being vulnerable. Their pattern is to avoid commitment and seek intimacy through sex. A sexual rendezvous is likened to winning. As self-esteem develops from within, competitors learn to love through respect. Developing intimacy with commitment can then become an expression of freedom to love as passionately as they work.

"To attain the success they crave, competitors must unmask the hidden fears of the unconscious. Overcoming the fear of being unworthy of the success they desire will bring competitors into the light of higher consciousness where they can begin to serve others for the betterment of mankind. Insight will also free the personality of the practice of living in a fantasy world. Understanding and expressing feelings spontaneously will free the personality to participate in life without distortion and unusual expectations. Exaggerated responses originating from past hurts will recede as self-mastery is experienced in a state of inner grinning."

The fairies cheered with the thought of inner grinning.

## Nature's Support for the Competitive Personality Traits

| | |
|---|---|
| Learning to be self-sufficient: | Borage |
| Fear of failure: | Lily |
| Overcoming difficulty: | Gaillardia |
| Life as a struggle: | Anemone |
| Direction or focus: | Bamboo |
| Self-appreciation: | Magnolia |
| Self-worth: | Red carnation |
| Self-image: | Basil |
| Shyness: | Daffodil |
| Introversion: | Narcissus |
| Realistically adjusting ideals and ideas: | Rose of Sharon |
| Overcoming burnout: | Shrimp |
| Self-discipline: | Wandering jew |
| Expressing strong emotions: | Meadow sage |
| Overcoming an exaggerated response: | White rose |
| Overactive, nervousness: | Stock |
| Need to be different: | Mexican bush sage |
| Indecision: | White petunia |
| Defining priorities: | Carrot |
| Responding to new situations: | Mexican oregano |
| Contemplation, learning from setbacks: | Silver lace |
| Inner conflict: | Snapdragon |
| Overreacting to stress: | Yarrow |
| Unique expression of talents: | Lady Eubanksia |
| Staying grounded to complete projects: | Viridiflora |
| Enhance public image: | Sweet Annie |
| Enhance public speaking, teaching: | Anise hyssop |
| Encourages longterm intimacy: | Marquis Bocella |
| Develop sense of touch: | Archduke Charles |
| Tune into the present moment of grace: | Bouquet of Harmony, a combination of vanilla and roses |

## How to Feed a Competitive Personality

As the fairies passed around flower essences, Flora asked Faith to describe the best diet for competitors.

"A good diet for competitors will accent low-stress proteins, such as soy, whitefish, chicken, and turkey to enhance stamina. Orange and yellow fruits and vegetables contribute minerals and vitamins to increase energy. Rich foods and dishes with several different ingredients tax digestion, slowing productivity. Highly spiced foods may be too stimulating unless served with mint and yogurt dishes."

"What about a tonic for competitors?" asked Vinnie, the only fairy who did not show signs of fatigue from the long lecture.

"Here's one that will relax even the most anxious fairy," she laughed.

### TONIC TO REDUCE STRESS FOR COMPETITIVE PERSONALITIES

Reducing stress will enhance immunity.

**Ingredients:**

1 cup water
½ teaspoon hops strobiles (*Humulus lupulus*)
1 teaspoon dried passion flower leaves (*Passiflora incarnata*)
1 teaspoon dried skullcap leaves (*Scutellaria laterofolia*)
½ teaspoon spearmint leaves, fresh or dried

In one cup of boiled water, steep the herbs for ten minutes, covered. Strain and sip at the end of a stressful day. Serves one.

As the fairies sipped their tonic, Faith began to brew the final tea for the day.

### TEA TO ENHANCE IMMUNITY FOR COMPETITORS

At the onset of viral symptoms or fever, sip this tea, cold or hot, throughout the day.

**Ingredients:**

2 cups water
1 tablespoon lemon juice
1 teaspoon honey
2 drops ginger juice

To two cups of water, add freshly squeezed lemon juice, honey, and two drops of freshly squeezed ginger juice from a garlic press. Serves two.

**Suggested supplements to correct imbalance and promote longevity:** Gaba amino acid; niacin; essential fatty acids, such as flaxseed oil and borage oil; potassium; beta-carotene; calcium; melantonin for insomnia for occasional use.

As Faith turned to pour some of the tea to the fairies, she found them fast asleep on their cushions. As she tiptoed out of the room, Faith noticed Vinnie's wings were still flapping in his sleep.

CHAPTER 13

# Subtle Body Healing
## Flower Essences and Herbal Tonics

*"Healing allows the mind, body and feelings to adjust to the changes."*
Judy Griffin, *The Healing Flowers*

The following day, Nimbus looked for Faith. He found her pruning roses, as Vinnie pulled weeds and shredded wood for the compost. Every time Nimbus politely tried to get Faith's attention, Vinnie would march between them while carrying another load of wood for the shredder.

"Do you need some help?" he asked Vinnie.

"Oh, my!" exclaimed Nimbus. "You are working faster and more efficiently than before, Vinnie. What are you doing differently to make such a dramatic change?"

"Working with flower essences and learning about the ego's personality traits made me realize that my biggest fear was being so powerful and brilliant that I would outshine even those that I admired," Vinnie explained calmly.

"And, then what?" queried Nimbus, with great curiosity.

"And, then I'd have an excuse not to be grown up and responsible for my actions," Vinnie stammered, as if the words didn't want to escape from his lips.

"Gee," mused Nimbus. "What's going to happen now that you've decided to let your light shine all the time?" Nimbus asked as he drew near Vinnie.

"I automatically give those around me permission to do the same," Vinnie nodded as he passed by his friend with another load of sticks.

As if on cue, Faith turned to the boys and added, "There's nothing attractive about a flower that doesn't bloom. Making the decision will bring the right opportunities for Vinnie to grow."

"Gee, it's taking me much longer to achieve my ideal weight than I hoped. Do you think I've done something wrong?" asked Nimbus.

"The greater the challenge, the longer it may take for fulfillment. Progress may come in baby steps rather than giant ones. This allows the mind, body, and emotions to have time to adjust to the changes," Faith replied as she cut spent blooms from her roses and herbs.

"It reminds me of a shooting star," offered Vinnie. "The faster it goes up, the sooner it falls."

"Well, I won't have to worry about progressing too quickly," laughed

Nimbus. "If anything, I'm too slow. I came to ask Faith if she could give me some examples of how the essences could help us."

## Clinical Research on Flower Essences

"Why, certainly," she replied. "For the past twenty years, I have used the essences with thousands of clients, many of whom came as a last resort.

"One client, under my care for nearly two years, came to me complaining of poor circulation, confusion, low energy, and an inability to cope with her life. As a recently widowed businesswoman, she had a lot of stress in her daily life and she was over seventy years old. I recommended dietary and herbal supplements initially, and some improvement was noted. However, it was not until the wisteria essence, to open the heart, was added that she began to feel at peace with herself."

"How did she know the difference?" Nimbus asked.

"She told me, 'The stress hasn't left me, but it doesn't send me into orbit like it did. I am able to make good decisions quickly, and I am able to turn off the outside world from time to time so that I can explore the world within. I take wisteria before retiring each night. More often than not I awaken refreshed and rested.'"

"So, the essence reduced the stress in her life and allowed her to handle her affairs, but what about her energy?" Vinnie asked as he hurried by.

"Her energy levels increased in proportion to a decrease in the stress," answered Faith. "Often, we experience a sense of inner calm when stress is significantly decreased."

"Do the essences help the immune system?" asked Flora as she walked into the garden and joined the conversation.

"Well, yes, because stress affects the immune system. The essences have been used to enhance the immune response in many ways," Faith explained.

"Often physicians refer terminally ill cancer patients to me for flower essence therapy. For a patient in Massachusetts suffering from prostate cancer, I chose a combination of essences to isolate the tumor; lilac to reduce tumor growth; marigold for sexual energies being imbalanced, as well as for sexual guilt; gaillardia to stimulate macrophage production; and meadow sage to reduce the growth enzymes of the tumor. African violet was added to help the patient experience a greater sense of fulfillment in his life. This is the only treatment he has used for more than five years, and the tumor has been contained to date. In his late seventies, he now says that he is looking forward to the best years of his life."

"When we finish in the garden, I'll show you the results of some research on several flower essences that were used during terminal illness," smiled Faith, as she reached to cut spent blooms from climbing roses.

## Female Essences

Later that day, Sweet Tooth helped Faith with her chores by distilling essential oils in the lab. When Sweet Tooth was finished, she met with Faith and the fairies that were still working in the garden.

"I noticed you make phytoestrogens and tonics for female problems," Sweet Tooth asked, as she returned from helping in the lab. "You make several female herbal tonics in your lab. Do you make a female essence, too?"

"The female herbal tonics are blended and cooked for a variety of symptoms. However, I have created a blend of flower essences for women that helps reduce stress and mood swings.

"One client came to me with menopausal symptoms, chronic headaches, neck pain, and aching shoulders. She was determined not to get caught in the 'estrogen fix,' but preferred to aid her body's transition with natural herbs and supplements. A searcher, she asked me if there might be some way to get a message to her body to relieve these symptoms, since nothing she tried had worked. I suggested that she have her husband put the mushroom essence on her back, and the pain eased. She became aware of her back, how she was sitting, when her shoulders were up, and when she was holding her head too low, causing strain on her neck. She felt her posture had become lax since the onset of menopause in her late forties.

"'My awareness came directly from the mushroom essence,' she said.

"The essence helped give her body a tool to send a message of hope for releasing those harmful patterns of posture. The hormone deficiency was corrected with my women's herbal tonic and a combination of essences I use for female balance."

"Interesting," mused Sweet Tooth. "What are some of the essences in the blend?"

"I use Japanese magnolia blooms for the dependent part of us that whines," chuckled Faith. "And, of course, Sweet Annie to help us age gracefully. Crepe Myrtle is included to help women use their creativity constructively, as well as speak their mind. Cherokee rose is added to help regulate the complaints of the female cycle. It also enhances opening the crown chakra to stimulate creativity in daily activities."

"Wow!" Sweet Tooth exclaimed, as her eyes grew larger. "I can understand why it helps women of all ages."

"Have you helped many people who are overweight?" Nimbus asked.

"Yes, I remember one young lady who reached several of her goals over a period of time," Faith answered, as her eyes looked up to the sky.

"Julia is an interesting case history, in part because of the complexity of the issues that occurred. She was referred to me with attention deficit and dyslexia. At thirty-six, she could not spell correctly and had poor memory and low self-esteem. I recommended white petunia to overcome the dyslexia, iris for mental stress, Blue Danube aster to increase concentration, and salvia to enhance self-esteem.

"Within three weeks, Julia was spelling words correctly for the first time in her life and she reported that her reading speed and comprehension had increased. She then felt confident to work on her weight problem. Salvia was continued, and pink rose was added for 'fat complex.' We also used ranunculus for childhood abuse. She lost ten pounds in one month and began to have vivid memories of sexual abuse. I added vanilla for protection, and she lost twenty more pounds over the next six months."

## Weight Loss Combination

"Well, that's very encouraging," Nimbus nodded. "Will you choose some essences to help me lose more weight?"

"Of course," Faith answered. "I would choose vanilla and pink rose again. Then, I would add moss rose for the personality who compensates his sense of inadequacy with comfort food."

"I'll take an extra dose of moss rose," Nimbus answered, under his breath.

Faith threw her head back and laughed before continuing. "Then I'd add a few drops of knotted marjoram to reduce the compulsive desire to eat. Often, this type of eating behavior is due to nervous energy."

"I get nervous just being around food. Will the knotted marjoram stop me from wanting to eat when I see food?" asked Nimbus.

"It should, but we can add a few drops of verbena to keep you calm and in the present moment. Then you can make a decision based on today rather than the person who couldn't say no to food," replied Faith.

"Well, is there a way to make this combination really strong?" Nimbus asked nervously.

"Sure," Faith nodded. "We can add one or two drops of yarrow to strengthen the formula."

"Where should I wear a combination formula of essences?" Nimbus asked, peering over Sweet Tooth's shoulder, as he spoke to Faith.

"Good question," she answered. "I recommend two drops of a combination be worn on the heart center, but I leave it to the individual to find the best placement.

"The essences are catalysts that encourage us to make the most of every situation. They work at an individual's pace to make constructive lifestyle changes.

They do not evoke a negative symptom to bring about healing; instead, they help promote inner harmony and peace.

"From the indigenous people of the world, I have learned how simple healing can be. As we return to the source, we will again express a passion for life in everything we experience. The flower essences have taught me that what is divine cannot be separated from its source, and that all true healing comes from the heart."

The fairies stood very quietly next to Faith, as she finished gathering flowers and dropping them into her apron. Then, Nimbus spoke. "Faith, you said earlier you would show us the results of some research on the flower essences."

"Oh, yes! Just follow me into the house and I'll show you another way flower essences are able to catalyze health," Faith answered as she walked toward the door.

The fairies followed her in single file. Flora nudged Vinnie and asked him to find Spider so they would be sure to have the information available when they returned to the Land of Thyme.

Vinnie flew off in a hurry to find the curious reporter. As he flapped, Vinnie thought to himself. "Gee, it seems odd to even think about leaving the Garden of Beauty. It seems as if I've been here my whole life. Or maybe it's because my new life seems to have begun here."

He found Spider patiently weaving a web around each disc he ejected from his computer.

"What are you doing?" asked Vinnie.

"I'm securing the information I've reported on discs. The web will keep any virus from entering the system when we return to the Land of Thyme," Spider replied dryly.

"Gee, everyone's talking about leaving, but we're not through here yet," replied Vinnie. "Flora needs you to return right away to record more research on the essences."

"All right, just let me finish this square knot and I'll join you," Spider sighed. "I'll need a ride from a winged god like you, though. This weaving takes a lot out of me."

As the two returned, Faith's lecture was just starting.

## Flower Essences, Herbs, and Essential Oils to Strengthen the Immune Response

"Some of the most powerful transformations have originated from people with terminal illness. The main essence I use is lilac. It was the first essence I used when I was told I had uterine cancer in the early 1980s. There is uterine cancer in my mother's family, and a history of women who sacrificed their creativity to raise a family. There was always a feeling of emptiness or lack of fulfillment in their personal lives. In search of healing, I learned lilac would release self-forgiveness and reduce the energy in the tumor. I promised to help others as I was shown the way of healing with flowers. Since then, I've taught at many hospitals, hospices, and cancer support groups and counseled individuals with a wide variety of illnesses for more than eighteen years.

"Let's begin with a look at how illness occurs on a subtle level. Dis-ease originates from suppression of emotions and desires. Thoughts, feelings, and will are suppressed to conform with society's rules. No alternate expressions of the desire are substituted. We are taught to obey society's rules and may be punished for honoring the self. As the emotional nature attempts to express spontaneously, the intellect puts the brakes on with a judgment call. Very often, this happens with a sexual taboo. For example, men do not often hug and kiss one another and women suppress angry feelings because these do not fit the image of a good woman. However, suppressing these feelings does not dissipate the energy. It concentrates in a chakra and expresses through an immune response, often an area of inherited or weakened immunity. As the energy concentrates, abnormal tissue growth may occur with the ability to build a blood supply to support tumor growth.

"If the immune system is well tuned, it will surround the area in an inflammatory response, releasing the tissue and the energy fueling it. The thymus gland, located above the heart, produces thymic lymphoid cells. These white blood cells travel to the site of inflammation. As the thymic *helper* and *suppressor cells* replace the thymic *killer cells,* the electromagnetic charge is reversed. New tissue growth will repair cellular damage, unless the immune response is weakened by repeated inflammation or fooled by a virus carrying the same protein sheath as the body.

"A weakened immune system will continue to protect the body by surrounding and sealing off what is now becoming a tumor. Without the inflammatory response, the growth and repair responses cease. However, the magnetic charge for new tissue growth will be used by cancer cells and converted into an unlimited growth substance. Since there is no signal to stop the energy flow, the cellular growth is uninhibited. It can metastasize into any tissue throughout the body which has a similar signal or origin. The emotions have found an expression. The path it takes from this point unravels the healing process of each individual. As simple as it may seem, it may be a long road to truly 'know thyself.' Any one of the essences may help. The following are the essences most associated with the healing of the personality and immune response. Use them singly, or up to five in combination on the subtle body centers."

| | |
|---|---|
| **Blue Danube Aster:** | Enhances antibody production targeted for diseased cells. These killer cells clean the internal environment. |
| **Bouquet of Harmony:** | Protects the skin, as an immune organ, from environmental pollutants, viral invasion and negative attitudes that can lead to disease. |
| **Christmas Cactus:** | Reinforces strengths and focuses on what is right. This helps to compensate for inherent weak organs that may be adversely affected by stress and disease. |
| **Dill:** | Enhances protective immunoglobulins that protect mucosa from bacterial invasion. This is the essence that helps us overcome abandonment and fear of death. |
| **French Lavender:** | Enhances immunity as a natural anti-viral; used in ancient times to combat intestinal cancers and growths. |
| **Gaillardia:** | Enhances macrophage bombardment of foreign matter and determination to become healthy. |
| **Iberis Candytuff:** | Enhances self-healing and regeneration. |
| **Indian Paintbrush:** | Promotes a success consciousness, affecting our health, prosperity, and well being. |
| **Lilac:** | Releases suppressed energy, letting go of past hurts. This is the essence I use for tumors and growths. |
| **Old Blush:** | Encourages stamina to keep going when the going is tough. |
| **Rose Campion:** | Aids those with inherited or predisposition for an illness. |
| **Wandering Jew:** | Overcomes discouragement. |

As Faith finished speaking, Flora immediately questioned, "Is there any place on the body we can put an essence, or combination of essences, and they will affect all the power centers of the body simultaneously?"

Faith thought a minute before replying. "Actually, there is. The ancients noted a place inside the ear, called *shen wen*. It is located in the right ear, just above the opening into the ear. This is where five cranial nerves converge into a ganglia. The ancients believed this is a communication center with the soul."

The fairies immediately began digging in their right ears to locate the spot.

"Ouch! I found it!" they called out one by one.

Suddenly, Snake appeared from deep within Vinnie's overall pocket.

"Hey! Will it do any good to just be around flowers, because I don't have an ear? I smell and hear with my tongue." Snake proceeded to demonstrate by wiggling his tongue. Flora and Faith moved away from him, cringing at the sight of Snake's tongue.

Vinnie took the initiative and petted Snake. "You can enjoy flowers anyway and still benefit from them," he advised Snake. "Mother Nature made flowers attractive and aromatic so creatures of all kinds will benefit from them."

"Thank you, Vinnie," Faith replied, quite surprised at his patronly manner. "I have some specific essences to help organ function and benefit those suffering from chronic and terminal illnesses. Let's start with the brain and neurological pathways."

The fairies stirred and settled in their cushions as Spider poised all eight legs for typing.

"The following studies were done mainly with people suffering from cancer and chronic debilitating illness. However, we can benefit from the selection of essences for any organ function, as well as self-actualization. I will now note the essence, essential oil, and tonic that helps to heal each part of the body, both physically and emotionally."

## Brain and Neurological Pathways

"Azalea enhances the creative imagination and latent talents to discover simple ways to solve complex situations. It is helpful for problems such as writer's block.

"*Echinacea pupura* purifies mental thoughts, encouraging a refined sense of judgment and understanding. It is indicated for slow thinking, poor memory, and neuropathies, when nerve cells die and cause numbness or tingling.

"Iris helps to reduce mental strain and stress associated with increased blood pressure, body temperature, and breathing. Its cooling nature reduces what I call 'heat' in the nervous system. It is indicated for predominately left-brainers, long hours on the computer, sudden angry outbursts, hyperkinetic behavior, and seizures.

"Rosemary helps release painful memories to remember better times instead. It is indicated for depressed thoughts and during difficult times of transition.

"Stock reduces nervous tension and anxiety and is indicated for the inability to sit still and relax. This is an excellent essence for those who lacked cuddling and nurturing during childhood.

"Lady Eubanksia balances energy affecting motor weakness, sensory loss, and demyelination of peripheral nerves. It is indicated for those who have learned through various experiences and are now able to teach others from the wisdom acquired."

When Faith finished the list, Flora asked, "Are there nutrients that work synergistically with these essences?"

"Yes," answered Faith. "I can think of a few, such as phosphatydl choline, phosphatydl serine, L glutamine, ginko biloba, inositol, and manganese as a gluconate. Safe dosages are suggested on the bottle."

"Can I use these essences and supplements if I just want to be smarter?" Vinnie inquired.

"Yes, I would recommend them for mental clarity," Faith answered smiling. "They also help hyper fairies," she added. Hearing this, Snake crawled out of Vinnie's pocket and nudged him. "Hey! Pay attention!"

"How about an herbal tonic?" interrupted Sweet Tooth.

"Oh, yes!" Faith answered. "We could brew a very relaxing tonic with schizandrae berries and lotus seeds."

## MIND TONIC

Faith turned to Vinnie and said, "In a short time, this tonic will sharpen the memory and promote mental clarity."

**Ingredients:**
   1 tablespoon schizandrae berries (*Schizandra chinensis*)
   1 cup cold water
   2 cups boiled water
   1 tablespoon lotus seeds (*Nelumbo nucifera*)

Soak the schizandrae berries overnight in cold water. Strain and discard water. Boil two cups of water, then add the lotus seeds and schizandrae berries. Reduce heat and simmer for twenty minutes. Strain, serve, and relax. Serves one.

"Are there any essential oil blends you've used successfully with these essences and tonics?" Sweet Tooth asked.

"Two drops of basil to one drop sandalwood in two tablespoons of carrier oil seem to work the best in my experience," Faith answered.

"I know you've worked for years with cancer patients in an integrated approach to medicine. Are there any blends you use successfully?" inquired Flora.

"I have one that I use in a major research hospital's healing-environment program. The hospital provides support to its patients though an integrated medical approach. With chemotherapy and bone marrow and stem cell transplants, patients are introduced to a variety of external therapeutic modalities. I provide a blend of the flower essences with lavender, sage, and synergistic essential oils to reduce anxiety, pain, and insomnia. Over time, it speeds recovery using less medication and heightens innate healing powers. The blend lifts quickly, which does not interfere with skin detoxification, so necessary for chemotherapy recipients."

"Gee, do you have to be in a hospital to use that blend?" asked Nimbus.

"Actually, family members of the recipients are using the blend to reduce their anxiety successfully," Faith answered. "If you're ready, we'll go to the next category."

## Bone, Joint, and Bone Marrow Pathways

"African violet touches the spirit to release self-nurturing and love that comes from deep within the soul. It is indicated when the deepest desires must manifest for us.

"Borage encourages self-sufficiency and is indicated for structural difficulties.

"Crossandra helps when fear and insecurity undermine major life changes. Fear can make us unable to move forward in the flow of life. It is indicated when environmental pollution and heavy metal toxicity, such as mercury from some car-repair preparations, are involved with bone and joint deterioration. If you are in a new situation and don't feel in control of your actions and reactions, crossandra is indicated.

"Black mushroom helps the energy affecting the spine and neck, reducing stress reactions during life changes such as marriage, divorce, illness, and death of loved ones.

"Viridiflora helps those who are very sensitive to the environment by aligning and maintaining the power centers. The essence helps ground sensory input by mediating impulses between sensory and motor neurons. It is indicated when we feel uncentered or dizzy or suffer from scoliosis and chronic problems with the feet, ankles, and hips.

"White rose works with the spinal cord's magnetic energy to open the channels and enhance the flow of impulses throughout the body. These positive-charged ions reduce stagnation which may cause aches and pain.

"Helpful essential oils include equal amounts of peppermint and lavender in two tablespoons of carrier oil or emu oil, available at health stores and grocers. Associated nutrients include potassium, magnesium and calcium citrate, pyridoxal phosphate ($B_6$), yucca root, folic acid, glucosamine sulfate, chondroitin, and emu oil used topically."

## BONE AND JOINT NOURISHING TONIC

This longevity tonic builds strong bones and joints.

**Ingredients:**
   1 teaspoon foti (*Polygonum multiflorum*)
   2 tablespoons *Rehmannia glutinosa,* prepared
   2 4-inch slices *Astragalus membranaceus*
   2 Zizyphus jujube red dates
   ¼ inch pinch cinnamon
   3 cups water


In three cups of water, simmer the above ingredients covered for thirty minutes. Strain and sip one cup daily. Serves three.

## Breast, Chest, and Throat

Faith continued with her lecture. "Chamomile releases past hurts and disappointments, the little things that build inside. It is indicated for lumps, cysts, and feeling mistreated or misunderstood.

"Crepe Myrtle releases the fear of expressing oneself. Inhibition reduces energy to the throat chakra, also closing the visual and the heart centers. The personality has a fear of expressing anger or being made to look like a fool and often withdraws to be alone. It is indicated for chest pain, tightness in the chest, inflammation and hypo-function of the thyroid and vocal cords, as an adjunct to therapy.

"Daffodil helps overcome shyness. It is indicated for palpitations and arrhythmias affecting the heart.

"India hawthorn opens the heart center to an impersonal love affecting group cooperation. It is indicated for restless sleep patterns.

"Lemon grass helps overcome the feeling of being rejected by parents and loved ones. It encourages self-nurturing and trust. It is indicated for those who feel slighted by their loved ones.

"Pansy helps transcend the loss of a loved one. It is indicated for grief, low adrenal function, chronic fatigue, and elimination of waste through the kidneys.

"Wisteria opens the heart chakra. It helps those who close down emotionally or feel separated from Nature and the environment. It is indicated for symptoms of coldness and poor circulation in the hands and feet.

"Zinnia benefits the inner child and those who were unable to enjoy childhood. It is indicated for critical behavior and arthritic or rheumatic discomfort with poor circulation.

"Helpful essential oils include three drops of eucalyptus to one drop of thyme or two drops of rose alone. Each blend combines in one tablespoon of carrier oil. The associated nutrients are selenium and vitamins E and C."

## HEART TONIC

This combination enhances circulation and relaxes and tones the heart muscle. It is safe and effective to use.

**Ingredients:**
    2 cups water
    1 tablespoon hawthorn berries
    1 tablespoon fresh or dried gotu kola leaves
    1 tablespoon rose hips
    1 teaspoon red raspberry leaves

In two cups of water, simmer the hawthorn berries and rose hips for thirty minutes. Remove from heat, strain and steep one tablespoon of fresh or dried gotu kola leaves, and one teaspoon red raspberry leaves, covered, for ten minutes. Strain and sip one cup daily. Serves two.

## FOR CONGESTED OR SWOLLEN BREASTS

This tonic will keep you from feeling top heavy.

**Ingredients:**
    1 cup boiled water
    1 tablespoon dandelion leaves, fresh or dried
    1 teaspoon of crushed fennel seed or 1 teaspoon peppermint leaves

Steep in one cup of boiled water for ten minutes. Strain and drink. Serves one.

## Colon and Low Back

Then Faith turned her attention to the lower body.

"Bougainvillea releases memories and feelings of guilt and shame. It is indicated for chronic pain.

"Garden mum releases critical thoughts. It is indicated for those who are slow to anger and hold onto grudges.

"Dandelion helps those who have restless sleep with fearful dreams. It is indicated for those who seek guidance during dreamtime.

"Mushroom offers help for those who miss opportunities or resist making major lifestyle changes. It is indicated for those who have feet, ankle, neck, and lower back symptoms of pain.

"Periwinkle clears memories affecting an organ function. It is indicated for those who want to clarify objectives and goals.

"Helpful essential oils include three drops of sage to one drop of pennyroyal in one tablespoon of carrier oil or emu oil for the low back. Associated nutrients are flaxseed oil capsules, devil's claw, dandelion root for constipation, yellow-dock root, Saint John's wort for low backaches, magnesium, pyridoxal$_5$ phosphate, B$_6$, and potassium."

## TONIC FOR LOW BACK FLEXIBILITY

This tonic will reduce pain and inflammation.

**Ingredients:**
    1 tablespoon cramp bark or black haw bark (*Viburnum prunifolium*)
    2 cups water
    1 teaspoon dandelion root (optional)

Simmer in two cups of water for thirty minutes. Strain and sip one tablespoon daily. Serves four.

## Immune Enhancers to Increase Vitality

"Essences and tonics can also be used to increase energy," Faith continued.

"Anemone releases the pattern of struggling through life. It is indicated for those who scar and form keloids easily.

"Dianthus releases apathy, and 'I don't care' attitudes. It is indicated for chronic fatigue and history of anemia.

"Jasmine balances a rebellious nature. It is indicated for those who are accident-prone.

"Red malva focuses on spiritual development. It is indicated when guidance is necessary.

"Wandering jew helps discouragement and low frustration levels. It is indicated when patience and tolerance are lacking.

"Yarrow is an essence that strengthens all essences. It is indicated when inflammation occurs or for autoimmune reactions.

"Snapdragon enhances discernment. It is indicated for balancing thymic helper and suppresser cells for allergy and immune deficiency problems.

"Essential oils include two drops each of sandalwood and rose in two tablespoons of carrier oil. Associated nutrients are bilberry, goldenseal, selenium, beta carotene, vitamin C, glutathione, zinc, and pyridoxal$_5$ phosphate, a coenzyme of B$_6$."

## VITALITY TONIC

This is a great tonic to boost energy and build better immunity.

**Ingredients:**
  4-inch slices of *Astragalus membranaceus*
  2 cups of water
  ½ ounce of *Rhemannia glutinosa* (use the prepared, black variety in the
      winter; the raw in summer)
  4 jujube red dates

Simmer in two cups of water for thirty minutes. Strain and add one teaspoon of blackstrap molasses. Drink one cup daily. Serves two.

## Kidney, Bladder, and Prostate

Faith paused briefly, then described tonics and essences for detoxification.

"Bachelor button releases past emotional trauma. It is indicated when localized edema is present and past experiences influence today's decisions.

"Lilac enables us to forgive others and ourselves. It helps us let go of unproductive situations, and is indicated for growths swelling.

"Marigold releases sexual guilt, identity problems and aids in balancing creative and receptive energy in the reproductive organs. It is indicated when creativity is blocked, such as frigidity, impotence, or prostatitis.

"Meadow sage helps us express strong emotions without feeling guilty or transgressing onto others. It can be beneficial for angry outbursts or the inability to express intense emotions. It is also indicated to enhance health of the mucosa of the eyes, intestines, reproductive organs, and lungs.

"Pansy helps transcend the grief over the loss of a loved one. It is indicated for low energy, situational depression, and elimination of toxins.

"Red carnation enhances a feeling of self-worth. It is indicated when hair loss occurs and to enhance lymphatic drainage.

"Shrimp helps overcome self-dissatisfaction and criticalness. It is indicated for the feeling of being overwhelmed and encourages self-healing.

"A helpful essential oil blend is three drops of lemon grass or orange blossom to two drops of spearmint in two tablespoons of carrier oil. Associated nutrients are zinc picolinate, vitamin C, grape seed extract, chlorophyll, polygonum multiflorum (foti), poria cocos, magnesium, $B_6$."

## KIDNEY TONIC

This tea is mildly diuretic and very soothing.

**Ingredients:**
>  2 cups water
>  1 tablespoon saw palmetto berries (*Serona*)
>  1 tablespoon marshmallow root (*Althea officinalis*)
>  1 tablespoon corn silk (*Zea mays*)
>  1 tablespoon fresh or dried dandelion leaves

In two cups of water, simmer saw palmetto berries and marshmallow root for twenty minutes. Strain and then add corn silk and dandelion leaves. Steep for ten minutes. Strain and sip one cup daily. Serves two.

## Liver and Gallbladder

"And, now, help for liver and gallbladder function," Faith said.

"Chamomile helps those who swallow little hurts and suppress their feelings. It is indicated for indigestion and symptoms related to gallbladder dysfunction.

"Garden mum releases critical thoughts. It is indicated for poor fat digestion.

"Pink geranium releases pent-up tension, anger, and frustration. It is indicated for muscle spasms and irritable bowel function.

"Silver moon subdues restless, obsessive thoughts and fearful dreams. It is indicated for those with exaggerated sense of importance who require extra attention.

"White petunia aids indecisive people. It is indicated for those who are uncoordinated and those who have difficulty acting on decisions.

"A good essential oil blend is two drops of marigold mint or fennel, three drops of lemon balm and one drop of rosemary in three tablespoons of carrier oil. Associated nutrients are pyridoxal$_5$ phosphate, coenzyme of $B_6$, magnesium, dandelion leaves, and sylmarin from milk thistle."

# LIVER TONIC

This is a mild tea to enhance detoxification.

**Ingredients:**
  1 cup boiled water
  1 tablespoon lemon grass
  1 teaspoon chamomile flowers
  2 teaspoons gotu kola leaves

In one cup of boiled water, steep ingredients, covered, for ten minutes. Strain and sip with meals. Serves one.


## Lymphatic Purification

"The lymphatics help remove acids and impurities from the blood," explained Faith.

"Cinnamon basil aids those who buckle under adversity. It is indicated for those who suffer from headaches and weak knees and ankles.

"Curry helps us think on our feet. It is indicated for lack of spontaneity, and for those who suffer migraines.

"Lobelia helps us define boundaries. It is indicated for those who need to say 'no!'

"Salad burnet releases disappointment from unfulfilled desires. It is also indicated when low blood volume occurs.

"Soapwort enhances lymphatic drainage. It is indicated for fatty tissue buildup or cellulite areas.

"Tansy is protective. It combats the effects of environmental pollution.

"Essential oils that can be used are two drops of cinnamon, two drops of curry, and one drop of basil in three tablespoons of carrier oil. Associated nutrients are pantothenic acid, $B_5$, vitamin C, pyridoxal$_5$ phosphate, coenzyme of $B_6$, niacinamide, $B_3$, echinacea root tincture, and red clover blossoms."

## LEMON THYME TEA

Enjoy this tea and benefit your lymphatic response.

**Ingredients:**
   1 cup boiled water
   2 teaspoons lemon thyme leaves, fresh or dried
   1 teaspoon lemon verbena leaves, fresh
   1 teaspoon spearmint leaves, fresh or dried

Steep herbs, covered, in one cup of boiled water for ten minutes. Serves one.


# Lung and Bronchial

"The lungs are very important. They purify the air we breathe from pollution and allergens," Faith said.

"Babies' breath resists implementing new ideas to maintain the status quo. It is indicated for people prone to lung and breathing difficulties, such as asthma, pleurisy, and bronchitis.

"Lantana helps oversensitive people who get their feelings hurt easily. It is indicated for those prone to allergies and seasonal sinusitis.

"Morning glory helps those who are uncomfortable in their present conditions and live in an illusion of happy memories in the past. It is indicated for those who sigh and feel heaviness in their chest with mucous congestion.

"Poppy helps us when we become demanding, selfish or possessive. It is indicated when tuberculosis is in the family history, and for those who suffer from breathlessness or dry cough and obstructed breathing.

"Spike lavender helps us practice cooperation with others. It is indicated when lung congestion and bronchial spasms occur.

"Thyme encourages us onto greater achievements. It is indicated for those who suffer from viral and bacterial invasion.

"White hyacinth helps reduce the effects of traumatic experiences. It is indicated for those who experienced a traumatic birth or suffer from a post-traumatic experience.

"Wild oats enhances a sense of humor. It is especially beneficial for children who pout and adults who brood.

"A good essential oil blend is two drops each of eucalyptus, thyme, and lemon grass in three tablespoons of carrier oil. Associated nutrients are vitamin C and selenium."

# LUNG TONIC

This tonic aids lung conditions with congestion and productive cough.

**Ingredients:**
- 2 cups water
- 1 tablespoon wild cherry bark (*Prunus serotina*)
- 2 teaspoons osha root (*Lingusticum porteri*)
- 1 tablespoon pleurisy root (*Ascelptias tuberosa*)
- ⅛ teaspoon ginger root, dried, fresh, or ground
- 1 teaspoon sage leaves (fresh is best)
- 1 teaspoon marjoram, fresh or dried (optional)

In two cups of water, simmer for thirty minutes, covered, the wild cherry bark, osha root, and pleurisy root. Strain and steep for ten minutes, adding the ginger root, sage leaves or marjoram. Strain, sweeten, and sip one cup daily. Serves two.

# DRY COUGH TONIC

Use this tonic for persistent, dry hacking coughs.

**Ingredients:**
- 2 cups water
- 1 tablespoon marshmallow root (*Althea officinalis*)
- 1 tablespoon pseudo ginseng (*Codonopsitis radix*)
- 1 tablespoon dried mullein leaves (*Verbascum thaspus*)
- 1 tablespoon yucca root, dried or ground
- 1-inch slice of licorice root (*Glycyrrhiza uralensis*), optional, but not if hypertension exists

Simmer in two cups of water for thirty minutes. Strain and sip one cup daily when symptoms occur. Serves two.

## Ovarian and Testicular Function

"The reproductive organs can affect creativity on a subtle body level, integrating talents and building self-esteem," explained Faith.

"Bluebonnet awakens us to fulfill our destiny. It is indicated when life calls to move forward to discover greater powers emerging from within.

"Gardenia integrates the personal life with long-term goals. It is indicated when personal relationships pull you down rather than awakening deeper values. This essence is often worn to attract a lifetime partner.

"Japanese magnolia creates an environment of security rather than dependency. It is indicated when premenstrual symptoms occur and for those suffering with headaches and fluid retention and feeling separate or different from their peers.

"Marigold aids us in accepting ourselves as we are. It is indicated when dissatisfaction with sexuality or personal appearance occurs. Marigold is indicated when the family history includes sexual or venereal disease and is generally helpful for diseases affecting the ovaries and testicles. Examples may include: cysts, pelvic inflammation, and social diseases.

"Salvia enhances self-esteem. It is indicated for warts, skin diseases, and acne related to hormonal imbalance.

"Carrot enhances initiative and organizes priorities. It is indicated when fertility or creative expression is stifled.

"Helpful essential oils are two drops of sage to one drop of cedar or pine in two tablespoons of carrier oil, or two drops each of rose, lavender, or geranium in three tablespoons of carrier oil.

"Associated nutrients are zinc picolinate or glycinate, pyridoxal$_5$ phosphate, B$_6$, niacinimide, B$_3$, polygonum multiflorum or foti."

## REJUVENATING TONIC

This tonic reduces heat or toxicity for the reproductive organs. It is considered safe to use on a regular basis.

**Ingredients:**
  2 cups water
  1 tablespoon *rhemannia glutinosa*
  1 tablespoon dendrobium stems (dendrobium orchid)
  2 lotus seeds
  1 tablespoon skullcap

Simmer in two cups of water for thirty minutes, covered. Strain and sip one-half to one cup daily. Serves two.

**Note:** The above herbs are available at Oriental groceries or bulk herb shops.

## Blood Sugar Regulation

"Proper pancreatic function aids digestion and blood sugar regulation," Faith continued.

"Mexican bush sage enhances the ability to be unique. It is indicated when peer pressure overrides better judgment.

"Mexican hat enhances our ability to be prosperous. It is indicated when we are feeling or experiencing lack or less than our potential.

"Moss rose aids those who feel the need to acquire more. Enough is never enough. It is indicated for those who experience poor digestion of starches, or those who love sweets.

"Evening primrose aids those who look to others to fulfill the need for love. It is indicated for those with a romantic need for love that is very idealistic. The essence is also indicated for those who have blood sugar fluctuations.

"For a good essential oil blend, combine two drops of lemon grass, bergamot, or vanilla in one tablespoon of carrier oil. Associated nutrients are alanine amino acid, chromium picolinate, zinc glycinate, borage oil, flaxseed oil, vitamin E, methionine, cysteine."

### SUSTAINED ENERGY TONIC

This tonic will enhance energy as well as correct blood sugar fluctuations for many of us.

**Ingredients:**

2 cups water
1 tablespoon foti (*Polygonum multiflorum*)
1 tablespoon *rhemannia glutinosa,* prepared
¼-inch cinnamon stick or 1-inch slice of licorice root

Simmer in two cups of water, covered, for thirty minutes. Strain and sip one-half to one cup daily. Serves two.

**Note:** Licorice root is not recommended for hypertensives.

As Faith finished the lecture, Spider collapsed from typing fatigue and Flora's forehead wrinkled in a questioning expression.

"How did you learn about all the flowers you grow? We grow and talk to flowers everyday, but for different reasons!"

"Nature is so very diverse," replied Faith. "The information is available as we need it and ask for it. All the personalities and indications of the essences were answers to specific needs of others or myself. They have been proven and researched by many doctors and practitioners, mainly in North America and western Europe, for nearly twenty years. However, essences are meant to help us become self-actualized through spiritual growth, which is very individualized. You don't have to go to a doctor or practitioner to benefit from essences."

"Well, I don't know how to become more spiritual," Vinnie thought aloud. "I imagine spiritual people being very tall and thin like angels."

"Speak for yourself," Sweet Tooth commented, as Nimbus jiggled with laughter beside her.

"But you and Nimbus are both in better shape and getting thinner," Flora quickly answered, defending the couple.

"Well, not for long," answered Sweet Tooth, as she reached Nimbus's hand.

"You don't mean you're giving up!" cried Flora, very distraught.

"Not exactly," Nimbus began to answer.

"We're going to divide our weight between three of us," Sweet Tooth finished, smiling.

"Does that mean I get to live with you?" asked Vinnie innocently.

"No, it means they're going to have a baby," answered Snake as he popped out of Vinnie's pocket. "Do I have to explain everything?"

"What are you going to name the little bundle of joy?" asked Spider as he stretched his tired limbs.

Before the happy couple could answer, Vinnie interrupted. "I think you should call the baby Kindness, because it's a child of love!"

The group caught their breath, then exclaimed their approval. "Great name! How did you think of the name?"

Vinnie stood up very proudly and answered, "Talent does what it can, genius does what it must!"

The group immediately applauded Vinnie and congratulated the happy couple, in single file. Flora was so excited she kissed Sweet Tooth, Nimbus and even Vinnie.

"Tomorrow we'll go over several new applications of flower essences and the safe use of herbal tonics," Faith explained, as she gathered the fairies around her. "But, for today, let's do what fairies and aspiring gods and goddesses do best—celebrate!"

And with that suggestion, the group enjoyed the evening celebrating in the moonlit garden.

# CHAPTER 14

# Fairy Potions
## Combining Herbs, Essential Oils, and Flower Essences for Optimal Health

*"Everybody is waiting for the Soul to be released"*
Vincent Ermis, *Train to Heaven*

### Reducing Stress

As promised, Faith joined the fairies the very next day to discuss the application of the flower essences. They were eager to learn and were bursting with questions.

"How can I explain flower essences to fairies of all varieties and ages?" inquired Flora.

"Think of flower essences as a way to create a healthy internal environment in the mind and body," replied Faith. "They are complementary to any therapy, supplement or medicine as a transformational practice that reduces stress."

"How do essences transform us physically?" asked Vinnie.

"Chronic and acute stress directly affects the immune system, weakening resistance to disease and the ability to make sound decisions," explained Faith. "Flower essences carry an imprint or memory of the flower's properties, which will match a memory or attitude imprinted in the mind. For every ailment and imbalance there is a remedy already produced by nature. Flowers heal by color, fragrance, texture, and biochemical nature, helping to transform us into our greatest potential. We only utilize a very small percentage of our brain's potential. Flowers have been used by every culture to transform their awareness and spiritual growth. It is best described by the mandalbrodt system, the mathematical equation that underlies the inner design inherent in all nature. The study of flower essences is the science of oneness," Faith concluded.

"How did ancient cultures make flower essences?" Sweet Tooth asked.

"They steeped flowers in full bloom in boiled water and inhaled the steam. They either bathed in it or drank the water like a tea. Later cultures steeped flowers in a medium like lard or made a conserve by cooking flowers in sugar water. Each culture found ways to prepare and ingest or wear essences," Faith replied.

"Is that how you make essences?" Spider inquired as he typed.

"I distill and extract essences. I concentrate the lipoic acid that makes flowers bloom under stress. Each essence has a unique formula I have worked out over the years. I may use various parts of the flower or plant," Faith answered.

"Then what do you do with them?" asked Spider, taking charge of the conversation.

"Some are worn like perfumes because they are very fragrant. For example, I grow antique roses like fimbriata and autumn damask, which make the finest aromas. The antique roses excite our passion for life and aid us in developing truly intimate and trusting relationships. Other fragrances, like vanilla, appeal to children, as well as to adults. The essence is very protective, sealing the aura and protecting the skin from viral invasion.

"Other essences I call 'natives' because they adapt to our environment and are worn on the waist or power center because they initiate an immune response. For example, Mexican oregano is a spicy essence initiating bacterial inhibitors to activate immune competency. It enhances the personality's ability to respond properly to new situations. The natives are excellent to add to a bath; try fifteen drops in a bathtub of warm water. The essences combine well with essential oils in a bath or skin care products."

"How do you combine them in skin care products?" Sweet Tooth inquired with great interest.

"Like adding essential oils to a product," Faith explained. "First I make the product, then I add five drops of essences. I like using them in shampoos and skin care products because we use them daily and it works into my routine easily."

"Can we overindulge in an essence or take the wrong one?" Nimbus asked with a furrowed brow.

"No, because they don't work like a drug. If you think essences can hurt you, then your mind can bring it to pass. Left on their own, essences affect us like music, revitalizing our spirit and moving us towards a positive emotional expression," Faith answered pointedly. "Rather than overindulge, we usually underindulge in their usage."

"How's that?" Vinnie asked puzzled.

"They often work better when we use them four or five times in an hour, especially during a crisis. Choose an essence from a flower you're attracted to, like I am to roses, or use African violet to release an endorphin response and lilac to let go of stress."

"Is there an essence I can take for itchy skin?" Snake asked as he wiggled across the floor and scratched himself against Faith's shoe.

"Of course," she answered, stepping back politely. "Salvia essence works very well for many skin conditions like dryness or even acne."

"Why don't you take a bottle outside with you and lay on a rock and molt?" suggested Flora.

"Why don't you lay on a rock with me and watch me shed for you?" Snake answered seductively.

"Well," Flora stammered, "because I have to stay close to Sweet Tooth…because she's pregnant. And, besides, I'd rather listen to a frog's heart beat before I…"

Vinnie suddenly flew to the rescue. "Well, maybe we should all take a break and join Snake outside a few minutes until he falls asleep." With that he scooped Snake into his arms and hurried toward the garden.

## An Essence for Flora

"Gee, you really have bad luck with partners, Flora," Nimbus remarked as he patted her drooping shoulder. "You ought to be able to attract someone more, umm, outgoing than Snake!"

"I've never thought about a relationship," Flora answered. "I've been very busy with my first major career opportunity since I left my apprenticeship with the star gods."

"Have you ever been in love?" asked Nimbus softly as he gently patted Flora's hand.

"Well, no, but I love my work," Flora answered. "And I'm beginning to appreciate my brother Vinnie," she stammered, smiling weakly.

"From my experiences with Vinnie that's a great accomplishment," Nimbus sighed.

Nimbus and Flora exchanged glances and began to giggle, first slowly, then uncontrollably. Nimbus giggled until his whole body shook, while Flora laughed until she cried. One by one, the fairies took notice and gathered around them eager to participate in the laughter.

Unable to think of an excuse, Nimbus blurted out, "Flora's a workaholic and needs an essence so she can fall in love!"

The fairies stepped back in surprise as their eyes popped open and they held their breath. Everyone looked at Flora to see what she would do.

Flora choked out an answer. "That's right! The only offer I've had so far is to lay on a rock with a molting snake!"

With that comment, the group joined in the laughter until Faith stepped into the conversation with advice. She couldn't pass a chance to teach such avid listeners.

"Dancing lady orchid is a great remedy to slow down a workaholic. And, there are two antique roses to help you attract a good relationship: Cecil Brünner helps those who hold back from entering a new relationship, and for the individual who never seems to have time for one. Then, there's Marquis Bocella to help attract a kindred spirit in a love relationship and gardenia to aid in planning a future with a partner."

By the time Faith finished speaking, Sweet Tooth appeared with a spray bottle of these essences and proceeded to squirt them on Flora. The fairies joined hands and danced in a circle around Flora enjoying the fine mist of essences.

## Essences for Animals and Pets

Sweet Tooth continued to spray the essences until the bottle was empty. She turned to Faith and asked, "Have you ever diluted the essences into a spray bottle?"

"Why, yes, I have, but not for the same reasons," Faith chuckled. "I dilute five drops in an ounce of distilled water and spray them on animals."

"Really? What type of animals have you worked with?" asked Nimbus.

"Mostly dogs, cats, horses, and pigs," replied Faith. "Today was my first opportunity to apply an essence on a snake."

"Give us some examples of what you have done with animals," Spider ordered in his journalistic fashion as he poised all eight legs over his laptop.

"Okay," Faith began. "The most successful essence is amaryllis, which is used for heartworms in dogs. It's also been used for many other parasitic infections."

"Would it be good to give to my friend Collie?" asked Nimbus.

"Yes, if I understand your question correctly," Faith answered. "Amaryllis has been used to prevent heartworms."

Spider then turned toward Faith and nodded to her, encouraging her to continue.

"Well, then, I've used lavender and vanilla to calm horses and dogs who were restless or upset. I either sprayed it on them or put some essences on my hand and petted their flank when possible."

"Tell us more," Spider implored impatiently.

"There was a kitten with liver disease showing signs of liver failure," Faith replied immediately. "It took three months of dandelion before the kitten's blood work showed complete correction. The drops were put in the kitten's water and applied to its abdomen.

"Then there was a piglet who wouldn't suckle. I suggested babies' breath until the piglet began to nurse. The owner applied the essence to its lips."

## Combining Essences and Herbal Tonics

"Do you ever combine or use essences with your herbal tonics?" asked Spider, jumping back to his laptop.

"All the time," answered Faith. "I especially use them with female tonics because I see a large percentage of women in my practice."

"That sounds like information we can all benefit from learning," remarked Sweet Tooth, encouraging Faith to continue. Faith hesitated briefly; shuffling through her papers, mumbling to herself about being more organized. Finally, she found what she was looking for and continued.

"Here are a few tonics and associated essences that have helped many women in times of need."

## FEMALE TONICS

The following tonics relieve symptoms. They can be safely used over a period of time and are enhanced by essences.

### BACK PAIN OR CRAMPS

For menstrual backaches with a feeling of heaviness, take this tonic only as needed to abate symptoms.

**Ingredients:**
  2 cups water
  2 tablespoons black cohosh root (*Cimicifuga racemosa*)
  2 teaspoons raspberry leaves
  2 teaspoons cramp bark (*Viburnum opulis*) or black haw (*Viburnum prunifolium*), which is more potent as an analgesic

In two cups of water, simmer the ingredients for thirty minutes, covered. Strain. Sip one-half to one cup as needed for back pain. Serves two.

**Associated essences:** Two drops each of mushroom, viridiflora, borage, and bougainvillea on the lower abdomen or back.

**Associated essential oil blend:** In one ounce of warm St. John's wort oil or emu oil, blend five drops of sandalwood, three drops of lavender, and two drops of sage. Allow to cure for three hours and then apply to the back.

## Irregular or Heavy Bleeding

Use these tonics to allay bleeding. Consult a healthcare professional to correct the source of imbalance.

**Ingredients:**
- 2 cups water
- 2 tablespoons shepherd's purse (*Capsella bursa-pastoris*)
- 1 tablespoon blessed thistle leaves (*Carbenia benedicta*) or milk thistle seeds (*Silybum marianum*)

In two cups of water, simmer herbs, covered, for thirty minutes. Serves one. For a variation try one teaspoon burnet root (*Sanguisorba officinalis*).

Strain; sip one to two cups daily to reduce or stop bleeding.
**Note:** This tonic works even better as a tincture.

**Ingredients:**
- 2 cups brandy, vodka, or gin

Steep the above herbs in two cups of brandy, vodka, or gin for two weeks in a covered glass jar. Dilute fifteen drops in four ounces of hot water every two hours until bleeding abates.
**Associated essences:** Wear two drops of each below the navel: salad burnet, dandelion, Cherokee rose, yarrow.

Flora described an aromatherapy blend to abate heavy bleeding.

**Associated essential oil blend:** In one ounce vegetable oil add two drops of yarrow, two drops of bergamot, and one drop of sandalwood. Blend and apply topically to pelvis.

## SWOLLEN BREASTS

"Swollen breasts can occur before menses begins. Here's how to alleviate discomfort," explained Flora. "Herbalists alleviate liver congestion to reduce the discomfort of swollen breasts."

**Ingredients:**
1 cup of water
1 teaspoon crushed fennel seeds
1 tablespoon dandelion leaves

Simmer one cup of water and add the crushed fennel seeds for five minutes. Remove from heat. Add one tablespoon of dandelion leaves and steep, covered for ten minutes longer. Strain. Drink one cup daily to reduce swelling. Serves one.

**Associated essences:** Wear two drops each of bachelor button, begonia, jasmine, and pansy on the heart center.

**Associated essential oil blend:** In one ounce of jojoba or sweet almond oil, add two drops rose and two drops jasmine. Optional: one drop of amber.

## CONSTIPATION

"It's important to keep channels of elimination working properly," continued Faith. "If constipation occurs, use this simple formula. This tonic is not habit-forming or harsh."

**Ingredients:**
1 cup water
1 tablespoon whole flax seeds
1 teaspoon dandelion root

Simmer the water and add flax seeds and dandelion root. Cook over low heat for five minutes, stirring the seeds with a fork. Strain. Drink one cup daily until regularity occurs. Serves one.

**Associated essences:** Wear two drops each of crossandra, bamboo, morning glory, or basil on the abdomen.

**Associated essential oil blend:** In one ounce of warm vegetable oil, add two drops of cinnamon or ginger. Blend and apply to the abdomen. Not recommended during pregnancy.

# CYSTITIS

Bladder irritation can be effectively relieved for most women with a simple tonic.

Put one teaspoon of uva ursi leaves (*Arctostaphylos uva urse*) in a cup of distilled water overnight. Keep refrigerated. Strain. Drink one cup upon rising. Consider using a diuretic tea. Serves one.

**Associated essences:** Wear two drops each of begonia, dandelion, or pink geranium on the lower abdomen.

**Associated essential oil blend:** In one ounce of warm vegetable oil, add five drops of pine, two drops of sage or clary sage, and one drop of pennyroyal. Apply warm to the abdomen.

# DIURETIC

For bloating and fluid retention, drink this tea to cleanse the system.

**Ingredients:**
   2 cups boiled water
   1 tablespoon dandelion leaves
   2 teaspoons of parsley leaves

In two cups of boiled water, steep, covered, for ten minutes.

**Associated essences:** Wear two drops each of pansy, bachelor button, rosemary, foxglove, and echinacea on the abdomen.

**Associated essential oil blend:** In an ounce of warm vegetable oil, add three drops of thyme or tea tree oil and two drops of lemon grass. Apply to the abdomen.

# EMMENOGOGUE

When menstruation is delayed or absent, use this tea for relief. It will also energize the blood to remove stagnation causing blood clots, throbbing, and migratory pain. Emmenogogues are not to be used during pregnancy or heavy bleeding.

**Ingredients:**
   2 cups water
   1 tablespoon safflowers (*Carthamus tinctorius*)
   2 teaspoons chamomile flowers
   1 tablespoon fresh tea rose buds, when available
   pinch of ginger (optional)

In two cups of boiled water, steep flowers for ten minutes, covered. Strain. Sip two cups daily until menses begins.

**Associated essences:** Wear two drops each of Japanese magnolia, Cherokee rose, fimbriata and dianthus below the navel.

**Associated essential oil blend:** In an ounce of warm oil, blend two drops of rose, three drops of geranium and one drop of lavender. Apply to the abdomen.

**Note:** See also female tonic for menopause (recipe on page 227). Drink one-quarter to one-half cup for two to three weeks to revitalize the reproductive system.

FERTILITY

Nature reproduces from a healthy body. These herbs build vitality and blood and nurture the reproductive organs.

**Ingredients:**
    2 cups water
    2 tablespoons *Angelica sinensis*
    1 tablespoon lovage root (*Ligusticum wallichi*)

Add above herbs to water and simmer for thirty minutes, covered. Serves two.

**Optional herbs:**
    1 teaspoon *rhemannia glutinosa,* prepared
    1 teaspoon peony root (*Paonia alba*) or false unicorn root
    (*Chamaelirium luteum*)
    Pinch of cinnamon or ginger

Strain, and sip one-half cup daily to complete two cups per week.

**Associated essences:** Wear two drops each of carrot, iris, azalea, or Madame Alfred Carriere on the lower abdomen.

**Associated essential oil blend:** In one ounce of warm vegetable oil, add three drops of rose and one drop lavender. Apply warm at night to the mid-abdomen.

# FETAL SECURITY

Herbalists assist in preventing miscarriage with a prepared tincture.

**Ingredients:**
  2 cups of brandy, vodka, or gin
  2 tablespoons skullcap (*Scutellaria laterifolia*)
  2 tablespoons false unicorn root (*Chamaelirium luteum*)
  2 tablespoons lotus seed (*Nelumbo nucifera*)

Soak ingredients in a glass jar for two weeks. Strain. Dilute fifteen drops in four ounces of hot water one to three times daily. Serves four.

**Associated essences:** Wear two drops each of knotted marjoram, tansy, vanilla, yarrow, and snapdragon on the heart center.

**Associated essential oil blend**: In one ounce of warm jojoba oil, blend five drops of lavender and two drops of vanilla.

# HEAT FLASHES

To reduce symptoms, use the following formula. Follow up with the menopause formula daily.

**Ingredients:**
  1 cup water
  1 teaspoon skullcap
  ½ teaspoon sage leaves
  ½ teaspoon hops

Add ingredients to boiled water and steep, covered, for ten minutes. Strain, and drink as the tea cools. Serves one.

**Associated essences:** Wear two drops each of sage, French lavender, Sweet Annie, or wild wood violet on the temples and neck.

**Associated essential oil blend:** In one ounce of jojoba oil, add four drops of geranium, two drops of rose, and two drops of sage. Apply to the neck and temples.

# HEADACHE

Hormone changes can cause tension and headaches. Use this tonic for female balance.

**Ingredients:**
   2 cups water
   2 tablespoons black cohosh root
   1 tablespoon vitex berries (*Vitex agnus castus*)

Bring two cups of water to a boil, reduce heat; simmer ingredients for twenty minutes, covered. Serves two.

**Optional:** Remove from heat and add two teaspoons of feverfew (*Chrysanthemum parthenium*). Steep for ten minutes, covered. Strain. Sip one-half to one cup daily to abate symptoms.

**Associated essences:** Wear two drops each of chamomile, pink geranium, garden mum, French lavender, or cinnamon basil on the temples or the back of the neck.

**Associated essential oil:** Wear lavender on the temples.

# INSOMNIA

Here's a great remedy for sleepless nights and anxiety.

**Ingredients:**
   1 cup brandy
   3 tablespoons black cohosh root

Tincture three tablespoons of black cohosh root in one cup of brandy for three weeks. Dilute fifteen to thirty drops in hot water thirty minutes before bedtime. For daytime anxiety, take eight to fifteen drops. Best not to drive. Serves eight.

**Associated essences:** Wear two drops each of catnip, chamomile, verbena, silver moon, or silver lace on the heart center.

**Associated essential oil blend:** Rub a drop of lavender inside the ear or put it on a cotton ball and place inside the ear.

## LACTATION

To increase milk flow, drink one-half to one cup daily of this tonic.

**Ingredients:**
   1 cup water
   1 tablespoon crushed fennel seeds
   1 teaspoon chamomile

Simmer crushed fennel seeds in one cup of water for ten minutes. Remove from heat. Steep one teaspoon of chamomile flowers for five minutes, covered. Strain and enjoy. Serves one.

   **Associated essences:** Wear two drops each of babies' breath, vanilla, or Mexican hat on the heart center.

   **Associated essential oil blend:** In one ounce of warm vegetable oil, add three drops of marigold mint, one drop of spearmint or peppermint. Apply to the temples or base of the neck.

   **Variation:** If hypertension exists, substitute dill for fennel. Simmer one tablespoon of asparagus root with dill seeds to increase body fluids.


## MENOPAUSE

Menopause is a time to express your creativity and talents in the community and environment. This tonic will bring renewed energy and a sense of well being and purpose to your life.

**Ingredients:**
   2 cups water
   2 tablespoons or 1 ounce of tang quei (*Angelica sinensis*)
   2 teaspoons of *rehmannia glutinosa,* prepared
   1 tablespoon of lovage (*Ligusticum wallichi*)
   1 tablespoon peony root (*Paeonia alba*)
   4 jujube red dates (*Zizyphus jujube*)
   1-inch slice of licorice root or substitute ginger, if hypertension exists

Simmer two cups of water and herbs, covered, for one hour. Strain and drink a half-cup daily. Refrigerate or freeze leftovers. Serves two.

   **Note:** These herbs are available through bulk mail order or Oriental grocers. *Angelica archangela* may be substituted for tang quei, but it is not as energizing.

   Tang Kuei contains phytoestrogens. Consult your physician if you are taking estrogen blockers, or as an alternative use the night sweats formula.

**Associated essences:** Wear two drops each of Champney's pink cluster, Cecil Brünner, fairy rose, old blush, or Maggie on the heart center.

**Associated essential oil blend:** In one ounce of jojoba or sweet almond oil, add four drops of rose and two drops of sandalwood and wear two drops on the heart center.

## NIGHT SWEATS

This tonic abates night sweats, thirst, demineralization of bones, anemia and symptoms of menopause, which increase at night.

### Ingredients:

    2 cups water
    1 tablespoon *Rehmannia glutinosa,* prepared
    1 tablespoon black cohosh root
    2 teaspoons *Atractylodes alba* to reduce involuntary sweating (optional)
    1 3-inch slice of astragalus root (a yellow center assures potency)
    2 jujube red dates

Simmer ingredients in two cups of water, covered, for one hour. Strain and sip one-half cup daily. Refrigerate or freeze leftovers. Serves four.

**Note:** Rehmannia, prepared, is a black, tarry looking herb. It tastes very sweet when cooked in a tonic. Cooking Oriental herbs dissipates sulfides added during processing. Red dates, also grown in Texas and parts of the southern U.S., and licorice root harmonize the formulas and reduce harmful effects.

**Associated essences:** Wear two drops each of purple garden sage, red malva, verbena, or rosemary on the neck.

**Associated essential oil blend:** In one ounce of water, add three drops of geranium, two drops of lemon balm, and one drop rosemary. Spray or apply to the face, avoiding the eyes.

# PREMENSTRUAL FORMULA

If premenstrual moodiness is straining your friendships, this is the formula to bring back your natural harmony.

**Ingredients:**
    2 cups water
    2 tablespoons of peony root
    1 tablespoon of vitex berries
    1 tablespoon cramp bark or black haw
    1 tablespoon wild yam root

Simmer two cups of water and herbs for thirty minutes. Strain, and sip one cup daily or dilute two tablespoons in four ounces of juice three times daily. Serves two.

**Associated essences:** Wear two drops each of Japanese magnolia, marigold, ranunculus, and salad burnet on the heart center and abdomen.

**Associated essential oil blend:** In one ounce of oil, wear on temples a blend of four drops of lavender, two drops of rose geranium, and one drop of sandalwood.

# PROLAPSED ORGANS

Use this tonic regularly for three months to increase the vitality and tone of the bladder, uterus and vagina.

**Ingredients:**
    2 cups brandy
    2 tablespoons of black cohosh root
    2 tablespoons astragalus root
    1 teaspoon suma (*Pfaffia paniculata*)
    1 tablespoon foti (*Polygonum multiflorum*)

Tincture in two cups of brandy for three weeks. Dilute fifteen drops in four ounces of hot water daily. Serves eight to ten.

**Associated essences:** Wear two drops of salvia, shrimp, red rose, Sweet Annie, or Marie Pavie across the lower abdomen or add to a bath.

**Associated essential oil blend:** In one ounce of warm vegetable oil, add three drops of peppermint, one drop of oregano, one drop of thyme, and one drop of eucalyptus. Apply to the lower abdomen.

## Understanding Herbal Blood Tonics

As Faith finished the lecture, Nimbus immediately questioned her.

"Can the essences and essential oils be combined and worn or added to a bath?" asked Sweet Tooth.

"Yes," she answered, "and you can still wear two drops of the combination," Faith added.

"Can the essences be combined?" asked Nimbus.

"Sure, be creative. You could try adding them to shampoos and lotions and wear them like skin care."

Flora waited for Faith to finish before changing the subject. "I have a question about the Oriental herbs used in some of the tonics, Faith. Why are herbs like tang kuei, rehmannia, peony root, foti and red dates so helpful?"

"These herbs are included in what the Orientals call blood tonics. They are widely used to maintain a healthy reproductive system. Both men and women can use them, although the percentage of ingredients may change. For example, tang kuei, also known as 'dong quai,' can be used for men and women. Larger amounts are used in female formulas for the estrogenic effect. For men, smaller amounts of the same herb act upon the blood only, nourishing the cells and removing waste.

"Oriental tonic herbs also nourish and moisten body fluids, such as blood plasma, spinal fluid, semen, lymph and mucosa. Tonic herbs also energize and move the blood. The Eastern approach to health is based on energetics, a balance of the movement and flow of energy. It is expressed as rhythm in the ebb and flow of opposing forces, allowing all organs to function synergistically.

"As you can tell from their properties, tonic herbs are very nutritious. They require special preparation in order to extract these qualities, such as cooking and tincturing in alcohol."

"Tell us some of their properties," asked Spider, looking over one of his shoulders.

"Well, okay, but keep in mind these are just a few examples," replied Faith.

"Go for it," prodded Spider.

"We'll start with the most-prized female herb," Faith said. Spider typed enthusiastically.


## Tang Kuei, *Angelica Sinensis*

Tang kuei is a blood tonic used to regulate menses, reduce menopausal symptoms and tone the reproductive organs. It can be used moderately before, during, and after pregnancy to improve circulation, tone the uterus, build hemoglobin, and relax pelvic muscles. It helps everyone utilize vitamin E and stabilize blood sugar. The energetics of tang kuei relaxes the heart muscle, reduces blood pressure, when necessary, and slows the pulse. It is an excellent herb for menopausal women with a high risk of heart disease. Tang kuei relaxes the heart muscle, reducing spasms and subsequent heart problems.

## Foti, *Polygonum Multiflorum*
In the orient, this herb is known as Ho Shou Wu and is used more than ginseng as a sexual and fertility tonic. It is a sedative tonic that is not as stimulating as ginseng. As a tonic, it fortifies the blood and reduces inflammation and hypertension. Foti is used to build stamina and restore vitality. I use it in tonics to reduce arthritic symptoms.

## *Astragalus Membranaceus*
Astragalus is known as "milk vetch" in the U.S. It regulates immune response and tones muscles. I use it to strengthen prolapsed organs and for weakness in the arms and legs. Astragalus regulates fluid balance and reduces bloating and edema.

## *Rehmannia Glutinosa*
Cooked rehmannia prolongs life as a heart and blood tonic. It nourishes bones, tendons, and marrow. Oriental women take it after childbirth. I use it to reduce night sweats, especially during menopause. It is non-estrogenic and safe for those on estrogen blockers suffering from heat flashes. Rehmannia nourishes the blood and fluids, often preventing kidney problems. In combination with other blood tonics, it reduces diabetic and blood sugar imbalances.

## Atractylodis
Atractylodis is used for weight control, anorexia, and fluid balance. It is a very safe diuretic that also reduces excess perspiration from weakness. Women use it to reduce appetite.

## Jujube Red Dates
Zizyphus jujube is a sedative, nutritive herb that regulates the dispersion of other herbs' energy. It relaxes smooth muscles, as a cardiotonic, and allows nutrients to be easily assimilated.

## Peony Root

The Orientals consider peony the most important female tonic herb. It restores balance to the liver, relaxing muscles and relieving cramps. Women who drink this tea have radiant, elastic skin, as beautiful as a peony flower. This herb aids all hormonal irregularities and moodiness.

As Spider finished typing, he turned to the group. "I know some female spiders who eat their males after mating that could sure use some of these tonic herbs."

"Maybe that's why they're called 'female longevity tonics,'" Nimbus giggled.

## Flora Decides to Return to the Land of Thyme

Finally, the group dispersed for tea. Flora noticed that Vinnie wasn't among them. Spontaneously, everyone started looking for Vinnie in every corner of the ceiling without results. Flora stopped in the middle of the room, thinking as she stroked her chin. The group encircled the goddess, waiting for her to act. Flora dropped her hand to her side and marched toward the back door. The fairies followed her in single file.

When they reached the garden, Flora found Vinnie right where she suspected — sound asleep on a rock beside the molting Snake, wings fluttering with each snore.

Spider tiptoed behind the group, commenting in a hushed voice.

"Well, I see not everyone is interested in female tonics. What we need to do now is document all the info on the flowers in the Garden of Beauty. I could broadcast a great television series live from my laptop on TV to the Land of Thyme."

"That's a great idea!" exclaimed Nimbus as the group gathered around Spider to congratulate him, shaking each of his eight hands.

Flora stepped apart from the group, a faraway look on her angelic face.

"I've been thinking about returning to the Land of Thyme," she announced softly.

The fairies looked shocked.

"Why?" asked Sweet Tooth with one eyebrow raised. "Are you missing someone?"

"Well, uh, yes, I mean sometimes," Flora stammered.

"And who would that be?" asked Nimbus softly.

"Well, it might be the captain of the Fairy Navy SEALs," Flora answered. "You know him. He was the Justice of the Garden for your wedding ceremony."

No one seemed surprised except Vinnie, who woke up just in time to hear Flora's confession. His face quickly wrinkled into a frown around his tiny nose.

"What in the Land of Thyme do you want to see that big showoff for?" Vinnie asked, in a demanding tone.

"Well, I just thought he might benefit from some of these essences," Flora answered quite defensively.

"You must have an essence for a showoff, don't you Faith?" asked Sweet Tooth, nudging Faith until she caught on.

"Uh, no. Oh! I mean, yes, yes, of course! That's, uh, well, I forget, but I do have one!" Faith looked around the circle to see if anyone really believed her.

"Well, I think it's an excellent idea," Sweet Tooth continued. "We've been gathering knowledge and experience for a long time and we should return. Anyway, I want to be home when the stork arrives."

## Vinnie's Decision

"But who's going to stay with me?" asked Spider. "This is a career opportunity of a lifetime! I can finally leap from being a desk reporter to a television anchor, and then, who knows? Maybe a talk show host!"

"I'll stay with you," Vinnie replied firmly. "I'm not ready to leave. In fact, I'm feeling quite at home here. What about you, Snake?"

Snake gathered his great length to raise his small head. "Well, since I've been beat out by a winged hero, I guess I'll stay here. I wouldn't want to make a grown fairy cry by slithering off with the prize."

"Okay, Snake," interrupted Spider. "Go molt a little longer. We'll let you know when we begin our research. Your help and wisdom will be greatly appreciated."

The compliment helped ease Snake's pain and even greater pride. He consoled himself with the thought that romance between Flora and the captain wouldn't last long. Then she'd be ready for the real love of her life. Until then, he planned to sleep. Vinnie was right beside him, petting his long, slender body.

Faith walked into the garden in time to hear the fairies' plans. She took this opportunity to approach Vinnie.

"I sure could use some help in the gardens, if you're interested in staying through the end of the harvest."

Upon hearing the invitation, Vinnie brightened and beamed from ear to ear. He jumped onto his feet and, in excitement, landed on Snake's back, adding injury after insult.

"Oof! Get off of me, you big ox!" Snake complained. "Pets shouldn't have to put up with such abuse! Where's the flower lady? I need a remedy!"

"Well, I do have ranunculus for those who suffered abuse," Faith thought out loud. "I gave it to a stray dog that had been beaten and she decided to move in with me," Faith smiled as she reached out to pet her dog, Mom, standing beside her.

"Oh, he'll get over it," decided Vinnie. "I'm as light as a fairy and Snake's just a little spoiled. Now, back to the garden invitation. I would be delighted to accommodate your organic needs. I even have my own gardening tools; I don't leave town without them!" Vinnie bounced all over Snake as he talked, while Snake moaned incessantly.

"Quick, lady, get me the ranunculus before my head gets permanently flattened!" Snake pleaded.

Snake sounded so pitifully convincing, Faith found herself running back to the house for the ranunculus with Vinnie flying right beside her, talking incessantly about his gardening experience, his love of flowers, and, well, just about everything under the sun until well into the night.

CHAPTER 15

# The Way Home
## History, Legend, and Lore

*"Healing from the heart embraces others through self love."*
Judy Griffin, *The Healing Flowers*

## Laptop TV Interview

The next day, plans were made for departure. Flora, Nimbus, and Sweet Tooth were ready to return to the Land of Thyme. Spider, Snake, and Vinnie would stay in the Garden of Beauty to research all the plants and broadcast live to the Land of Thyme via Spider's soon-to-be-infamous laptop. The group stood around chatting and making small talk, each feeling a little insecure about separating. All, that is, except for Spider, who was hurrying from one person to the next trying to set up interviews. Then he explained, "When the laptop screen flashes on, you'll hear an okay from the station. Just look directly into the little camera above the screen and answer the questions. Here we go!"

The screen flashed as the fairies stared in amazement. Suddenly, a voice could be heard through the static.

"Standby, you're on the air! Come in, Spider, can you hear me?"

Without hesitation, Spider answered, "This is Spider reporting from the Garden of Beauty at the end of the rainbow. I hear ya loud and clear, John."

"Can you briefly tell us what you're doing in the Garden of Beauty?" John asked Spider.

"We're here learning about the therapeutic qualities of local herbs and flowers from a totally different culture," Spider answered in an authoritative voice.

"And what can we learn from the flowers and herbs blooming in the Garden of Beauty?" asked the anchorman, John.

To answer this question, Spider shoved Faith in front of the laptop.

"This is Faith, our hostess in the Garden of Beauty to answer your questions for our listeners."

Faith peered into the little camera, as if she could really see her audience as she began to speak.

"Flowers and herbs help us bloom under stress. They catalyze our creative potentials by keeping us strong in our approach to external situations, yet open and receptive to guidance from within. Flowers and aromatic herbs directly affect the way we feel about ourselves and help overcome the personal problems blocking or slowing personality development."

"How did you develop this rapport with flowers?" asked John.

"Through listening," Faith answered. "Just like the ancient seers and Native American healers. The information is stored in the genetic memory of the plant and comes to me through intuition. I was drawn to my flowers in my garden to help my children's health and later my own. The twins had 105° temperatures and suffered from asthma, febrile convulsions, prophylactic shock and eczema. I used flower essences to strengthen their immunity and observed their recuperation on a daily basis. I received an answer to my prayer, in a different way than I expected. With every challenging situation, an essence would come to me to offer psychological support for myself and my children, clients, and students."

"Why do you feel that stress is a problem that flower essences can solve?" asked John, digging deeper for answers.

"Because life is very complicated," Faith quickly answered. "For example, I went through school with a tablet and a pencil. Kids today need computers and expensive calculators that may be obsolete before the school year ends! It's stressful to keep up with everyday demands and choices. These type of stressors adversely affect the immune and nervous systems."

"Why, I feel stressed just thinking about all these things," answered John. "Let's ask the visiting fairies how flower essences reduced stress in their lives."

Nimbus surprised everyone by volunteering to go first.

"Flower essences helped me lose weight by reducing compulsive eating caused by internal stress. I have more weight to lose, but I feel like I can handle my eating patterns now," he chuckled as he patted his tummy. "Enlightenment has made me lighter!"

"You do look like you've slimmed down a little," commented John. "How about you, Sweet Tooth?"

Sweet Tooth blushed as she faced the screen.

"I realized my passion for chocolate was fulfilling a desire for my dad's attention," she began. "Flower essences are helping me open my creative ability to find nurturing within. And, I don't seem to need extra weight to feel powerful or protected anymore, so I guess my weight will adjust to my new image. With a baby on the way, I want to take good care of my body."

"Excellent!" Spider clapped with all eight hands. "Now, let's hear from Flora, the goddess whose knowledge has impacted the Land of Thyme in every way," he said as he positioned Flora in front of the laptop.

"I learned about healing from the heart, when self-love embraces others to benefit all concerned."

"How did flower essences do that?" John asked emphatically.

"They opened my heart and moved beyond my work ethic and goals. Now, I just want to come home and get to know everybody. Then, along with my knowledge in diet and nutrition, I can really impact the Land of Thyme," Flora answered humbly. "More than results, I care about the fairies."

"Wow! We're looking forward to your return!" John commented as he leaned forward in his chair, smiling broadly. "Who else is there with you today?"

Before Spider could answer, Vinnie pushed his way in front of the screen.

"I have self-esteem!" he cried into the microphone, pressing his face against the camera and grinning from ear to ear mischievously.

"Well, my goodness," sighed John. "It's Vinnie and he's hyper and he's happy!"

"Yes! I learned to like myself just the way I am," Vinnie answered while smashing his nose against the screen to make everyone laugh.

Spider's voice could be hard in the background. "And I have to live with him! He's staying with me to broadcast about flower remedies."

As the group chuckled, Vinnie turned and put his arm around Spider and continued. "We're staying in the Garden of Beauty to research and document the flowers' healing qualities. Then, I can show you how gaining self-esteem has helped me."

"So, you'll have a reprieve from Vinnie in the Land of Thyme," Spider added. "We'll be broadcasting the information daily in a series called 'Flower Remedies from the Garden.'"

"Great news, Spider! We'll be looking forward to the series," John commented. "We'll be back after this brief message from our sponsor."

## The Departure

As the broadcast faded, the fairies flew around congratulating one another. Shortly, they became quiet and pensive as the time drew near for the final good-byes.

"We'll watch you everyday on TV," promised Flora earnestly.

"I'll return before you run out of Melba toast!" assured Vinnie.

"That's because you're the only one who eats it," laughed Flora with tears in her eyes.

As tears were shed and hugs were shared, the group parted with promises to reunite soon.

## Digging into the Past

Spider and Vinnie immediately began to prepare their research for the series. Vinnie compiled historical facts and uses for every flower Faith made into an essence. Spider tackled this volume of material with superb editing skills after interviewing Faith on the subtle healing properties of her flowers.

Vinnie became so absorbed in his work, he had less time to spend with his pet, Snake. When Snake approached Spider about being abandoned, Spider put him to work looking for the Latin names of the flowers. Vinnie and Snake then worked as a team. They were so busy meeting Spider's TV deadlines that Vinnie forgot to fly around and talk incessantly. Within a week, they loved the challenge of their work. Within three weeks, Spider was ready to go on the air.

"This is Spider ready to begin the series of 'Flower Remedies from the Garden.' Can you hear me, John?"

"We hear you loud and clear, Spider. Everyone here in the Land of Thyme is ready to learn about flower remedies. What have you got for us today, Spider?"

"I have for you today, John, the symbolic meanings of a flower's soul, expressed in legend and lore, followed by the meaning of its essence, related to us by Faith in the Garden of Beauty. These flowers come to us from all over the Old World."

As the listeners pulled their leaf cushions closer to the television set, Spider began to weave a web linking the past and present for each flower in Faith's garden. He proudly presented the following chronicle of floral myths and historical and traditional uses of flowers used for healing from the heart.

## African violet essence, *Saint Paulia,* East African origin

African violet releases endorphins from the subtle body, fulfilling the desire for love that can only come from within.

The vibration touches a chord within the spirit to release nurturing and love from the soul. African violet helps one express a peaceful, mindful state of being, allowing a general good feeling about oneself. This will enhance the entire positive vibrations and talents in each individual.

*I am lifted up on the Petals of Love.*

### Historical uses

The flowers can be candied and eaten like violets. (See Pressed Violet recipe on page 115).

### Legend and lore

The African violet was believed to spring from the graves of virgins. In Hindu mythology, it represents the lingam, a phallus symbol associated with Shiva, the Hindu destroyer god.

## Amaryllis essence, *Hippeastrum, leopoldii,* Peruvian origin

Amaryllis raises the vibration of the individual to overcome fear and anxiety about the unknown. One will become clear about the path to follow in the future and begin to move in the direction talents lead, integrating all positive aspects of the personality. In the physical body, the vibration aids parasitic and fungal growth to turn to ash. It is used often for pets and owners.

This personality has the potential of being naturally intuitive as he opens and allows his true Self to emerge.

*I step out in faith to achieve the Greatest Good.*

**Historical uses**

The red flowers make a beautiful dye used to color paper and ink.

**Legend and lore**

The amaryllis is haughty, very proud, and showy. It likes to bloom at a different time than other flowers so it will receive the admiration due such a beautiful bloom. Legend tells us this beauty refused fragrance because it didn't want anyone getting too close.

## Anemone essence, *Coronaria coccinea,* Greek origin

Anemone aids the personality who believes that "life is hard and a struggle." To really experience pleasure in its fullest seems impossible because this personality is always waiting for the ax to fall. Phrases mentioned in conversation with this person might be "it's too good to be true," or "it can't last."

Instead of having his ideals and desires nurtured during infancy, this child was raised with the attitude that you can't have what you want and believes it.

In the physical body this may manifest in scarring, slow wound healing, or adhesions. The inability to enjoy life will block the flow of healing energy and regeneration of healthy tissue growth in wounds.

The anemone personality is a natural with children, sports, advertising for pleasure vacations, and creating excitement in an otherwise dull environment.

*I realize the fullest melody of Joy lies within me.*

**Historical uses**

Anemone flowers have been used to treat ringworm. Oriental cultures used them to treat tuberculosis of the lymphatic glands, more common in Asian countries.

**Legend and lore**

Anemone is the windflower, springing from the tears of Aphrodite. During rain, the flowers close and drop their heads to protect their pollen. Fairies were believed to cause the petals to close as they curled up inside them for protection.

The English wore anemones around their neck or arm to ward off disease, and believed it was bad luck to run through a field of anemones.

## Aquilegia columbine, *Aquilegia skinneri,* Mexican origin

This variety of columbine enhances the ability to think and act independently of others.

Aquilegia will also help drop the role others have chosen for you. Columbine will encourage us to tour life as a unique individual. We will develop a sense of knowing rather than feeling or intuiting in the decision-making process. In the body, this may correspond to becoming independent from the mother's genetic role to claim autonomy. Research points to its ability to enhance lymphatic drainage.

*I drop the roles others have given me to become autonomous.*

**Historical uses**

Native American tribes used columbine flowers in love potions. They are known as hummingbird flowers, bringing joy to the household. In homeopathy, the flower is used to reduce nervous complaints. The seeds are *toxic* in any form.

**Legend and lore**

Aquilegia is named after Aquia, the eagle, and columbine is a dove. It was also known as "herba leonis" because lions allegedly ate them. Thus, if you rub your hands on the flowers, you will gain the courage of a lion. Aphrodite, the goddess of love, was associated with both lions and doves in ancient Greece. Touch one if you dare.

## Anise hyssop, *Hsopus anisum,* Mediterranean origin

Anise hyssop enhances public speaking and teaching abilities, alleviating the "butterflies" one feels in the stomach before a performance. It is indicated for those who have chronic headaches, dizzy spells, or stomachaches characterized by a stabbing or fluttering pain.

For those who are overcoming a speech impediment, anise hyssop combines well with daffodil and silver moon.

*I encourage honest and sincere communication.*

**Historical uses**

In colonial America, flowers were pressed into prayer books to increase alertness during church services. The flowers contain an essential oil that is strongly antiseptic and aromatic. Bees make a delicious honey from the flowers. The Romans brewed a wine with the flowers for coughs and respiratory problems. American colonists made an oil from the flowers to heal infected wounds.

**Legend and lore**

The Hebrew word *esob* (hyssop) means "holy herb" and it has been used since recorded times to clean and purge.

## Aster, Stoksia, *Blue Danube,* originated in Bombay China

Aster promotes a consciousness of being strong within and gentle in the outreach to others. A personality may increase the power of concentration. In business and personal relationships, one will use the power of encouragement rather than intimidation to promote an environment of loyalty and honesty. The personality will enjoy a more nurturing attitude towards his own internal environment and be better attuned to others' desires.

In the immune system, this attitude enhances the body's ability to produce its own toxins, monoclonal antibodies. The T lymphocytes killer cells inject helper cells into diseased cells, virus and tumors to clean up the internal environment.

*I encourage others to bloom with me.*

### Historical uses

The flowers are a favorite of "he loves me, he loves me not" fantasies. For healing broken bones, a poultice of asters was applied locally to facilitate regeneration.

### Legend and lore

Aster is sacred to Aphrodite, a flower of love. The Chinese have given aster the attributes of beauty, charm, and elegance.

## Azalea, *Rhododendron species*, originated in the southern U.S. preceding the Civil War 1860–1865

Azalea essence induces creative imagination, releasing energy to balance the chakras. The feeling of personal power is enhanced, aiding the individual in controlling his life. One will feel more capable of integrating all aspects of the personality with available talents. Latent talents will be recognized.

Although everyone will benefit from azalea essence, the personality who will have the most dramatic results will be the individual who is unable to see past statistics and logic. The personality is usually defined as a left-brain thinker. Azalea will aid in integrating facts and figures to uncover simple ways to solve the complex situations challenging humanity today.

*I am the flower of Creation, blooming into my fullest Creative Expression.*

### Historical uses

Azalea is grown by the Japanese for its great beauty, color, and grace. It represents the transitory nature of beauty and helps perceive life as a fleeting moment of beauty in the cosmos. Azaleas attract hummingbirds, a symbol of joy.

### Legend and lore

Azalea grew from tears of blood from a young boy turned into a cuckoo by his jealous stepmother. It represents great talents and abilities born from adversity.

## Babies' breath, *Gypsophilia paniculata elegans,* originated in Eastern Europe and southern Russia

The individual most likely to benefit from the essence of babies' breath will reject new ideas because, "It won't work!" There is a certain amount of fear and resistance to change or incorporating new ideas into proven methods. Behind this idea is the attitude of "don't rock the boat, things may become worse than they are." This person may be trading off some of the good things in life to keep the status quo.

Babies' breath may be especially useful to people prone to conditions affecting the lungs, such as pleurisy and asthma, or angina as it encourages the thoracic area to relax.

This personality has a childlike innocence bringing new life into most any situation. The person will be most likely to be invited to parties and remembered as a true friend.

*I am the beauty of innocence.*

**Historical uses**

The flower blooms in a white haze in semi shade. It is known as the "florist's flower," and is used as sprays in arrangements, especially at weddings to ensure fertility.

**Legend and lore**

Babies' breath is believed to shelter the cradles of newborn fairies.

## Bachelor's button, *Centaura cyanus,* originated in the Near East

Bachelor's button will most accommodate the personality straddling the fence, afraid to release the past and unable to formulate a plan for the future.

Other than feeling trapped in an uncomfortable emotional situation, this personality may experience edema in a localized area of the body or generalized throughout the body. The personality using bachelor's button will benefit by completing projects and using goal-planning objectives to carry through thought processes.

Fluid excesses are often associated with tears. Releasing the past and the need to hold onto past pains will aid the body in correcting fluid imbalances.

Once the bachelor's button personality makes a decision, the person will quickly bring these desires into reality. The personality will have beginner's luck in achieving goals and has a talent for making money work for himself and others.

*I stand firmly in Truth, flowing in the Present Moment of Grace.*

**Historical uses**

Bachelor's buttons were decocted to treat inflamed eyes. The flower juice mixed with alum makes a blue ink. Native Americans used bachelor's buttons to draw out snake poison. The Romans burned the flowers to drive away snakes. And the Jamaicans mix the flowers with alum and apply them locally for toothaches. The flowers are mildly stimulating to the immune system. A flower infusion has been used to stimulate digestion and alleviate arthritic complaints as a folk remedy.

**Legend and lore**

*Centaurea cyanus* was named after an ancient Greek centaur believed to be the "Father of Medicine." He covered wounds with bachelor's buttons to make them heal.

## Bamboo, *Bambusa,* originated in Asia

Bamboo will most assist the personality who needs to be directed in life. The bamboo personality will often ask, "Where do I go now?" or "What do I do next?" He will often be searching and attracting someone to take him by the hand, anywhere.

The individual looks to others for guidance, unable to access his/her own inner wisdom. Physical symptoms may include intestinal distress, such as irritable bowel syndrome.

While using bamboo essence, one should concentrate on planning career goals and lifestyles around activities and talents that are most enjoyable. As a result, this person will most likely become a prominent leader, and will be active in community and fund raising projects.

*My direction is ever inward.*

**Historical Uses**

Local compresses were used to treat rheumatism and increase circulation.

**Legend and lore**

Bamboo is one of the three friends of winter, along with plum and pine. It is an emblem of Buddha, the perfect man who bows to the storm to rise again. It is a sign of longevity and lasting friendship. The seven knots on bamboo stems indicate seven degrees of initiation into the spiritual life and invocation.

## Basil, *Ocimum basilicum,* originated in the Mediterranean and India

Basil enables one to achieve self-love and worthiness by releasing the negativity of past experiences. This personality would consider himself and his achievements not good enough. Oftentimes, this person is a perfectionist with an inferiority complex.

A lack of self-worth and love is comparable to toxicity in the bloodstream. One might consider this person to be a "type A." He will likely be a high achiever and measure self-worth by financial success.

While using basil, this person would benefit from finding new ways to feel good and allow self-nurturing habits to form.

The basil personality is capable of organizing projects, developing businesses, consulting, and planning large-scale projects and bringing order into chaotic circumstances.

*Perfection and Achievement shine before me.*

**Historical uses**

Basil flowers are high in camphor and used to treat virus and repel insects. The distillation is added to liquor. As an inhalant or compress, basil flowers treat headache, nausea, and vomiting. Its properties are classified as a digestant. A compress may be applied topically from the flowers to facilitate healing wounds. An essential oil of the flowering stems stimulate the adrenal cortex, increasing stamina, alertness, and intelligence.

**Legend and lore**

Basil was associated with the legendary Basilisk, half bird and half reptile, whose breath or stare could kill one instantly. Basil later became known as protector of evil and symbol of love. In the language of flowers, a sprig of flowering basil was put on a windowsill to encourage a suitor. The Latin name, *Ocinum,* means "to smell."

## Begonia, *Begonia odorata,* originated in Jamaica as a nontoxic variety

Begonia allows one to feel more trusting and secure in life. The personality may feel tense and threatened by general life experiences. Holding tension within oneself may affect the bladder by causing cramping or by withholding fluids. Bladder infections may occur. Begonias are for people who tend to be pack rats and store things in drawers and closets like little squirrels.

The question which should be asked of a begonia personality is, "What are you afraid to let go of?" When in control of one's life, externals won't seem as threatening and the ability to relax and let go can be achieved. Life can be seen as a challenge as one realizes that fear can become an adventurous experience without limitation.

Once the belief in limitations and insecurity of life is removed, the begonia personality will become useful in tackling situations such as food shortages, space conquests, and uncovering the secrets of the Universe.

*I am the will to create through love and cooperation.*

### Historical uses

The flowers attract beneficial insects in the garden. Third world cultures have used the flowers topically to reduce inflammation and swelling.

**Legend and lore**

The flowers of begonias are believed to be replicas of angel wings.

## Bluebonnet, *Lupinus texenis,* native only to Texas

The Bluebonnet personality is awakened by the call of destiny. A greater force is now leading and calling the individual to move forward with a new consciousness.

The individual may ask silently: "What am I here to do?" The search for a true identity will discover great powers emerging from within. The person works within to create truth, beauty, peace, and prosperity in every aspect of life. With bluebonnet, there will be a call from within to make some important changes in career, relationships, and health. The call will also be to serve the many. The only choice is to follow.

*I bloom from my inner awareness.*

**Historical uses**

Bluebonnet is only native in Texas and is as unique as Texas is big! There are actually six native bluebonnets. All six are state flowers in Texas. Considered the most beautiful is *Lupinus texensis.* Large varieties attract hummingbirds. These wildflowers spread carpets of blue-violet color throughout the vast Texas landscape in early spring, dazzling the imagination center with their color.

**Legend and lore**

Bluebonnets were once bluebells growing wild in the English oak forests. After traveling to America, they settled in what is now Texas's open fields waiting for the trees to grow around them for protection. When that day comes, they will turn in their sunbonnets and become bluebells once again.

## Borage, *Boragio officinalis,* originated in the Mediterranean

Borage aids those who must be self-sufficient and stand alone in their career or personal life. It is indicated for those with structural difficulties affecting the feet, ankles, and hips. Borage combines well with viridiflora and mushroom to enhance balance and agility.

*I learn to stand on my own.*

**Historical uses**

Borage flowers steeped in wine was a Medieval cure for melancholy. Bees make honey from borage flowers. A poultice can be made to soothe itchy red skin and a tea cures sore throats. Celts and, later, Roman soldiers drank a wine made with borage flowers to enhance their courage. The flower seeds contain omega 3 essential fatty acids, protecting the heart with anti-inflammatory properties. A flower infusion makes an adrenaline tonic that reduces stress and depression.

**Legend and lore**

Borage flowers were eaten in salads to drive away sorrow and comfort the heart. It is known as the "star flower" and believed to be a sign from heaven that aid is forthcoming.

## Bronze fennel, *Foeniculum vulgare* bronze variety, originated in the Caucus

Bronze fennel helps overcome limitations by stimulating the imagination and planning centers. It aids those who want to create a much greater reality through visualization. Bronze fennel strengthens mental and psychic abilities, enhancing clarity and direction. It combines well with azalea, autumn damask, and echinacea to enhance creative pleasures.

*I can see clearly now.*

**Historical uses**

Bronze fennel is grown as a bee plant for a delicious licorice-flavored honey. The blooms contain anethol, an essential oil with an anise flavor. It is anti-spasmodic, a carminative digestant, that increases milk flow and treats coughs and urinary disorders.

**Legend and lore**

The Greek word for fennel, *Maraino,* means to grow thin. It is believed to suppress the appetite, reduce adipose tissue, and improve vision. Fennel was introduced from the Mediterranean by a Spanish priest and naturalized around the missions in North America. Its Latin name, *foenum,* means "hay." During the Middle Ages, fennel flowers were hung over doorways to repel evil spirits and the bulbs were served often during the Lenten season. It was cooked with fish in the Middle Ages to offset any toxicity believed to be in the fish.

Fennel is sacred to Sabazios, a Greek god. Wreaths of fennel were worn during the sacred rites.

## Bougainvillea, *Nyctaginacceae,* originated in Brazil

The personality of bougainvillea lives in fear of being punished for every wrong thought or mistake ever manifested. The individual may be feeling so guilty that rewards pass by.

The individual lived in fear of "when daddy gets home" or "mama's going to get you." This child not only experienced physical pain, but emotional suppression for fear or reprisal at home, church, or institutions.

While using bougainvillea, this person should establish habits that are rewarding and pleasurable and see each day with more distance from a painful past.

The bougainvillea personality is most appreciative of life's every pleasure and can aid others in feeling comfortable and welcome, even in the most difficult situations. The individual is a natural politician and a true representative of the people.

*Unconditional love shatters the illusion of guilt.*

**Historical uses**

The flowers are protective to butterflies. Their shape resembles the body of a butterfly.

**Legend and lore**

Bougainvilleas grow wild in the Costa Rican jungles and are very attractive to butterflies. They are believed to grow along the butterflies' path of migration.

## Bouquet of Harmony, antique red and white rose blend with the vanilla orchid

Bouquet of Harmony aids the conscious mind in harnessing Universal authority, taking control of emotions. As the mind conditions itself to order its thoughts, attention, goals, and direction, the emotions are channeled constructively to move in peace, harmony, and good will. The mind in tune with the Present Moment is also in tune with the All-Powerful Infinite Source. The combination of three harmonious essences disciplines the imagination with the Faith to look within, to contact the hidden source of power, and to move into Truth with the confidence of one direction. Truth is the Law of Creation, blessing but never condemning. As we step forward in faith, we accept the communion of life, which blesses the responsibility for creating our environment, the living thoughts and images of the mind. We cease to condemn ourselves and others and find freedom in forgiveness. Outer conditions conform to the spiritual awakening within the source of the divine center, where there is no order of difficulty. Through the feeling of faith, spiritual enrichment leads to the conscious communion of the divine mind.

*I am the Melody of Creation.*

**Historical uses**

The roses are antiques, over one hundred years old, original vegetative cuttings. The essence works with the unnamed chakra, divine union, reversing psychological denial, fears and balancing the *tridosha* (the three primary life forces) neurological, immune, and endocrine systems, allowing every part of the body to coordinate and talk to one other. When all else fails, harmony helps those suffering from anxiety, traumatic injury, bruising, and hysteria and simply enhances peace of mind. It is fragrant and often worn as a scent. This essence crosses over into aromatherapy in that it directly affects brain chemistry and neural transmission. Present research includes hospital studies helping bone marrow-transplant and stem cell-transplant patients.

*When in doubt, use Bouquet of Harmony.*

## Carrot, *Daucus carota,* originated in Greece

The individual aided by carrot essence excels in developing organizational priorities and healthy personal disciplines to reach ambitions and goals. Physically, the essence aids those with upper respiratory symptoms and low fertility by enhancing the competency of hair-like cilia cells in muscosa tissue.

*My ambitions bloom from my inner confidence.*

**Historical uses**

The flower heads were eaten to prevent epileptic seizures. When allowed to reseed naturally, the plant returns to its ancestry as Queen Anne's Lace and is identified by a tiny red flower in its center. Children were treated for digestive disorders and tonsillitis with a tea, while bees enjoyed its flavor for honey.

**Legend and lore**

Carrot flowers, leaves, and roots were used as a treatment for infertility in the Greco-Roman times.

## Catnip, *Nepeta cataria,* originated in Europe and Asia

Catnip brings people closer together, enhancing friendships and common bonds. It is indicated for those who feel inhibited socially, or are in unfamiliar social situations. Catnip softens perceived boundaries, eliminating apprehension and promoting contentment. It combines well with India hawthorn to encourage a sense of oneness around others.

*I attract enduring friendship and love.*

**Historical uses**

Catnip flowers were used in a tea to alleviate insomnia, colic, colds, menstrual cramps, and fever. Its properties are basically antispasmodic. Native Americans brewed the flowering tops to soothe a sore throat. The generic name, *Nepeta,* is from Nepeta, Italy, where it was cultivated.

**Legend and lore**

During the Middle Ages, women sat over the steam of catnip tea to take away barrenness (infertility). Directly seeded plants are said to be of no interest to cats; only cuttings attract them.

## Chamomile, *Anthemis nobilis or chamaemelum nobili,* originated in Egypt

As a flower essence, chamomile aids the person who is most likely to swallow hurt and suppress true feelings. Instead of letting the offender know that feelings are hurt, this person applies an attitude of "What's the use?" and gives way to apathy or indifference.

The chamomile personality may feel very misunderstood, as if nothing one does or says can be appreciated. Upon using chamomile essence, one may become more confident and assertive in relationships. This person has the ability to become an excellent marriage counselor and mediator with the ability to encourage others to work in harmony, even under the most adverse circumstances.

*I am the Blossom of Faith.*

### Historical uses

Chamomile has long been used as a Mexican herbal aid for gallstones and a sluggish gallbladder. Chamomile flowers are brewed into a delicious, relaxing beverage for insomnia, headaches, spasms, muscular pain, and delayed menses. The tea can be used topically to reduce swelling and inflammation as well as a hair rinse for blondes. An essential oil of the flowers is crystal-blue azulene, which can be used in skin care to reduce wrinkles. "Manzanilla tea" in Latin cultures is used to flavor sherry and is the first drink given to babies.

### Legend and lore

Chamomile means "ground apple," referring to its fresh scent and flavor. It was used to treat malaria in ancient times.

## Christmas cactus, *Schlumbergera, bridgesi,* originated in Chiapas, Mexico

A tropical plant sharing its joy at Christmastime, Christmas cactus gives us psychological support by helping us focus on what is right about others and ourselves. In the healing arts, people often focus too much on finding something to correct. By reinforcing our strengths, we will all grow stronger and healthier, and our paths will be peaceful. This will give us much better direction and balance on our journey together.

Christmas cactus goes well with azalea because it inspires our creative nature. In the body, Christmas cactus will support our genetic strengths and natural talents to enhance our well-being.

*I focus on my inner strength.*

### Historical uses

Christmas cactus received its name because it blooms at Christmastime. In Mexican folk culture, it blooms to remind us of the return of Christ.

The Christmas cactus learned to bloom at Yuletide to allow the desert flora to celebrate Christmas.

## Cinnamon basil, *Ocimum basilicum cinnamon,* originated in India

Cinnamon basil fortifies those who buckle under adversity or feel they can't go on under their present circumstances. It is indicated for those who suffer from weak knees and lower back pain. To enhance new potentials and personal growth, combine it with Gaillardia and Madame Louis Levique.

*Adversity brings out the best in me.*

**Historical uses**

The flowers are used by Southeast Asians to reduce fever and heat from the body. They can be used to reduce high blood sugar in diabetics as a tea, flower essence, and culinary flavoring. The stems and flowers are a deep purple color.

**Legend and lore**

Cinnamon basil flowers are laid on the graves of loved ones in Malaysia to assure peace and happiness in eternity.

## Crepe myrtle, *Lagerstroemid indica,* originating in the Near East and known since biblical times

Crepe myrtle will enhance the individual who is unable to speak his mind or who has been suppressed vocally since childhood. The individual may be afraid of incorrect expression and feeling foolish.

Oftentimes, behind these fears is real rage. The crepe myrtle individual needs to be aware of this and focus energy on constructive ways to release anger. The individual will also realize that anger can be creative when it makes one conscious of the need for change.

*My voice is meant to express the Love within me.*

**Historical uses**

The bruised leaves and flowers are used by Brazilians to heal cuts and bruises. A tea was brewed to cleanse the kidneys.

**Legend and lore**

The myrtle is a symbol of abundance and a sign of joy and peace. The lacy, bright flowers are believed to be used to dress fairies.

## Crossandra, *Infundivuliformis,* originated in India and later in South America

The crossandra personality is insecure and fearful of any major changes in life. This would include changes in the lives of those close to him. The individual not only doesn't want to rock the boat, but he won't allow anyone to paddle.

This personality is prone to gastrointestinal stagnation and toxicity. The desire to still the waters is so intense, it may affect energy in the gastrointestinal tract. Heavy metal toxicity may also contaminate the gastrointestinal tract. Living in a heavily polluted environment and using aluminum cookware may also contribute to heavy metal toxicity.

Realizing life is change may help the vibration of crossandra to encourage this personality to GO FOR IT! The individual will find success lies in solving economic and social situations that plague society. Any new situation that is not under control may be helped by the crossandra essence. This includes having a new baby or moving to a new job or environment. Crossandra helps us to adapt to inevitable changes.

*I am the joy of an answered prayer.*

**Historical uses**

Natives in tropical areas of the Far East, who believe the vibrant color will increase sexual potency, eat the flowers.

**Legend and lore**

The firecracker plant, a native tropical plant in Ceylon and India, grows three feet tall. The orange blooms attract birds year round, and are believed to be a beacon for migrating birds. Natives believe the flowers encourage the gift of prophecy.

## Curry essence, *Helichrysum italicum x angustofolium,* originated in the Middle East

Curry aids those who have to think on their feet with no time for quiet thought. It enhances new talents and potentials by freeing the mind of linear thought patterns. For those who want to figure out their life in advance or lack spontaneity, curry combines well with Christmas cactus and Mexican oregano. It is also indicated for migraine headaches resulting from tension and decreased circulation.

*I look within to discover hidden talents.*

**Historical uses**

The flowers are cut for everlastings in arrangements. The aroma clears the air of stale smoke and negativity. Flowers and leaves taste like the curry spice blend. The flowers yield an essential oil, Immortelle, employed by aromatherapists to abate bacterial and fungal infections and lethargy from depression.

**Legend and lore**

The curry plant acquired its unique taste by pollinating bees from India.

## Daffodil, *Narcissus naegelia,* originated as a hybrid from Portugal

The daffodil personality is quiet and often considered timid or meek. The individual often feels intimidated by explosive and outgoing parents. This personality will go out of his way to avoid an emotional scene.

The individual tries to make everyone happy. In so doing, the daffodil personality hopes to be happy also. This may be one way to manifest heaven on earth, if one enjoys putting out fires. However, the constant tension and anxiety this personality can create within can cause symptoms such as heart palpitations. He's become dependent on being a people-pleaser. Daffodil will help the person feel more at ease with himself and others while releasing some of the pressure from suppressed anger.

The daffodil personality will discover a natural ability to heal others and help dysfunctional families.

*I am the Compassion healing all wounds.*

**Historical uses**

Daffodil flowers have been made into a tea or syrup for respiratory congestion.

**Legend and lore:**

Daffodil is Greek for *narke* (numbness) because the bulb contains toxic alkaloids that cause paralysis and death. The common name "Daffodil" refers to the Greek work *asphodelos,* a flower that was believed to bloom in the afterlife.

## Dandelion, *Taraxacum officinalis,* originated in Europe

Dandelion frees the psyche from fretful dreams and aids those who wake up with a feeling of falling into their body. It enables one to receive answers in dreams and to remember dreams. It combines well with fairy rose, verbena, and Madame Alfred Carrier.

*My dreams set free the best in me.*

**Historical uses**

The flowers are brewed into a delicious wine and are also a favorite for honeybees. They are used as a yellow dye and have a long history of culinary and medicinal use for liver complaints and gout. Drinking a cup of dandelion flower tea was used as preventative for rheumatism. The flowers can be cooked into syrup for a cough suppressant and to detoxify the blood. The flowers are slightly diuretic.

**Legend and lore**

Dandelion flowers have long been used as an oracle. If you blow off all the seeds on the seedhead, your wish will come true. This later evolved into the celebration of blowing out all the birthday candles to receive a wish.

## Daylily, *Hamerocallis aurantiaca,* originated in China

Daylily helps those who are planning major changes in their personal life or career. It is indicated when one's job affects the future of many individuals.

Daylily can help those who are brainstorming to overcome social, economic, and political problems. Daylily is beneficial for those who suffer from chemical sensitivities and environmental pollution. It combines well with bamboo, carrot, and Cecil Brunner.

*I have faith in my future.*

### Historical uses

The blossoms are gathered before they open by Asians and Native Americans to cook as a food. They are gathered in the fall when they have the most nutrients. Daylilies are believed to soothe the heart as well as satisfy the stomach.

### Legend and lore

Daylilies were worn in the girdle of a pregnant woman in China to cause the birth of a boy. In Europe, they were believed to cure melancholy by causing the loss of memory.

## Delphinium, *Ajacis* variety, originated in Switzerland and the northern Mediterranean

Delphinium aids those who cannot focus and complete projects. It is indicated for adults and children who are forgetful or have attention deficit. Delphinium helps those who suffer from low blood sugar, affecting attention span and memory. It has been used to eradicate the affects of parasitic infections when combined with amaryllis. It may be combined with Alfredo de Damas for hand-to-eye coordination problems. Delphinium combines well with silver moon for palsy.

*I focus on perfecting my skills.*

### Historical uses

The flowers were used in Medieval times to kill external lice and parasites. They were issued to Wellington's British troops during the Battle of Waterloo (1815) as a delousing remedy. The Union soldiers used delphinium to delouse during the Civil War (1860–1865). It is considered toxic internally with alkaloids adversely affecting the nervous system. The flowering stalk attracts bees, butterflies, and beneficial insects.

### Legend and lore

Delphinium is a Greek word meaning "dolphin plant." They thought it resembled a dolphin.

## Dianthus, *Caryophyllaceae chinensis,* originated in China

A dianthus personality is most easily described as apathetic. The individual was never allowed to release anger and has passed anger into apathy. His favorite expression is: "I don't care."

What the individual is really trying to tell us is nobody cares about him. This feeling of separation from humanity causes disinterest in life. Life is no longer worth living. So, the individual becomes anemic and withdrawn and finds nothing to ignite a passion for life. This individual rarely laughs aloud or squeals with enthusiasm.

Taking dianthus and recognizing the limitation of apathy will aid the personality to view life on a brighter tone. The person will find ways to nurture and love oneself, and ultimately others.

*Inner Joy is all I know.*

### Historical uses

Dianthus flowers were used as a substitute for cloves, an expensive import in Elizabethan times.

### Legend and lore

Known as "pinks" or "gillyflowers," dianthus flowers represent the pursuit of perfection. During the French Revolution, Chevalier de Rougeville tried to rescue Marie Antoinette, the deposed Queen of France, by concealing his plans in a gillyflower. The jailer found the message and Marie Antoinette was soon beheaded.

## Dill, *Anethum graveolens,* originated in the eastern Mediterranean and western Asia

Dill essence releases the fear of abandonment and the ultimate fear of death. The personality may experience self-alienation or denial of feelings and bodily experiences. Dill flowers help bring us into autonomy through a deeper connection with our body. The first "self" we experience is voiced through the body. Our physical body is the foundation for autonomy and the source for effective thinking and channeling. Through subtle energy, dill increases the body's ability to produce the most protective immunoglobulin. It is most prevalent in mother's milk, and protects muscosal surfaces from pathological, bacterial invasion. Dill is the tiny flower of a culinary herb, not a pickle.

*I am never alone.*

### Historical uses

The name is Norse, meaning, "to lull." Dill flowers are hung over a baby's cradle for protection and a tea is brewed to alleviate colic. It was known to the Egyptians as *imset* and was found in the tomb of Tutankhamun to prevent an upset stomach on his journey to the afterlife. The flowering stalk promotes milk flow and has a tranquil effect.

**Legend and lore**

The ancient Greeks used dill seeds to stop hiccoughs, a practice that brought dill to North America with the Puritans. They were later named "meeting seeds," believed to ward off evil spirits during church services. The evil eye could be "stayed" by dill. Magicians used dill seed to break spells and old maids brewed them in love potions.

## Echinacea, *pupura,* originating in Kansas, Louisiana, and Texas

This herb is the most widely known nontoxic blood purifier in the herbal kingdom. The flower essence, known as the "purple coneflower," will be most beneficial in purifying our mental thoughts. A refined sense of judgment and understanding will prevail in the personality.

*My thoughts are pure.*

**Historical uses**

The Native Americans squeezed the flowers to produce a juice applied to burns. The three-year-old root is antibiotic. The seeds are toxic and can be hallucinogenic.

**Legend and lore**

Echinacea is grown in the garden to attract butterflies and bees. It is so beloved by the Native Americans, it's known as the "rose of the plains."

## Foxglove, *Digitalis pupurea,* native to Europe

Foxglove attracts fulfilling personal relationships, enhancing compassion and sensitivity for others. When the heart is right, for and against are forgotten. It is indicated when the heart beats out of control or poor circulation is detected. For cardiovascular congestion or irregularity, it may combine well with daffodil. To attract good working relationships, combine foxglove with India hawthorn and wisteria.

*My soul cries out for that which fulfills me.*

**Historical uses**

The flowers have a slightly diuretic effect. The leaves are both medicinal and toxic as a heart stimulant (digitalis).

**Legend and lore**

The freckles on foxglove flowers are believed to be the footprints of fairies, which loaned the blooms to wily foxes to cover their paws. Thus, the fox could sneak into the chicken house without alarming the prey.

## French lavender, Lavendula hybrid Reverchon, originated in France

French lavender helps us appreciate and focus on the blessings in our lives. It also helps release the need for "bigger and better," a bigger house, a better car. French lavender steers the focus away from the material world into the gifts of the heart and spirit. Combine French lavender with Christmas cactus and apply it to the temples for headache or the outside of the ears to decrease congestion and earaches.

*I find pleasure in simplicity.*

**Historical uses**
The flowers are used as a disinfectant for topical wounds and as natural smelling salts. The essential oil blend of several lavenders is used in European hospitals as aromatherapy to replace sleeping pills. In China, it is called "white flower oil." The aroma is sedative and relaxing. The flowering stalks can be rolled in ribbon to make a decorative sachet and moth repellent. French lavender blooms frequently.

**Legend and lore**
French lavender is the herb of love and was thought to be an aphrodisiac. However, wearing lavender on the head was believed to keep one chaste. The conquering Romans planted it throughout Europe to remind them of loved ones. The scent is both romantic and healing for the heart.

## Gaillardia, *Pulchella,* originated in North America, native to Texas

This Texas wildflower enhances our determination to succeed despite obstacles. Gaillardia lightens the "stubborn" personality with the joy of overcoming. The essence can be associated with the oldest part of the immune system, the macrophage activity. When these "dinosaurs of the immune system" move into action, nothing can stop them. They can change shapes, squeeze through tissues and intracellular spaces, and engulf foreign or damaged cells. Macrophages disintegrate their foe by showering them with strong enzymes and hydrogen peroxide made within the body.

Gaillardia promotes our latent ability to overcome opposition and difficulties no matter what obstacles confront us. We will take with us the joy of completion.

*I meet every challenge.*

**Historical uses**
The flowers are used as a dye plant in Native American weaves.

**Legend and lore**
Settlers named gaillardia "Indian blanket" because it was used as a dye plant

and woven into beautiful blankets. The design of the flower was replicated in the blankets.

## Gardenia, *Rubiaceae uasmincides,* originated in China

The gardenia personality desires to integrate the personal life with future goals. This harmony includes healthy personal habits, supportive relationships, and freedom from emotional complications. Vision now stimulates long-range planning. A powerful spiritual force has awakened deeper values that can be used to benefit many. The desire to uplift humankind brings out talents in teaching, writing, and speaking.

Concepts are translated into reality, where only ideas had previously existed. This visionary is inspired into constructive action. The personality is now aware of what has been holding him back.

This creativity extends into the home and family. A loving atmosphere nourishes inspiration and achievement for all concerned. Existing commitments are deepened. The personality becomes more aware of the family's needs and desires and acts upon them. It is the essence used to attract a soulmate.

The gardenia personality envisions plans to make dreams come true.

*I can plan and fulfill my future.*

### Historical uses

The flowers are used to reduce inflammation in the intestines and heat in the body. Gardenia is called the "happiness herb" in China and is used as a mood elevator.

### Legend and lore

Gardenia is known as a flower of grace and artistic merit. The scent alone is a legend.

## Garden mum, *Chrysanthemum morifolium,* originated in China

Garden mum essence relates to the occasional critical nature of the personality. The essence helps remove blocked energy and lighten critical thoughts.

The garden mum personality may be wishing the worst would happen to everyone — under his breath, of course. Whatever may not have pleased this person is always someone else's fault. This part of the personality is looking for a scapegoat or feels revengeful due to an unfortunate situation. Critical and bitter thoughts may affect the liver and gallbladder, blocking energy otherwise used to secrete the enzyme bile, to separate fats.

Garden mum will enhance the feeling of love for mankind, including oneself. It will then allow one to accept everyone as they are and encourage people to manifest their true human potential. Garden mums are natural researchers as well as counselors.

*I am the channel of Love.*

**Historical uses**

*Chrysanthemum morifolium* flowers stimulate blood flow, improve vision, and treat liver weakness. They help relieve night blindness, menstrual disorders, nervous complaints, and digestive disorders. And improve potency. In Japan, chrysanthemum treats skin infections and hypertension.

The Orientals eat the *morifolium* variety, blanched and seasoned with vinegar in salads.

**Legend and lore**

The yellow garden mum was cultivated in China prior to 500 B.C. It was the imperial flower of Japan and was symbolized in the rising sun emblem on their flag. The Japanese call it the "flower of long life and happiness." Mums have decorated Buddhist altars for more than a century.

## Iberis Candytuft, *Sempervirens,* originated in southern Europe

Iberis candytuft essence encourages regeneration and self-healing by activating the light inherent in each cell. This will enhance a balanced mineral pattern within the cell, allowing the tissues to be bathed with nutrients. It works well with crossandra to facilitate transition and lifestyle changes.

**Historical uses**

The dazzling white flowers are believed to attract fairies and beneficial elementals.

**Legend and lore**

The tiny flowers of candytuft are believed to house families of fairies.

## India Hawthorn, *Raphiolepsis indica,* originated in southern China

Pink India hawthorn works with group karma to help us love in deed and by example to *all* living things. It accents an impersonal love and helps dispel confusion in our mind. This one works well with yellow rose and wisteria to facilitate our actions to flow from the Heart that beats as One. Combined with Kolanchoe it will help us love all as One. It also helps attract those who will enhance our career, home life, and community.

*I accept unconditional love.*

**Historical uses**

The flowers were steeped in wine to increase cardiovascular circulation. White varieties contain quercetin, and the effect is vasodilating and hypotensive. Due to its action on the heart, it is not recommended in large doses as an infusion or tea. A little goes a long way to control high and low blood pressure by improving the pumping action of the heart.

**Legend and lore**

Hawthorns were named "Mayflower" because they bloom in May. In fact, the Mayflower ship that brought colonists to America was named after the hawthorn. Ancient Greco-Romans believed hawthorn brought hope and placed it in babies' cradles to keep evil away.

## Indian Paintbrush, *Castelleja,* native to Texas

The Indian paintbrush personality is ready to bring the Light of the Unconscious into everyday life. The eternal self and personality have joined together to celebrate the divinity of the ordinary. Every challenge is met with a consciousness of success.

Health, career, and relationships change and accelerate from the experience of enlightenment. The person is alive with childlike joy and innocence. He has traveled through the fear of external changes to know that success shoots from the fountain of life within. This individual takes every day and makes it a miracle.

From darkness, light is born. Freedom has burst from a liberated consciousness as a positive attitude transforms into one of wonder. The individual knows what it wants to attract and creatively express. An Indian paintbrush personality goes within to plant and nurture the seeds of truth from an attitude united with meaning and purpose. Life becomes a vision from within as action is balanced with the wisdom of a sage; success is the natural outcome.

*I make every day a miracle.*

**Historical uses**

This is a Texas wildflower of many colors and varieties. In central Texas, it blooms orange in May, right after the violet bluebonnets. The flowers are difficult to naturalize in the garden from seed because they are parasitic on grass roots. Grow them in a field or near an ornamental grass.

**Legend and lore**

The Indian paintbrush was originally purple until a young Native American child went from field to meadow painting them orange, yellow, and red to attract hummingbirds. And they do!

## Iris, *pallida,* originated in Asia (the bearded iris originated in Germany)

Iris essence releases energy to balance the mental strain of incorrect creative expression. The personality can then become clear on how to use his talents for financial success in a way most beneficial to humanity.

The iris personality can be most easily defined as predominately left-brain, logical, and analytical. He has an explanation for everything.

Iris essence stimulates the pleasure center of the hypothalamus, balancing the energy in the posterior hypothalamus to reduce violent behavior and regulating blood pressure, temperature, and breathing.

The iris personality will then release latent creative abilities and feel free to entertain associates with his carefree, humorous personality. An uninhibited iris personality will discover it is a natural entertainer with all the qualities of a celebrity.

*I bloom, therefore, I am.*

**Historical uses**

Iris flowers have a delicate scent that attracts birds and flying insects to the garden. Irises are cultivated in romantic gardens.

**Legend and lore**

Iris is named after Isis, the Greek goddess of the rainbow, bringing messages from heaven. The French royalty chose it for their emblem, the *fleur de lis*.

## Japanese magnolia, *Magnolia verbanica,* originated in Japan

The essence of Japanese magnolia aids the dependent part of the personality to create an atmosphere of security. It helps the personality accept responsibility for its talents and dispense with a feeling of being used. The victim becomes the victor as separateness is replaced by a feeling of independence.

*I blend the opposites within me.*

**Historical uses**

Japanese magnolia is a longevity tonic flower used to reduce pain in Oriental medicine. The flowers are brewed as a tea.

**Legend and lore**

The Japanese call this the "tulip tree" or "cucumber tree" and use the beautiful February buds in Chabana flower arrangements.

## Jasmine, *Jasminum nudiflorum,* originated in India

The jasmine personality is the loner of society. The individual may have been the black sheep of the family as he or she rebelled against authority, finding it difficult to get along well with others.

A rebellious nature may result in bone fractures due to accidents, osteoporosis, or deficiencies in nutrients, such as vitamin D and calcium. Jasmine essence allows the feeling of alienation and dualism in the personality to be replaced by a larger overview of life. As the individual develops the perspective of a sage, he is likely to find peace in his environment, as the tension of isolation and opposition gives way to diplomacy. Jasmine essence may be beneficial when inner conflict overcomes the natural rhythm of an individual.

*Where Order reigns, I am.*

**Historical uses**

Jasmine flowers are prepared as a tea to reduce tumorous growths in Ayurvedic medicine. The fragrance of the flowers is used both as an antidepressant and aphrodisiac. The flowers are also used to scent desserts and green tea. An infusion of the flower in distilled water can be used as eyewash.

**Legend and lore**

Jasmine is the symbol of sweetness and grace in Christianity. In India, it is called the "queen of the night" because of its alluring aroma released after dark.

## Kalanchoe, *Blossfeldiana,* originated in Madagascar

This essence helps correct the ingrained image of dualism creating the illusion of opposites. This is the good-or-bad, black-or-white consciousness. The split consciousness then creates a self and a not-so-good self, or non-self. The personality will compensate by either trying to escape or to control the environment. The result is separation where a complement is necessary for polarity.

The personality may accept only one side of life that corresponds to his ideals or desires. This preconceived illusion can replace the inner vision of continuity. Kalanchoe will aid a receptive mind to polarize logic and intuition. Kalanchoe works well with Indian paintbrush and onion to mend illusions and preconceived notions. It helps us see our own blind spots.

*I see only Beauty.*

**Historical uses**

This is a tropical pot plant grown to brighten every room. The flower attracts butterflies when it's aired on patios and porches. The orange and bright pink colors are native to the tropics.

**Legend and lore**

The broad lobed leaves were named "elephant's ears" or "Napoleon's hat" due to their shape.

## Knotted marjoram, *Marjorana hortensis,* originated in the Mediterranean

In our personality development, marjoram enhances forethought and working out details when change is indicated. Specifically, marjoram enhances clarity that can avoid premature actions when the situation calls for a calculated transformation. It's beneficial in overcoming compulsive eating habits.

Knotted marjoram essence works with the skin's ability to produce intereukin. Interleukin signals mass production of helper T cells, an antibody in the immune system's external defense. Marjoram has antiseptic properties in its volatile oils that are protective to the skin.

*I think before I act.*

**Historical uses**

Wreaths crowned a marrying couple for prosperity and fecundity in Greek and Roman times. During colonial times, the flowering plant was brewed to bring on menses and was worn in the bosom to calm the senses. Today, the essential oil of flowering stalks is used for female complaints, aches, sprains, and melancholy. The flowers attract butterflies and bees; the seedheads feed the birds.

**Legend and lore**

Marjoram was a favorite of Aphrodite, the goddess of beauty and love. It was known as the "herb of a happy marriage."

## Lantana, *Camana,* is native to the southern U.S. and Texas

Lantana essence aids the oversensitive personality that is easily hurt and basically shy. The individual is often sensitive to common allergens. As a child, the personality often withdraws into mental and artistic pursuits.

Lantana essence will vibrate with the hidden dynamic side of his personality. The personality is likely to become more assertive and feel less threatened by sensitivities. The person may continue to be quiet and artistic, but his opinions will command respect. Any anger that is disguised by sensitivity will abate and sneezing may cease.

*I am as dynamic as a newborn star.*

**Historical uses**

The flowering plant was made into a tea to bathe scabies and leprosy. The flowers and leaves can be brewed into an effective insect repellent. The berries are toxic. The medicinal property of lantana is lantanine, and is used in minute quantities as a tea for fever, bronchitis, and bronchial spasms.

**Legend and lore**

The unpleasant scent of lantana flowers tells birds the berries are harmful.

## Lemon grass, *Cynopogan citratus,* originated in Southeast Asia

Lemon grass essence will aid the individual who feels rejected by its parents. By releasing the need to be nurtured by parents, an adult will begin self-nurturing in the ways only the individual can discover.

Very often the lemon grass personality will expand rejection from parents into a general "love hurts" belief and manifest painful relationships throughout life. Lemon grass essence will not only ease the pain, but also change the attitude of the individual. Perception of love and choice of those to love deeply will become more refined. As the personality learns to trust on an individual basis, it will reach out to love and embrace humanity.

*I am the Child of the Universe, a Starburst of Joy.*

**Historical uses**

It treats coughs, colds, and coughs that produce blood. It yields a very anti-septic essential oil that improves circulation, muscle tone, skin renewal, and digestion. It can be diluted in water to reduce airborne virus and bacteria and treat athlete's foot and acne. Lemon grass oil is the source of commercial lemon flavoring in the food, cosmetic, and household product industries. The scent repels mosquitoes and fleas.

**Legend and lore**

In India, lemon grass is planted in long rows to keep tigers away.

## Ligustrum, *Oleacea privit lucidum,* originated in Japan, Korea, China

Ligustrum addresses the inability to assert oneself and express anger often manifesting as apathy or haughtiness. The deep grief that accompanies such emotions may cause a leakage of the vital life force, resulting in fatigue and lack of spontaneity.

Ligustrum essence helps release repressive feelings, allowing the personality to be assertive and express anger constructively and without guilt. Expression will become spontaneous, instead of thinking of an appropriate answer hours later. The personality will eventually become more naturally optimistic and encourage others in their time of need.

*I am a Symbol of Creation, self-confidence, and self-esteem.*

**Historical uses**

Ligustrum is a fragrant flower used in love potions.

**Legend and lore**

Bees have their first honey-making lessons on the fragrant blooms of the southern ligustrum.

## Lilac, *Syringa vulgaris,* originated in southeastern Europe

Lilac essence will allow a person to be forgiving. In other words, a lilac personality may hold grudges. The typical expression of a lilac vibration would be, "I'll forgive you, but I'll never forget what you did to me." So, by taking lilac, one is able to release the past and progress into a future without revenge. Both for and against are forgotten.

To truly forgive is an act of love. The result of taking lilac is that it also promotes self-love. We can only love others as much as we love ourselves.

The lilac personality expects too much from itself and is very unforgiving. The individual usually suffers from stress patterns prone to perfectionists. Lilac will change this attitude and start life on a more fulfilling and constructive basis, seeing all of mankind as a reflection of oneself.

*I am the tenderness of First Love.*

**Historical uses**

The flowers have been used to reduce fever. The heady scent is said to attract a first love.

**Legend and lore**

The lilac was once a bulb that grew to reach the heavens and colored its flowers from the rainbow.

## Lily, *Liliaceae longiflorum, Japanese L. gignanteum,* originated in Japan

One is likely to recognize the lily personality by the absence of fingernails. This individual is always biting them because of anxiety about the future.

The lily personality has not realized that present thoughts and actions create the future. It feels fearful because it is not aware of being in control. The personality is likely to be first in line to watch the Dow Jones dip, wringing his hands, and wishing he had some nails left to chew. The lily is not anxious about the undefined or unknown future, but the outcome of everyday affairs.

The greatest fear is losing control. Releasing anxiety about the future will boost the immune system of the individual and build better resilience.

*I am the self-control that holds the key to my future.*

**Historical uses**

The flowers are cooked in soups and teas to nurture the nervous system and reduce hysteria.

**Legend and lore**

Lily is the flower of purity and innocence, the joy of resurrection. It represents angelic powers and trust in God. In Greco-Roman myth, the lily sprang from the milk of Hera and is the flower of Diana, representing chastity.

## Lobelia, *Inflata,* originated in South Africa

Lobelia teaches us to create boundaries with others. It is indicated for those who have difficulty saying no. Combine it with snapdragon for discernment and with Country marilou to reduce the need to please others or be liked by peers.

*My boundaries allow me to say no.*

**Historical uses**

The flowers are steeped in vinegar or alcohol to make a compress for bruised and itchy skin. The leaves were smoked by Native Americans to relieve asthma and whooping cough. It is toxic even in small doses and should be handled only by professionals.

**Legend and lore**

Lobelia was named "Indian tobacco" and is believed to be similar to nicotine. Native Americans laid flowers in an arguing couple's bed to rekindle love.

## Magnolia, *grandiflora,* originated in the southern United States

Magnolia represents the personality who lacks self-appreciation. Magnolia will encourage the person to enjoy and know oneself as a fully integrated personality. The magnolia personality can often be recognized by an "I don't deserve it" attitude.

It is no surprise that a person with this attitude fails to assimilate nutrients and proteins in the small intestine. The individual doesn't believe it deserves to be healthy.

Once the attitude change begins, this personality will begin to prosper and grow like a breast-fed infant. The appearance and manner of dress will improve, as the personality becomes extroverted. Life will become a game one can skillfully play and achievements will be all of our reward.

*I appreciate myself for what I am.*

**Historical uses**

Flower buds increase menstrual flow and decrease facial neuralgia and pain. The open flower is used to strengthen the stomach and liver and improve digestion.

**Legend and lore**

Magnolia is the first fossilized flower and may be the first bloom of the angiosperms. The shape and color of the flowers have not changed in more than one hundred million years.

## Marigold, *Tagetes patula*, originated in Africa

Marigold essence will release guilt, identity issues, and confusion around sexuality.

Marigold essence can also aid those affected by frigidity and impotence, although other attitudes should be acknowledged, such as an inability to give oneself to another and fear of failure.

Marigold also aids people who had confusion about their sexual role or identity in childhood. Marigold will balance both the male and female aspects in each personality, allowing creativity and receptivity to flow uninterrupted.

*Through Knowledge, I recognize my identity.*

**Historical uses**

Marigold flowers are being used to treat certain cancers, especially those affecting the skin and lymph nodes. They can be infused to stimulate bile flow and have been used to treat alcoholic sclerosis. All flowers of the tagetes species can be used to make a yellow dye.

**Legend and lore**
Marigold is the flower of Krishna and a Chinese symbol of longevity, "the flower of ten thousand years." "Ten thousand" represents the Tao, the source of heavenly blessings and all existence. The marigold was sacred to the agricultural gods of Ecuador and Peru before the Inca ruled.

## Meadow sage, *Salvia clevelandi,* originated in the northern Mediterranean

This essence helps us express strong emotions, such as anger, without transgression or vindictiveness. A true sage is not afraid to express emotions or feel with the senses, but is ever watchful not to be caught up in their extremes. By balancing extremes, we are constantly renewed. Meadow sage essence enhances enzymes that dissolve and break down bacteria's protein sheath, allowing natural immunity to respond appropriately.

*I choose my words wisely.*

**Historical uses**
Native Americans steeped the flowers of blue meadow sage in boiled water and the steam was inhaled to alleviate a throbbing headache.

**Legend and lore**
In Texas, this plant is called "mealy sage" due to the silver fuzz covering the stem and leaves.

## Mexican bush sage, *Salvia leukantha,* originated in Mexico

Mexican bush sage enhances our ability to be unique. It is indicated for those adversely affected by peer pressure. Mexican bush sage gives us permission to be who we really are, combining well with Aquilegia columbine to help us drop the roles others give to us. It is also indicated for red, itchy skin, when combined with *salvia.*

*I enjoy being unique.*

**Historical uses**
Flowers bloom into a beautiful purple plume that attracts bees and predator insects.

**Legend and lore**
Mexican bush sage naturalized in Texas by following its friends, the bees and butterflies.

## Mexican hat, *Ratibida columnaria,* originated in Mexico

Mexican hat helps bring in prosperity, combining well with Indian paintbrush for a success consciousness. Mexican hat will work on an unconscious level to activate latent talents or dissolve financial blocks to success.

*I bloom with the abundance of nature.*

### Historical uses

Flowers were used in love potions by Native Americans. The bright orange flower was also worn to attract a lover.

### Legend and lore

Mexican hat used to be a daisy until it pulled down its petals to prevent its face from freckling in the hot sun.

## Mexican oregano, *Poliomentha longiflora,* originated in Mexico

Mexican oregano essence enables us to quickly respond to new situations, grasping what is necessary and responding properly. In the body, Mexican oregano initiates chemical bacterial inhibitors, such as lactic and oleic acids, to lubricate and cleanse the skin by activating sebum and sweat. It activates the skin's immune response to ward off bacterial, fungal, and viral invasion.

*I quickly respond to new situations.*

### Historical uses

The blooms attract hummingbirds and produce an essential oil similar to oregano in aroma and use. It is a native in Mexico and Texas with beautiful tubular, lavender flowers that can be soaked in water (covered) for several hours, strained, and enjoyed in a refreshing bath or foot soak.

### Legend and lore

When Texas seceded from Mexico, many Mexican families were split apart. They grew this fragrant herb in Texas in remembrance of their loved ones far away who loved the color of the beautiful lavender flowers and used the leaves to flavor their meats.

## Morning glory, *Convolvulacea,* originated in South and Central America

Morning glory aids the personality living in the illusion of the golden age of the past. This is often the result of feeling confined to an unpleasant reality in the present. The personality is unwilling to change the unpleasantness of the present situations, so he or she reverts to happier memories of the past. No matter what the present environment, the morning glory personality wants to romanticize a better past.

The only way to change the illusions of this personality is to have something to look forward to with enthusiasm. Morning glory is the essence that will fire the flame for the future through progressive thoughts and faith in oneself that change will always allow opportunity for advancement.

As enthusiasm increases, circulation in the physical body will increase and flow with regularity, as all channels for elimination will release the past and regenerate.

*I welcome change as the challenge of the present moment.*

**Historical uses**

Morning glory is grown in romantic gardens, on a trellis, or near a doorway.

**Legend and lore**

The morning glory represents the season of autumn and rebirth. In the garden, it never seems to die. The Latin name *convolvare* means to "entwine" or "bind." It is also known as "bindweed" in its most common genera, and the flower of obstinacy.

## Moss rose, *Portulaccea floreplens,* originated in Brazil

Moss rose essence affects the personality who can't get enough in life. It may pertain to money, love of another, or possessions. This is a person who believes needs will be provided by other people or possessions. Once the individual acquires something or someone, it becomes very possessive.

The need to acquire more will produce anxiety and a feeling of lack. It may also produce overweight since this is the type of person who can't push himself away from the table until satisfied that the plate is clean. In the physical body, this person may be affected by irregular glucose regulation and poor digestion of starches and fats. Moss rose will enable this personality to look within to provide sufficient needs.

*I am the abundant source of wealth.*

**Historical uses**

Moss rose only blooms in sunshine. Brazilians wore the flowers during the day to increase energy.

**Legend and lore**

The colorful moss rose carpets the floors of fairies. They are rolled up at night to be laid fresh again when the sun comes out.

## Black mushroom, *Shitaki,* originated in Japan

Black mushroom essence affects everyone who may resist the flow of life. This insecurity causes people to plant their feet firmly on the ground and stay there. Everybody and everything else seems to be changing.

The most likely physical symptoms would manifest in stiffness of the feet, calves, ankles, and spine, including the neck. Emotionally, one may be resisting leaving a marriage or changing careers.

Black mushroom will enable the person to become more open and clearly perceive what is best in life, without anxiety. This person will then become an example to others, showing how easy it is to adapt to change without missing an advantageous opportunity.

*I am the free-flowing Abundance of Life.*

**Historical uses**

Shitaki is an immune-stimulant fungus that improves circulation and lowers blood pressure. It reduces free radical damage and is beneficial for cancer treatment. In China, it is used for anemia, diabetes, and allergies. The therapeutic property is found in the substance known as lentinan.

**Legend and lore**

Mushrooms growing in rings were called "fairy rings," the place believed to be where fairies danced. To the Chinese Taoist, shitaki was the "elixir of life" associated with longevity.

## Narcissus, *Cyclamineus,* originated in Portugal

The narcissus personality is withdrawn and introverted. The individual is usually artistic and talented in many ways, but lacks the desire to share with others. This person has a tendency to "freeze" people out of life and live in another world.

Balancing the energy in the emotional limbic center will release more energy to the cerebellum of the brain. This controls warmth and affection, and allows one to experience more pleasure, due to a mediated pathway to the neural connections in the cerebellum.

Often, the narcissus personality was deprived of touch and rocking movement during early infancy. Utilizing touch and movement therapy will enhance the feeling of pleasure and security desired by the narcissus personality, and will aid in fully integrating with society.

*I am a Peacemaker, harmonizing the efforts of man.*

**Historical uses**

Narcissus is a flower associated with Christmas. The bulbs are forced to bloom six to eight weeks prior to the holiday season by planting them in a dish or pot.

**Legend and lore**

The Orientals grow narcissus for the New Year celebration as a sign of good fortune. It is sacred to Narcissus, Hades, and Demeter. The intoxicating scent caused death to the vain.

## Onion, *Allium cepa,* originated in Egypt

Onion essence reduces prejudices of the personality, limiting potentials from narrow-minded opinions. Onion will allow the individual to become more tolerant and compassionate towards others and less critical of others' views and habits, becoming a better listener. Becoming more emotionally supportive will allow the outspoken nature to mature into a natural champion of the people.

*With an open mind, I become more tolerant of others.*

**Historical uses**

Onion was cut, warmed, and applied to burns or to the chest to abate colds. The flowering stalks were cut and put in the room of a convalescent as an antiseptic. Men bathed in onion juice as a contraceptive.

**Legend and lore**

Frontiersmen located Native American camps by following the smell of onion. The onion is considered unique because it flowers in the waning of the moon. Onion flowers best in drier climates and represents unity, the cosmos, and the many as one.

## Orchid, dancing lady, *Oncidium spacelatum,* originated in Mexico

The orchid personality needs to make peace with the past. This is the personality with all the skeletons in the closet, silently punishing itself for the past, yet unwilling to admit misdeeds to oneself and others. The person is usually a high achiever, always trying to compensate for past failures by putting an emotional bandage on them. The biggest mistake is accepting others' judgments of oneself and one's deeds.

The orchid personality may suffer from numbness and nerve degeneration. Orchid will release the feeling of past inadequacy and allow the spinal energy to activate and consistently flow to all areas of the body. Then, the orchid personality will see past "failures" as steps to success.

The individual will become less of a workaholic and more interested in loved ones and the community. A naturally high energy level will then be enjoyed by the entire environment.

*I make peace with the past and I accept the Grace of the Present Moment.*

**Historical uses**

Oncidium treats skin rashes and is used to reduce arthritic pain and as a tea the flowers have been brewed to treat impotence.

**Legend and lore**

The orchid is a symbol of harmony, the Perfect Man, and the reclusive scholar.

## Pansy, *Viola tricolor*, wild pansy of Central Asia

Pansy essence aids one with a deep sense of grief over the loss of a loved one. Grief often affects the kidney and adrenal function and the elimination of waste products. Pansy essence aids in transcending grief, which then adds energy to the kidneys for the elimination of toxins.

Although there is no way to completely replace a loved one, the personality will learn to transfer the love to someone else or a worthwhile project. The personality needs to love and feel appreciated. Pansy personalities have a generous, loving nature and should look for several outlets for their compassion. The pansy personality should also seek ways to replace the part of themselves they feel has been lost with their loved one.

*I choose to bloom in Faith and transcend the illusion of Death.*

### Historical uses

Pansy flowers were brewed as a tea for upper respiratory congestion and to prevent infantile convulsions from high fever. For external use, flowers were steeped in oil and applied to skin ulcers and cancers. As a folk remedy, the flowers were also used as a sedative and blood purifier, brewed as a tea, or made into a wine. The Celts made a tea from the petals for a love potion.

### Legend and lore

The French word *pensee* is the word for thought. The three colors, yellow, white, and purple represented memories, loving thoughts, and souvenirs of separated lovers. It became known as "heartsease," and was used in love potions for forlorn lovers. The heart-shaped petals were believed to heal a broken heart. In early Christian times, the pansy, originally yellow, white, and purple represented the trinity.

Long ago, pansies had an aroma that would bring admirers from all over to smell them. It upset the pansies that the admirers trampled the surrounding grass. In answer to a prayer, God took the aroma and left the pansy great beauty.

## Penta, *Pentas lanceolata,* originated in Africa and Arabia

Penta essence affects the personality prone to withholding love. This person is often thought to be inconsiderate of others or selfish. The individual has learned through a painful past experience to be self-reliant, feeling no need for others.

The penta personality may suffer from lower blood pressure, vertigo, or stress. The past experiences of "love hurts" suppress the energy flow from within. Penta essence is designed to ease the pain, and allow a feeling of well-being and love for oneself.

Once the penta personality feels safe about loving, this personality can be a delightful mate. The personality will be an ideal example of how to depend more from within for his or her needs, without draining loved ones for nurturing.

*I am lovable and it is safe to love.*

**Historical uses**

Penta flowers attract butterflies and beneficial insects.

**Legend and lore**

Pentas are known as the Egyptian "star flower," believed to be fallen stars from the heavens.

## Peppermint, *Mentha peperita*, is a cross-hybrid from the Mediterranean

Peppermint aids the individual who believes in loss and lives in fear of losing loved ones, possessions, health, and security. The individual usually has an inner conflict related to an incomplete relationship with the mother. The emotions are dependent on external conditions, over which there is little control.

Absence of control in one's life can result in an incomplete digestion of protein, the building block of life. Energy in the intestine can become blocked and locked into a pattern of pain. Essence of peppermint will build an attitude of confidence and control, which will affect all aspects of life. The personality will be able to visualize a future with desires fulfilled. Life experiences will feel safe, enabling one to plan a future without lack and limitation.

*I am the realization of my heart's desires.*

**Historical uses**

Peppermint treats nausea, upset stomach, and colic. The flowers were decocted into an oil-based ointment for sore muscles. Europeans chewed the flowers to freshen their breath. The aroma and volatile oils are very stimulating. It is best used at least two hours before bedtime as a digestant, analgesic for muscle pain, headaches, and nausea, and to increase concentration. The properties are antiseptic, antiviral, and diaphoretic, inducing sweat.

**Legend and lore**

Mentha was once a nymph loved by Pluto. His jealous wife, Prosperine, turned Mentha into a mint we now enjoy as tea.

## Periwinkle, *Vinca rosea,* originated in Asia Minor

Periwinkle essence is valuable to anyone who wishes to clear past experiences. Past experiences may affect the energy in any organ. Therefore, what we focus on in spirit will become the past with which we identify. Periwinkle will clear the vibration from any experiences that may be holding us from completing the evolutionary changes destined in this time. Our goals will become clearer as we begin to have a larger overview of life and the destiny of humankind.

*I am complete in the present moment.*

**Historical uses**

The purple flowers are pellatized and made into the chemotherapy agents vincristine and vinblastine. The flowers were used in Europe as a hemostatic, arresting bleeding, as well as an antihypertensive and hypoglycemic agent. In Cuba, Puerto Rico, and Jamaica, an extract of the flowers has been used for eye-wash for many centuries.

**Legend and lore**

"Violette des sorciers" is a protective flower hung in doorways to ward off evil spirits. It is associated with death and grown or strewn on graves. In Tuscany, it covers graves of children and is called "death's flower." The flower was once believed to increase fertility and was used in many love potions. Children tied the flowering plant around their calves to prevent cramping as they walked.

## Pine, *Pinus sylvestes,* originated in Japan

The pine personality only remembers the mistakes of the past and experiences guilt, punishment, and pain. This reaction to life will create unusual stress in the body, resulting in symptoms of hypoadrenia. Fatigue (due to lack of absorbed minerals and proteins), aches, nervousness, and mood fluctuations are payments on the debts for not forgiving past mistakes. What is lacking is admiration for achievements.

As the pine personality realizes the way to overcome the past is in present positive thoughts and actions, nothing and no one will impede progress. This individual is conscious of how to help others. It has truly learned valuable lessons from past misfortunes. Inner strengths and tenacity will lead to a future of fulfilling destiny. The individual will become someone who will encourage his fellow men to overcome limitations.

*I bury the past and look forward to the future.*

**Historical uses**

Male cones are dried and rubbed between the hands, releasing pollen to increase blood cell production. The cones have been used to flavor beer and wine, such as the Greek *retsina.* The needles were used as mattress stuffing to repel lice and fleas.

**Legend and lore**

Pine represents a sacred tree of paradise, decorated at Christmas with gold and silver bells and ornaments with a sacred bird in the branches. Pine is sacred to Attis, Cybele Atargatis. The cone is a symbol of fertility in Eurasian cultures and the emblem of Confucius.

## Pink geranium, *Pelargonium x hortorum,* originated in South Africa

The pink geranium personality is tense and appears wired. One can readily imagine this person clenching his fists. However, the anger and intense emotions are sometimes so suppressed that the individual is totally unaware of them. The person may experience spasms in the colon or liver and gallbladder trouble.

Pink geranium will ease the emotional pain and enable the personality to laugh and enjoy life again. The individual will become aware of who (or what) is causing anger and takes steps to rectify the situation. Then it will learn to constructively release tension and anger without transferring anger to others. The energy will be used in leadership and organization. This is a very honest and straightforward person, reliable in carrying projects to completion.

*The decision is mine; I am created perfect.*

**Historical uses**

The flowers bloom best when watered with cool tea.

**Legend and lore**

Pink geraniums were originally brought to England from Reunion Island off the Coast of Africa. They are believed to have originated from the prophet Mohammed. One day he washed his clothes and spread them over a common mallow, which miraculously turned into a beautiful geranium as the clothes dried.

## Pink rose, a blend of *Rosa chinensis,* originated in China

The person most able to benefit from the pink rose essence has a "fat complex." The individual is forever trying a new diet, but unable to lose those last five pounds before putting on another five.

The personality often stuffs hurt feelings in its mouth. This individual often seeks love from others since there is little love for oneself. When love from others is lacking, the scales begin to tip in favor of the junk food economy.

Even if weight is within the normal range, this person may be obsessed with the thought of being fat.

Pink rose will support the individual to "think thin." Consequently, the individual will begin acknowledging and focusing on what can change. The pounds are likely to gradually fall off and stay off. When the negative energy is not fanned with more fuel, it will consume itself and the attitude will change.

*I am secure in my beautiful new image.*

**Historical uses**

Pink rose petals were steeped in animal grease by Native Americans to treat mouth ulcers and sores. American colonists as well as natives of India made a jam to treat anemia and fatigue. Flower petals were distilled to treat eye problems. The petals contain the bioflavonoid quercitin and a powerful anti-inflammatory antioxidant.

**Legend and lore**

The aroma of fresh roses is believed to enchant a lover. Cleopatra strew rose petals to win Mark Anthony's love.

## Poppy (Texas), *Hunnemannia fumaraefolia,* originated in Mexico

The poppy personality is both selfish to the degree of being demanding, and possessive to the point of hoarding. This type can be jealous and want what everyone else has, but is not very willing to share. The first spoken word was probably "mine!" It is natural for the personality to transition stages of possessiveness. However, this person may be plagued by confusion due to the way it perceives the environment. The personality feels a need to guard the territory and goods.

Poppy essence can aid the individual to perceive life as a window instead of a mirror. Selfishness will be replaced by a more constructive action, such as service to others in the community. This person has the potential of being just as generous as possessive.

*I am free to share myself.*

**Historical uses**

Poppies were used by Mexican Americans to attract unresponsive lovers. They also simmer the leaves and flowers in olive oil and apply it to make their hair shine and grow very thick.

**Legend and lore**

*Dormidera,* the "drowsy one," closes its flowers at night. Poppy is sacred to all nocturnal deities and represents fertility. The Greco-Roman period honored poppy as the emblem of Demeter, Ceres, Persephone, Venus, Hypnos, and Morpheus. It is also the symbol of the Great Mother.

## Evening Primrose, *Primulacceae,* native to the U.S. and Canada

The primrose personality is the most likely to reject love and be rejected because it is "not good enough." Lack of love may develop physically into diabetes and true hypoglycemia. Often, this personality felt rejected by a parent at a young age and doesn't understand why no one else can quite fulfill the needs in love.

This personality often has a very Byronic romantic and idealistic view of what love should be. Being loving to oneself is the best way to attract acceptable love from others. This joyfulness will naturally overflow into the environment. The personality will become more appreciative of love offered.

The primrose personality is naturally dynamic and, with the acceptance of love, finds success in any project, career, or relationship of interest.

*I am the vessel receiving every kind and loving thought.*

**Historical uses**

Flowers are used as a cough suppressant, cooked into syrup. They are used externally to soothe inflamed skin as a compress. The petals are sedative and soothe free radical-damaged skin and sunburn. A face wash will abate wrinkles and acne.

**Legend and lore**

The primrose is a Celtic fairy flower. It is a symbol of youthful purity. At night the primrose exudes a perfume that attracts the nocturnal sphinx moth as a pollinator. By daybreak, the flowers fade.

## Purple garden sage, *Salvia officinalis pupuracens,* originated in the Mediterranean

Purple garden sage helps us focus on what is valuable and true in love relationships. It is indicated when relationships are tested by external conditions. Sage is also helpful when sinusitis, viruses and profuse sweating or heat flashes occur. It combines well with onion and thyme to counteract viral complaints.

*I experience the true value of love.*

**Historical uses**

Flowers were steeped in wine to stop heavy menses and reduce menopausal symptoms and profuse sweating. In ancient times, sage flowers were used to reduce palsy (shaking), fever, and epilepsy. It was laid on graves with parsley as a promise of resurrection.

**Legend and lore**

Sage was believed to make men immortal. Sage growing on one's property foretold prosperity. It was sacred to Zeus in Greece and Jupiter in Rome. When Christianity overthrew the pagan gods, the power of sage remained.

To reveal the identity of a future lover, pick twelve sage leaves at night on Halloween and his or her shadow shall appear in the moonlight.

## Rain lily, *Cooperia pendunculata, zephyranthes candida* (fairy lily), originated in Argentina

Rain lily helps reconcile lovers and rifts in friendships. It is indicated when one feels slighted or left out in a relationship. Combine rain lily with Marquis Bocella to encourage a long-term relationship.

*I reconcile with friends and lovers.*

**Historical uses**

Rain lily blooms pure white and turns pink over several days. It is a summer flower destined to bloom after a rain.

## Legend and lore

Rain lilies only bloom after a summer rain to shelter the earthworms that were washed up by the rainwater.

## Ranunculus, *Asiaticel,* originated in Asia

Ranunculus essence assists the body to balance the energy from the central nervous system to the brain. It particularly affects the cerebellum and smooth muscle movement in the body. Imbalanced energy in the brain can manifest in many ways, such as muscle spasms, temperamental and emotional outbursts, and chemical imbalances.

During infancy, the child may have been deprived of movement and TLC. The child could have been abused or even born premature, but it is touch that will balance the nervous system.

*I am the Restoration of the Mind.*

### Historical uses

The flowers are grown in the garden each spring for their rich, colorful blooms. They attract pollinating, beneficial insects. An ointment of the flowers and stems is made to treat wounds and skin ulcers.

### Legend and lore

Ranunculus is the Persian buttercup. It traveled to Holland before finding its way to western Europe and America. When applied to rheumatic joints, it was believed to make them blister, producing a cure.

## Red carnation, *Carophyllaceae,* originated in Southern Europe and India

Red carnation has a profound effect on the individual feeling unworthy. The personality may desire success, love, and appreciation, but at some hidden level feels unable to accept it. This is the individual whom no one takes seriously. The vibration of the personality attracts the very response from others it does not desire. The individual is lonely and sets goals higher than talents can achieve. The personality has several great ideas and plans, but never quite follows them through to completion.

The red carnation personality's lymphatic system may be clogged with impurities, which adversely affects circulation. One result may even be hair loss or baldness. Toxicity in the blood, due to an impaired lymphatic system, short-circuits the electrical system and drains the body of its vital energy and blood flow. Stagnation leads to infection or growths.

Red carnation essence will enable the personality to manifest more through greater self-worth.

*I am worthy of having what I want.*

**Historical uses of red carnation**

The flowers were used to reduce fever and spice wine.

**Legend and lore**

Carnation is the flower of admiration, representing the Divine Mother. The flowers sprang from the tears of Mary as she saw her son, Jesus, carrying the cross. They are the flower of marriage and passionate love, the favorite of Greeks and Romans. Carnations were named "Jove's flower" in honor of the Greco-Romans' most revered god.

## Red malva, *Malva sylvestris mauritanica x hibiscus rosa chinensis,* originated in China

Red malva helps us stay centered and tuned in to receive guidance and chan-neling. This guidance will be focused on spiritual development. It combines well with dill and verbena to calm the desire to withdraw from others or "run away" from the challenges of society.

*My guidance comes from within.*

**Historical uses**

The flowers can be brewed as a tea like hibiscus or added to cold punch for color and flavor (red fruit punch!). Like other mallow, it is a favorite humming-bird and butterfly plant native to southern United States.

**Legend and lore**

Red malva was grown around graves in ancient Greek times, symbolizing safe passage to the underworld. Malva is a derivative of the Greek word *malays,* referring to its emollient or softening properties. It was eaten often by the Greek peasants who could not afford wheat for bread. It is a relative of the hollyhock, which originated in China.

## Red rose, a blend of *Rosa chinensis,* originated in China

Red rose essence affects all who have negative thoughts, but especially those who suffer from the many causes of depression. If standing in front of a mirror and observing the sad reflection doesn't lift gloom, then red rose will.

Red rose will aid people who even suffer only occasionally from depression. The time to stop using it is when negative thoughts no longer are a part of the normal thought process. Red rose often helps our moods as we complete transi-tions.

When enthusiastic action and joy in life replace sadness and gloom, humani-ty will no longer have excuses for not manifesting heaven on earth in abundance. Joy will no longer depend on external situations, but will come from the internal spring of Joy which dwells in each of us.

*I am the Joy of a full bloom.*

**Historical uses**

Red rose treats irregular menses and lower intestinal pain as a tea, jam, or syrup.

**Legend and lore**

The red rose is a universal symbol of love and war, romance and union. Its central point is the heart.

## Rose campion, *Verbascum thaspus rosa,* originated in Asia

Rose campion helps consolidate the bodily essence. It works for those with inherited weakness, strengthening the natural bodily defenses. Character development is completed by uprooting an old ingrained pattern that has been holding one back.

*I am liberated from outdated habits.*

**Historical uses**

The flowers were believed to heal bladder cysts or cystitis, and were brewed as a tea. The brackets holding the flowers looked like a bladder; therefore, it was used to heal the same. This was practiced in the Doctrine of Signatures, in which a plant was used to heal a part of the body it resembles.

**Legend and lore**

In colonial times, a traveler returning home could find no roses to bring his lady, only the roadside weed called campion. Upon picking it, the white flower turned into a beautiful rose hue and has attracted women ever since.

## Rosemary, *Rosemarinus officinalis, arp x Hills hardy,* originated in Texas

Rosemary encourages an endorphin release associated with pleasant memories. It helps release past painful memories when combined with bachelor's button and morning glory. When others misunderstand us, rosemary will bring out the best in us.

*I remember to share my joy with all forms of Nature.*

**Historical uses**

Flowers were distilled for eyewash. An oil was made to rub onto rheumatic limbs. The flowers were believed to make the old young again. They were decocted into an infusion for a bath. Bathing in rosemary water three times and anointing the head was believed to return youth to the aged. The flowers were also steeped in white wine for a facial. The steam distillation yields an essential oil that stimulates the central nervous system, increasing circulation and memory. The essential oil is also antifungal and antibacterial, stimulating an immune response and reducing muscle aches.

**Legend and lore**

Rosemary has been known for remembrance since early Greek times. Students wore it around their heads to help them study. In later times, brides wore it to remember their family, and the dead were buried with it as a symbol of remembrance. It is sacred to Ares, the Greek god of war, now referred to as Mars. During plagues, it was burned to cleanse the air.

A biblical myth states that rosemary's flowers turned blue when Mary spread the baby Jesus's clothes across it to dry.

Today, the flowering wreaths are worn by lovers at weddings and celebrations. In many cultures, it is burned as incense in a sick chamber to facilitate healing.

## Rose of Sharon, *Althea officinalis,* originated in Asia

The Rose of Sharon personality is highly creative and successful but finds it hard to stay on this planet. Sometimes life and the responsibilities just don't seem to be worth the effort. The personality's real desire is to transcend to a higher plane. Idealism often makes it difficult to adjust to the grosser aspects of reality, as the Rose of Sharon personality has high standards and is straightforward and honest.

Rose of Sharon essence will aid attraction to a worthwhile cause and utilize genius, manifesting heaven on earth before he travels on his endless journey to a higher plane. The Rose of Sharon personality can be prone to heart disease, which can be overcome with realization of rewards for efforts.

*Through selfless action, I attain the fulfillment of my Heart.*

**Historical uses**

The flowers are astringent and soothing to the skin. The flowers and petals can be made into a colorful tea that soothes the digestive tract and throat.

**Legend and lore**

The Greek word *althea* is derived from the verb "to heal." The name "Rose of Sharon" comes from the Song of Solomon, "I am the Rose of Sharon," the beautiful bride in the mystical union of humanity with the soul.

## Salvia, *Salvia coccinea,* scarlet sage of Texas

The salvia personality dislikes itself so much that one has manifested these beliefs physically. There is nothing essentially wrong with this person, except that he believes there is. The salvia personality will learn constructive attitudes about personality and physical appearance. The subconscious mirrors the beliefs of our perceptions into the body as well as the world we live in.

Salvia will enhance the individual's ability to change the self-image for the better. The joy will be contagious.

Physically, maladies such as acne, warts, and birthmarks will begin to heal as the individual learns to see itself as a worthwhile individual. The essence of salvia will support this attitude change; the body completes the rest.

*I am the Silhouette of Beauty.*

**Historical uses**

The flowers treat enlarged organs, parasitic infections, malaria, and dropsy. In Asia, the whole plant may be used in healing as a tea. In Texas, scarlet sage is grown as a groundcover. It's hardy and drought-tolerant in the dry regions and has to be mowed in the coastal, rainier regions. The flowers attract hummingbirds.

**Legend and lore**

Where the sage flourishes, so does the family.

## Salad burnet, *Poterium sanguisorba,* originated in Europe and the former Soviet Union

Salad burnet helps overcome depression from unfulfilled desires in relationships. When the romance fades, it's time to surrender to the nurturing essence of salad burnet. Melancholy lifts and nutrient uptake and dispersion increase, enhancing blood volume and neuromuscular response. It combines well with fortune's double yellow, daffodil, and chamomile as an anti-inflammatory heart tonic.

*I am calm and relaxed as life flows through me with ease.*

**Historical uses**

The flowers have been used to stop bleeding. It is a member of the rose family that is soothing to the skin. Traditionally, a wash was used for sunburn.

**Legend and lore**

The Latin name, *sanguisorba,* means blood absorber because it stops bleeding and heals wounds. Its unusual cucumber flavor was thought to stop plagues and pucker wounds.

## Shrimp, *Belaperone guttata,* originated in Mexico

Shrimp essence is designed for the individual who is searching for the expertise and opportunity to create a better life. On a deep level the individual is very self-competitive and attracts situations that encourage change. Shrimp essence will speed the process of change and allow creative ideas and actions to flow. This personality is not highly critical of others, but he is often more aware of others' achievements and assets.

Physically, the adrenal cortex is most affected by self-competition. The healing and aging processes are most impaired, while the immune system is unable to handle everyday stress. Shrimp essence will help the adrenals to function with maximum energy and release hormones into the bloodstream as needed.

*I like myself the way I am.*

**Historical uses**

The orange brackets look like a shrimp and produce a tiny white flower. The flower tastes very sweet and feeds hummingbirds and children alike.

**Legend and lore**

There's adequate nectar in one bloom to feed a large family of fairies (or Nimbus).

## Silver lace, *Polygonum auberti,* originated in the Himalayas of northern India

Silver lace is a relative of the famous Chinese herb Ho Shou Wu. It works with the body's ability to synthesize interferon, a protein that inhibits viral attacks against our character development. Silver lace helps us contemplate and learn from setbacks. Otherwise, we could confuse setbacks with failure and give in to difficulties. Growth is not linear, but cyclical. Silver lace helps us ride the waves of advance and retreat.

*Adversity spurs me on to greater accomplishments.*

**Historical uses**

This vine yields its beauty in the fall with curls of lacy white flowers. It attracts butterflies, wasps, and hummingbirds.

**Legend and lore**

The flowers of the silver lace vine are used to make bridal gowns for fairies smaller than Sweet Tooth.

## Soapwort, *Sporangia officinalis,* originated in central and southern Europe

Soapwort opens the channels for inner hearing to increase, uniting the personality with the inner wisdom of the "still, quiet voice" within. The essence helps the body detoxify fatty deposits, affecting cardiovascular health and lymphatic drainage. It combines well with pink rose to reduce cellulite or a feeling of heaviness.

*I bloom to the melody of Nature.*

**Historical uses**

The flowers were used by the Pennsylvania Dutch to make their beer foam.

Medicinally, it was used externally to treat skin eruptions, eczema, acne, and boils.

**Legend and lore**

The nickname "Bouncing Bet" is derived from an Old English pub, where barmaids (called "Bet") washed beer bottles with the soapy compounds of this plant.

## Spike Lavender, *Lavendula latifolia,* Originated on Mediterranean Coast

Spike lavender is a sedative. An essence from blooming stalks of spike lavender aids in practicing the art of cooperation. It is indicated when one or more individuals try to control a relationship or organization and for those who want to cooperate in group efforts. The essence is also indicated for those who sigh frequently or feel heaviness in the chest. It may help reduce bronchial spasms and lung congestion with its aromatic essence.

*Cooperation will attract the best for me.*

**Historical Uses**

The scent is used to cure insomniacs and make lions docile. It was used especially to "comfort the brains" during the sixteenth century. Queen Elizabeth I ate a conserve of the flowers with sugar for that purpose. A wine was made with the flowers to comfort the stomach and toilet water was used for cosmetic purposes. The flowering stalks repel flies and moths when laid in a drawer or hung from a closet. The essential oil of flowering stalks is used in lacquers and china paintings as well as aromatherapy.

**Legend and lore**

*Lavore* means "to wash," referring to the clean scent of lavender's perfume. It has been used as a perfume since early Phoenician and Egyptian times. Loving parents tied lavender flowers to a child's bed for protection during the night.

## Snapdragon, *Antirrhinum majus,* originated in northern Africa

The spring blooms of this flower increase the perception of judgment and discernment. It also helps us to recognize what brings us into alignment with others and to define guidelines that will clarify and refine our plans with reasonable expectations. Within the immune system, an attitude of discernment may enhance the regulation of T cells. T cells can become helper or suppressor cells, dependent upon the internal demands. An imbalance may lead to various autoimmune responses. Snapdragon can enhance our internal and external judgment, raising the consciousness of our immune system.

*I see with the Wisdom of discernment.*

**Historical uses**

The spring blooms herald the coming of yellow butterflies.

**Legend and lore**

When dragons breathe out the last of their fire, they turn into brightly colored snapdragons and cease to roar.

## Stock, *Matthiola incana rosea,* "gillyflower," originated in the Canary Islands

The person who will benefit from stock essence is tense, nervous and kinesthetic. The individual is often defined as being hyperactive. The stock personality desires movement, action, and pleasure, but its energy is easily distracted. Exhaustion is inevitable because the stock personality doesn't know how to pace its time and energy. Stock essence will help to slow the individual down to experience pleasure.

Kinesthetic people respond well to touch and may have been abruptly treated in infancy, or lacked sufficient soft, cuddly nurturing attention. As the individual learns to channel energy, it is able to complete fulfilling projects and takes time for relaxation. Stock individuals do well in jobs and hobbies requiring action. They feel grounded when exerting themselves in activities such as gardening, sports, and taking jobs that keep them moving or outside of an office.

*I am calm and relaxed and allow life to fulfill me.*

**Historical uses**

The flowers are hardy annuals that survive through the winter to bloom in the spring. They reseed to return to Mother Nature during the heat of summer. Grow them in fragrant or romantic gardens.

**Legend and lore**

Stock is an old-fashioned garden flower with a light enchanting fragrance that returns the busy mind to happier times. The fragrance is believed to be released by the fairies at night to bring lovers together.

## Sunflower, *Helianthus annus,* native to the southwestern U.S.

The sunflower personality feels separated from God and Nature. God is somewhere far away. The individual feels lonely and left to defend itself in an unfriendly world. The personality has not experienced the oneness connecting all creation and perceives itself through the eyes of separation.

Sunflower will enable this individual to find and experience the common denominator in all of creation and take responsibility for one's place in it. Sunflower is indicated whenever loneliness or separation from others is experienced. When this harmony is established, the sunflower personality will be able to fulfill its greater purpose in life.

*I am One with the Spirit of Life.*

**Historical uses**

Sunflower seeds and petals were a sacred food of the prairie Native Americans. The sunflower was cultivated by Native Americans before 1,000 B.C. The flowers were used to treat malaria. Dried flower heads are used as a diuretic, reducing inflammation, diarrhea, and stomach distress. The flower buds were often boiled like artichokes or pounded into flour.

**Legend and lore**

The sunflower represented the sun god to the Incas. Sunflowers made from gold were carried by virgins to the temples of the Sun. The Chinese believe it has magical powers associated with longevity. In ancient Greece, it was the emblem of Daphne. The nymph Clytie turned into a sunflower when Apollo rejected her. Hospice nurses, who care for terminal cancer patients, have chosen the sunflower as their international emblem to remind us to thrive under adverse circumstances.

## Sweet Annie, *Artemesia annua,* originated in the Mediterranean

Sweet Annie will benefit those who wish to enhance their public image. It is indicated to bring out the best during personal appearances. The personality may find itself in the public eye unexpectedly and may not be a natural in the lime-light. Sweet Annie can also help those who want to be more socially active and to feel and act gracefully in public. The essence of Sweet Annie also aids in aging gracefully, accenting the beauty originating from self-confidence and poise.

*I move with the simplicity of grace.*

**Historical uses**

The flowers have a heavenly fragrance. They can be distilled as an essential oil from the flowering stalks to make a skincare cream, to alleviate wrinkles, stretch marks, and scars, as well as fragrance to attract a lover. The essential oil and all parts of the plant are toxic if ingested and should only be used externally. The flowering stalks can be dried in flower arrangements that remain fragrant for years. The artemesia family is easy to grow and can be burned, strewn, or hung inside to repel moths. Sweet Annie is often referred to as sweet mugwort or sweet wormwood.

**Legend and lore**

Sacred to Artemis, artemesias represent the lunar, nocturnal feminine side of life. In ancient China, it represents one of the eight precious gifts in life, dignity. Westerners know it as the "lover's plant" or "lad's love" because young men give sprays to their sweethearts.

## Tansy, *Tanacetum vulgare,* originated in Asia

Tansy protects the aura from environmental pollution and radiation. It has been worn for centuries by spiritual warriors and advocates of progressive change. Mother Nature has a way of taking care of her own. Tansy combines well with old blush and verbena to enhance energy and muscle tone.

*I am the protector of gentle souls.*

### Historical uses

The flowers repel insects of many varieties. They were hung from rafters, strewn on floors, and placed between mattresses and bedding. Meat was rubbed with tansy leaves and flowers to repel flies while it roasted. Tansy is now planted near nuclear waste sites. When it flourishes, the land is considered safe to re-inhabit.

### Legend and lore

Tansy is believed to be a variation of the Greek word for immortality, *athanasia.* It was a favorite strewing herb and had the honor of paving the way for kings. Tansy's ability to live for decades in one area made it seem immortal and be the perfect carpet for kings.

## Thyme, *Thymus vulgares,* originated in the Middle East

Thyme attracts all those who will inspire, aid, and encourage our greatest achievements. The flower essence also attracts unseen beneficial elements, such as griffins, devas, nymphs, and fairies. Thyme combines well with onion, sage, and lavender essences to guard the immune system against viral invasion.

*I attract the magical qualities of Nature.*

### Historical uses

The flowers were brewed into a tea and inhaled to prevent epilepsy and depression. Syrup was made for coughs and respiratory infections. Flowering thyme was used as a strewing herb. The essential oil, thymol, is a very effective antiseptic used commercially in mouthwashes and cough and cold medicines. Sheep were once grazed in fields of wild thyme, *Thymus serphyllum,* to produce tasty meat. Egyptians used the oil for embalming and to treat hookworm.

### Legend and lore

Thyme flowers attract fairies. If you pick the flowers of thyme and put them over your eyes, you will be able to see fairies.

In medieval times, thyme was a symbol of courage. Crusaders received a scarf with a sprig embroidered into it from their loved one. Thyme was brought to America on the wool of sheep to naturalize and later was served in beer to cure shyness. The drink was served to children to prevent nightmares.

## Tiger's jaw cactus, *Faucaria tuberculosa,* originated in Cape Providence, South Africa

This is a personality who likes to sit. The individual is quite comfortable watching someone else work or observing everyone else play.

This may sound like the Monday-night TV jock, but in reality, this is the individual immobilized by fear of failure to the point of apathy or laziness.

Tiger's jaw cactus will light a spark under the tiger jaw personality's feet, allay fear, and put creative thoughts into action. All good things take time to mature, but with a little encouragement, the individual will turn into a productive and confident person.

*I am the Self-discipline of action.*

**Historical uses**

The flower can be brewed as a tea for a mild energy stimulant.

**Legend and lore**

It is believed to be unlucky to grow cactus inside a home since the natural habitat is outdoors.

## Vanilla, *Planifolia fragrens,* originated in Mexico

Vanilla essence offers protection against the influence of scattered or negative energy from others and ourselves. Since each thought is living, we need protection from overloading our circuits and draining our energy that could be used creatively.

This negative energy may affect an individual in several ways. One could feel tired, depressed, or irritated for no apparent reason. The individual may suddenly feel the desire to withdraw from a situation or individual and may not understand why. Vanilla essence will calm inner turmoil and relax the individual.

Vanilla essence will allow us to stay clear and in control of our individual environment without unnecessary interference. It is a favorite of children who enjoy the nurturing protection of the fragrant vanilla.

*I am protected by the arm of Mother Nature.*

**Historical uses**

The flowers must be hand pollinated to produce the delicious bean.

**Legend and lore**

Vanilla bean pods were an ancient Aztec flavoring believed to be a food of the gods.

## Verbena, *Hortensis hybrids,* originated in Brazil and Chile

Verbena induces the meditative state accompanying the peaceful feeling of spiritual reality. Thoughts do not go beyond the present. Inner turmoil is replaced by inner polarity as the ego is transcended and the personality is centered in enlightenment. Impulsive action fades. Verbena will allow the mind and body to relax and regenerate, as the true meaning of life comes into perspective. Motives will cease to be self-serving, as the true reality of spirit will come in tune with the family of man.

*Enter my kingdom of Peace.*

**Historical uses**

In medieval times, people bathed in verbena flower water to foresee the future and to make a wish come true. Verbena water was also used to ward off evil spirits, prevent dreaming, and produce a love potion.

**Legend and lore**

To dream of verbena means your wish will be granted.

## Wandering jew, *Setcreasea purpurea,* originated in Mexico

The wandering jew personality is easily discouraged. A lack of inner discipline allows the personality to give up easily and not complete a project. The individual doesn't need an excuse. A low frustration level is reason enough. Physical complaints may include neuritis, an inflammation or irritation of the nerve endings.

Wandering jew can aid this personality to achieve greater self-discipline and confidence to carry on to a point of self-satisfaction. As a bonus, the individual will learn patience and tolerance.

This is the personality who often has great ideas. Therefore, with the help of wandering jew essence and a little effort, the individual will be able to combine creative and analytical thought into logical and well-executed action.

*I am encouraged by the light within me.*

**Historical uses**

Wandering jew is easily established from a cutting and has traveled to all parts of the world to naturalize on many soils.

**Legend and lore**

In Buddhism, the wandering is symbolized by samsara, the condition of being caught in the life and death cycle until enlightenment and liberation is attained. The word "jew" refers to one who has traveled to many lands.

## White carnation, *chinensis,* originated in China

The white carnation personality is best known for willfulness, otherwise known as stubbornness. Tenacity is helpful in times of need; however, the white carnation personality doesn't always understand when to turn it off.

Being headstrong can upset the balance of the adrenal hormones and can manifest in a variety of symptoms. The individual may be in a constant state of anxiety and tension, resulting in adrenal exhaustion and mood fluctuations.

White carnation will ease the fears behind the anxiety of the individual. As the tension eases, the personality will balance desire and release anxiety. A complacent personality can then manifest support and a peaceful environment. The white carnation personality has the strength to focus energy on that which is desired and the patience to teach others to do the same.

*I am peaceful, empty of all desires.*

**Historical uses**

The flower has a red dot in the center because it was genetically hybridized from the red carnation. It represents purity in love relations of every kind, and is considered good luck when given to a woman.

**Legend and lore**

The white carnation is used to foretell the future in Korea and to decorate graves in Mexico.

## White hyacinth, *Hyacinthus orientalis,* originated in the Mediterranean

White hyacinth is an essence that releases trauma such as during birth. Since birth is considered uncomfortable regardless of the circumstances, everyone may benefit from using it. However, the energy is most beneficial to those who were delivered under adverse circumstances, have experienced an injury due to an accident, or suffer an emotional shock.

The emotions involved are uncertainty and insecurity, which can also result from the loss of the mother. The essence is used to enhance the individual's sense of self-reliance. Therefore, the idea of rebirthing is to give the individual a new sense of strength and awareness of control in a continued existence.

White hyacinth releases the shock of imbalanced energy throughout the subtle body. Shocks can be emotional trauma or physical trauma such as accidents, operations, and violence.

White hyacinth will also help correct the attitude to allow the individual to adjust to a more secure environment.

*I experience only pleasure.*

**Historical uses**

The flower is grown in mass to produce a profusion of fragrant blooms heralding spring and the cycle of rebirth.

**Legend and lore**

The hyacinth sprang from the blood of Hyacinthus, accidentally killed by Apollo's discus. It is an emblem of Cronos, representing resurrection in the spring. It grew wild in Biblical lands and was taken to Holland in the early six-teenth century to evolve into the highly bred Dutch bulb.

## White petunia is a hybrid of the nightshade family, *solanum,* originated in South America

White petunia is for the individual who can't quite get thoughts, concentration, and body movement synchronizing.

This personality has difficulty making decisions and even more difficulty acting on decisions. Often, this individual is uncoordinated and cannot draw a straight line with a ruler. A misfiring in the brain's neurochemistry can also cause stuttering, another form of uncoordinated activity.

The essence of white petunia will harmonize and unite the creative energy between mind, brain, and body. The analytical and logical left brain will synergize with the creative right brain. The mind will begin to overcome past negative programming with constructive actions and the physical body will utilize this energy for healing and coordination.

*My body and mind work as one.*

**Historical uses**

White petunia is grown in fairy gardens because the flower shimmers in the moonlight.

**Legend and lore**

The alluring scent of the petunia is released at night by the souls of forlorn lovers. The generic name, "solanum," is derived from the Latin word *solamen,* meaning quieting. It alludes to the poisonous qualities of the nightshade family.

## White rose, *Rosa chinensis alba,* originated in China

White rose will protect an individual from jealousy and negative thoughts. The individual often feels uncomfortable around others. White rose will allow the individual to attract and create sufficient positive energy to feel comfortable with anyone.

The personality will realize that fears once defined are in the past and freedom is unlimited. Natural attraction will produce those of similar interest and positive attitudes.

White rose will help us view life objectively and live in the present moment of total conscious awareness.

*My self-confidence shields me from criticism.*

**Historical uses**

The native Texas white roses are unusually hardy, disease resistant, drought tolerant, and insect resistant. They grow into dense thickets of fragrant blooms.

White antique roses have been cultivated since 3,000 B.C. in the Orient and naturalized in the western world during the last century.

**Legend and lore**

White rose is the flower of Venus, representing the union of opposites and protector of darkness.

## Wild oats, *Avena fatua,* originated in Mesopotamia

Wild oats enhances and develops our sense of humor. We can easily let go and laugh our way past imperfections and inhibitions holding back natural growth. It is also indicated for the "blues" and for children who pout. Combine wild oats with dianthus, red rose, and fimbriata and let the good times roll.

*Laughter is my medicine.*

**Historical uses**

Wild oats is an ancient remedy for depression and muscle spasms. A wine steeped with oats was a remedy for nervous exhaustion for writers, speakers, and lawyers. Externally, a compress was applied to psoriasis and skin problems, such as poison ivy. Applied to the face, a compress made from ground oats will promote a beautiful, radiant complexion.

The grain is a source of protein, B vitamins, calcium, potassium, iron, and carotene. As porridge, it is used to treat diarrhea. As a tea, it stimulates the appetite, soothes the nerves, and relieves anxiety and chest pains. Oat straw can be brewed to add to the bath for rheumatism, skin problems, and sciatic pain. In Australia, a decoction is made from the aerial parts, crushed and pounded, to reduce fever and symptoms of chest colds. In Ayurvedic medicine, oats are used to cure addiction, shingles, and multiple sclerosis.

**Legend and lore**

Eating oats was believed to give one courage and strength.

## Wild wood violet, *Viola odorata,* originated in southern Europe and North Africa

Wild wood violet will help one instinctively choose endeavors that benefit society. This path of modesty and non-interference allows the mind to enter the wholeness of the universe and predict the evolution of events to follow.

*I look within for answers.*

**Historical uses**

Violets were cultivated in ancient Persian gardens to make a drink called sherbet. The flower later became the emblem of Athens, available year-round for wreaths. The Romans enjoyed making a sedative wine and served violets with orange and lemon.

White wood violets were also used to abate anger and insomnia as a tea. The Celts made them into a facial cosmetic with goat's milk. A syrup was given to English children as a laxative during the sixteenth century. Today, the blossoms are used in colognes and cough syrups.

**Legend and lore**

Romans wore the flowers around their heads to alleviate dizziness and headaches. Napoleon promised to return from exile in Elba with the violets in the spring. The violet became the symbol of loyalty to Bonaparte and was worn in his honor throughout the Second Empire. His son was buried with violets in 1879 in honor of the deposed hero, which finally ended the cult of the violet and the Bonapartists.

## Wisteria, *Macrostachya,* originated in Japan

Wisteria essence draws subtle energy into the heart chakra. This helps the individual who is not aware of loving feelings, or not feeling love at all. Love may be defined simply as a joyful, unattached, unconditional love. While using wisteria essence, an individual will begin enjoying everyone. The person often becomes very talkative and cordial.

Wisteria aids in opening humanity to the spiritual, creative energy that connects us all in an impersonal love. The essence is meant to allow humankind to work with creation as one, raising consciousness for constructive thought and action. A deeper connection with all Nature will also transpire. This is a wonderful aid for those working in alternative health practices and the service fields.

*I am the Love that teaches by example.*

**Historical uses**

Texas wisteria is less aggressive than the Asian variety and blooms after the leaves appear. Asian varieties bloom on bare wood and then leaf. Be sure to buy one blooming to assure color. Wisterias grown from seed can take ten to fifteen years to bloom.

**Legend and lore**

In the Orient, wisteria blooms as a reminder of the orderliness of the seasons. An early bloomer, wisteria heralds the coming fertility of springtime.

## Yarrow, *Achilles millifollium,* originated in Neanderthal times

Yarrow is used to accent the strength of other flower essences. Add two or more drops to any flower essence combination. Yarrow reduces autoimmune reactions and inflammatory responses adversely affecting the immune system and central nervous system. It has natural antiseptic properties to enhance healing.

*I am an advocate of peace, attracting all those who will inspire, aid and direct me to attain the greatest good.*

### Historical uses
Flowers were brewed into a tonic for dysentery, colds, and lung hemorrhages. Yarrow flowers were plucked one at a time to produce a vision of a future lover in Old England. Yarrow was often grown near graves and associated with death in dreams and visions. Flowers have been used to flavor liquors, reduce blood pressure, and abate allergic eczema and catarrh.

### Legend and lore
Culpeper recommended yarrow, the herb of Venus, to treat gonorrhea, relating the disease to the careless worship of the goddess. It was used in magical potions and named the "Devil's plaything." English physicians applied yarrow soaked in oil to the head to prevent hair from falling out. Yarrow is native to the British Isles.

## Yellow rose, a cross between *Gloria Dei* and *Meilland Gioia,* originated in France
The yellow rose personality desires to serve society with an unselfish commitment of talents. Intuition is attuned to the times and existing conditions. The individual wishes to benefit the established order by working to improve it.

The yellow rose personality is a reformer who has chosen a life of service. Imagination and intellect enlarge the possibilities of life and inspire those who work side by side. High goals only enhance the personality's affectionate nature. The yellow rose lives by the old adage "Love isn't love, till you give it away."

*I am the Service of Love for Mankind.*

### Historical uses
Yellow roses originated in the fertile regions of the Middle East. The true species was produced by Mother Nature in the subgenus *pimpinellifoliae.* Vegetative propagation by compassionate gardeners kept the species from dying out like the blue roses.

### Legend and lore
The yellow rose is a symbol of peace and is the state flower of Texas.

## Zinnia, *elegans,* originated in Mexico
Zinnia most affects the personality who is feeling unloved. The hurt and anger this produces manifests as criticism of oneself or others. The zinnia personality is most likely to be affected by arthritic pain or chronic aches and pain.

This personality is feeling some bitterness from being deprived of nurturing attention. Zinnia will help release the bitterness and aid the individual to be more self-nurturing. Loving oneself attracts love from others and the circle is complete.

The zinnia personality can direct others to their greatest good, being able to view individuals objectively, and is generous with advice and guidance.

*I become the love I share with others.*

**Historical uses**

Zinnias are grown to attract pollinating insects and lure slugs away from the vegetable garden.

**Legend and lore**

Zinnias are daisies that shortened their skirts.

CHAPTER 16

# Mysterious Origins
## Healing with Antique Roses

### Vinnie Introduces the Antique Rose Collection

The information Spider reported was vast and a bit overwhelming, yet the response from the Land of Thyme was very positive. Indeed, the fairies wanted even more information on flowering plants. Spider looked for Vinnie and Snake to provide research from the garden. He found them occupying a rock deep in thought.

"What are you two doing?" Spider asked frantically. "We need more data on flowering plants for the broadcast."

"We're stumped," answered Vinnie. "We haven't been able to locate the origin of the old roses in Faith's garden."

"Some of the roses don't even know who their parents are!" complained Snake. "The roses are hybrid plants derived from cross-breeding original rose stocks growing in the Orient, the Middle East, Europe, and the Americas hundreds or thousands of years ago. Many have naturalized, especially in the southern U.S. prior to the Civil War, from 1860 to 1865. Roses have become the national flower since then."

"Wow! This sounds really interesting, even more so since the rose's origin is mysterious," Spider replied. "What is the best way to convey the information to the public?"

"They're known for their history and growing conditions," replied Vinnie with his hands cupping his face.

"Well, let's give them what we've got," answered Spider, throwing all eight hands into the air.

"That makes my job easier," agreed Snake as he slithered back into the garden.

"Vinnie, I want you to introduce the old roses tonight on the broadcast," Spider nodded as he instructed Vinnie.

Immediately, Vinnie's eyes brightened at the idea of being a star on laptop television. He grabbed his pen and note pad and flew off to interview Faith.

Later that evening, Vinnie appeared at the broadcast introducing the old roses as if he knew everything about them.

"Ladies and gentlemen, I bring to you tonight a collection of old roses so ancient and unique that I will refer to them as antique roses. Little is known about their origin and background. Most are without a formal Latin name, but what we do know is that their genetic memory allows them to enhance our ability to communicate with one another on an intimate level. Yes, fairies, this collection of antique roses senses our deepest hopes, dreams, and fears about truly intimate relationships with one another and even within ourselves. They understand our need for love and fear of commitment. Each provides an essence encouraging the subtle body to receive direction from within, and to give and receive love freely with one another in appropriate ways."

As Vinnie spoke, the fairies in the Land of Thyme watched in total amazement. First, an old timer shook his head and jiggled a flower inserted into his ear as a hearing aid.

"I knew I had a hearing challenge, but am I seeing whom I think I'm seeing? He sure looks like that hyper little fairy who used to fly around here getting on everyone's nerves."

"That's him," yawned Jason as he stretched. "I recognize his elfish grin." Petite nodded in agreement as she nuzzled into Jason's shoulder and stroked his hair.

"I'm so glad he helped me find you," Petite whispered into Jason's ear as he turned to pet his friend, the German shepherd.

"It's perfect that he's introducing love essences," agreed Jason shyly.

Suddenly, Flora jumped into the conversation, unable to conceal her excitement.

"It's him, it's him!" she cried. "That's my hyper twin brother! I saw him transform with flower essences right before my eyes!"

"He acts so mature!" commented Rosie.

"That's just one of the results of healing from the heart," added Flora. "Vinnie calmed down and I opened up my heart!"

"If I didn't know you so well, I would think you were the hyper fairy," laughed Collie.

With that comment, Flora flopped down into her cushion to quietly watch the program. As the broadcast continued, she passed a plate of freshly baked Melba toast, which everyone politely refused.

Nimbus was the only fairy that was speechless that night. His heart was bursting with pride for this newborn star. The little imp had finally grown into his potential. He felt like a proud father watching Vinnie at his best. His eyes only left the television once to kiss Sweet Tooth, who was fast asleep with her head on his shoulder. Pregnancy agreed with Sweet Tooth like broadcasting suited Vinnie. Nimbus enjoyed the best of both of their worlds that night.

After a brief message from the broadcasting sponsor, Vinnie introduced twenty-two antique roses, adding the following information.

## Archduke Charles

Archduke Charles enhances intimacy, allowing one to feel safe when being touched. Archduke Charles may help those who pull away from others or push people away who get "too close." The personality may move in and out of intimate relationships too quickly, avoiding total commitment, always finding a reason to move on. Archduke Charles touches the heart where true intimacy grows unhindered by intellect and desire. In the body, it encourages regeneration of the structural stability of the skin, arterial lining, and stomach lining.

*I delight in your touch.*

Origin: This hybrid of *Rosa chinensis,* prior to 1837, originated from China and Asia. It blooms pink and turns red. As summer heat progresses, it blooms only red. As an essence, it aids those who avoid touch and intimate commitments.

## Alfredo de Damas

This essence helps assert power of command over body and mind to affect constructive habits. It may enhance memory and reduce disorientation, confusion, and complications from alcoholism or sensitivity to alcohol.

An individual may have chronic polyneuropathy with exaggerated reflexes or complain of weakness in the lower limbs. Mind and body seem to be at odds with one another. The mind races, leaving the body lagging behind. Alfredo de Damas essence grounds the personality, allowing what he envisions to channel through writing, horticulture, architecture, and the healing arts.

*I renew myself through constructive changes.*

Origin: *Rosa x centifolia,* parentage unknown, and blooms creamy pink fragrant multi-petal flowers from early spring through the fall.

## Autumn Damask

Autumn Damask develops constancy in faith. The personality has often experienced many disappointments in past relationships and is hesitant to become involved again. The essence of Autumn Damask helps the personality to learn from past disappointments and become more discerning in intimate relationships. Developing the faith to work through patterns concerning intimacy will attract fulfilling relationships and enhance nutrient uptake in the body cells.

*Faith resides in my heart.*

Origin: *Rosa x damascena bifera* is one of the most ancient roses of the Middle East; the scent is one of the finest. Autumn Damask later parented the fragrant Bourbon and Hybrid Perpetual roses. In an essence, the scent heals the wounds of disappointing relationships, encouraging cellular nutrient uptake. It is instrumental in working through depression related to disappointment in intimate relationships.

## Cecil Brünner

Cecil Brünner encourages those who withdraw or hold back from entering new relationships. The essence also helps overcome fear arising from new challenges and situations. In relationships, it aids in defining comfortable boundaries and realistic goals. Until a balance is reached, the individual may awaken feeling exhausted and have difficulty starting the day. When ability to love is unhindered, it can attract those who will assist in achieving the highest goals.

*I feel safe to bloom.*

Origin: The Sweetheart Rose from China. It is a hybrid of *Rosa chinensis,* aiding those who hold back from entering new relationships.

## Champney's Pink Cluster

Champney's Pink Cluster is the rose of integrity. The essence teaches us to love through respect rather than through passion alone. We learn to connect with divinity by recognizing and honoring the love that created each person. Seeing through the eyes of love allows us to accept others and ourselves and allow love to lead us to share with others in the best way possible. The essence of Champney's Pink Cluster enhances the resting potential of nerve cells, encouraging the muscles to relax and regenerate.

*Share my joy.*

Origin: This hybrid of *Rosa chinensis x Rosa moschata* is an American creation of two very important China roses by John Champney of South Carolina. It teaches us to love through acceptance and allow others' influences to transform us. Through trust, passion is born and cellular regeneration occurs. Champney's has a relaxing neuroinhibitor effect.

## Cherokee Rose

Cherokee Rose is a China rose and the child of Lady Eubanksia antique rose. The essence opens the crown chakra to stimulate creative ideas in daily activities. It enhances endocrine balance of the pituitary, pineal, and hypothalamus to regulate menstrual cycles and reduces fluid retention from female complaints. For men, Cherokee Rose often enhances protein metabolism and subsequent muscle strength as a new vision of oneself is created.

*I remember the best things in life.*

Origin: *Rosa laevigata* is a China rose naturalized in southern climates. The essence opens the crown chakra and balances the trinity of master endocrines:

pituitary, pineal, and hypothalamus. It can be used to enhance protein metabolism and regulate menstrual cycles. It grows twelve to twenty feet tall and several feet in width with large thorns that discourage predators.

## Country Marilou

Country Marilou unlocks inner joy to promote vitality and regeneration. It releases the beauty of inner strength and security. It knows no age or order of difficulty. The essence helps an individual to release uncomfortable feelings and perceptions from the body. It may be beneficial for those who form nodes of neuronal tissue and suffer from neuritis.

Origin: *Rosa centifolia* originated in the Middle East. It is the rose that brings out inner strength and beauty.

## The Fairy Rose

The Fairy Rose promotes a passionate connection with every life form, linking the first and seventh chakras. This is a transpersonal experience, often witnessed in a dreamlike experience. The personality may see nature spirits, leaving the safety of everyday experiences to learn, think, feel, and see life in a beneficial way. You can bloom with the roses or fly like an angel, but your life will never feel ordinary again. The Fairy Rose is often indicated for those who tap Mother Nature's power to heal others.

*My blooms set free the magic in me.*

Origin: *Rosa chinenesis minima,* 1815, began the line of miniature China roses. By connecting the first and seventh chakras, it enhances a transpersonal experience allowing one to see Nature Spirits.

## Fimbriata

Fimbriata encourages a passion for life. The essence is indicated when an individual needs to release nonproductive relationships. Fimbriata opens the mind and heart to new possibilities, setting the law of attraction in motion. Even in friendships, Fimbriata enhances an enthusiasm that is contagious, forming new alliances with those of like minds. The essence may also encourage pathways to develop and to enhance the synergistic harmony of organ function.

*My passion attracts the best to me.*

Origin: *Rosa rugosa x Mme Alfred Carriere* is a French hybrid dating to 1811, and is also known as Dianthaflora. The essence kindles a passion for life, setting the law of attraction in motion.

# Fortune's Double Yellow

Fortune's Double Yellow calms excessive desires and attracts the greatest good. Double Yellow gently reminds us we always have what we need. What we claim will return to us, just as we return to our Source. The essence discourages envy and feelings that we won't get what we want from life. It may aid those who have a tendency for hypertension and tension headaches, and nurtures those who are separated by distance from loved ones. Double Yellow will soothe an aching heart with a feeling that time is on our side.

*A river of peace flows through me.*

Origin: This hybrid of *Rosa chinensis* was discovered in China by Robert Fortune in 1845 and naturalized in Europe. The essence calms excessive desires, envy, and jealousy and also aids in attracting the greatest good.

# Fortuniana

This essence aids realization and penetration into the universal truths of man. As leadership qualities emerge, the personality is able to perceive what is best for those who serve and inspire cooperation. This essence will help integrate the Universal Soul desires with personal desires. In the body, healing of symmetrical dysfunction of motor and sensory nerves will be enhanced. There may be a generalized regeneration of all nerves, and an increase in the ability to smell.

As the nervous system fully develops, a sixth sense is acquired that is beyond intuition. The level of security expands to include an inner communication or "understanding" on the electromagnetic level we call the aura.

*My creativity integrates me with the Universal Soul.*

Origin: A cross between Lady Eubanksia and Cherokee Rose from China.

# Grüss an Aachen

Grüss an Aachen encourages us to withdraw from partnerships and relationships that require us to settle for less than what we know in our hearts is best. Quality, not quantity, will open the heart to fulfillment. During the transition or recovery time, an individual may awaken frequently during the night or experience food cravings. Grüss an Aachen encourages us to walk with a good heart so we'll run with success.

*I know who is best for me.*

Origin: *Frau Karl Drushchi x Frans Deegen* is the original rose of the Floribunda cluster roses bred from the Hybrid Perpetuals. The essence helps us withdraw from relationships that require that we settle for less.

## Lady Eubanksia

Lady Eubanksia encourages a reclusive or loner individual to join the community and teach from the knowledge gained through many years of experience. It also helps balance motor weakness, sensory loss and degeneration of the peripheral nerves affecting the limbs by enhancing circulation.

*I bloom from Wisdom and Understanding.*

Origin: *Rosa banksiae lutescens* is a Chinese vining rose appearing in 1870. It blooms once in the early spring with tiny, single fragrant white or yellow roses. She climbs twenty feet high and ten feet wide on a wall or fence in a spectacular display of cascading flowers and foliage.

## Louis Philippe

Louis Philippe offers hope to those who feel love has passed them by. Hopelessness can only be overcome by surrender to the love within. Affirm the truth, that all of your needs are provided, and call on your heart to receive its greatest good. Louis Philippe encourages growth of receptor sites activating cardiovascular flow, enhancing the feeling we describe as love. This warmth not only provides new life for the blood, but also new loves to bless your life.

*I surrender to the Love within me.*

Origin: This hybrid of *Rosa chinensis* was introduced in France with an unknown parentage in 1834. The flowers are deep crimson semi-double blooms. It prefers loose, humus soil and blooms profusely during the spring and fall.

## Madame Alfred Carriere

Madame Alfred Carriere encourages prophetic dreams, encouraging the individual to seek answers in dreamtime. This essence enhances parasympathetic responses to encourage the body to heal itself, transcending time and difficulty. Since dreamtime allows us to leave the illusion of opposites, the subtle body is able to function without inner conflict. The spirit seeks freedom like a bird seeks flight. Madame Alfred Carriere invites you to allow your intellect to rest and seek answers from the depths of the unconscious.

*I am the rose of devotion.*

Origin: This hybrid of *Rosa chinensis* is another China rose where exact parentage is unknown. She blooms continuously with large white, highly scented flowers with a hint of pink.

## Madame Louis Levique

Madame Louis Levique increases the desire for service and devotion, surrendering the need to be in control. The energy can help neutralize toxins affecting the nervous system and blocking the free flow of chi. By letting go, we also let go of insecurities and defenses. Madame Louis Levique encourages us to take an active part in nurturing the environment as we learn to take responsibility of our lives.

*I surrender to the Present Moment of Grace.*

Origin: *Rosa centifolia muscosa* is another French introduction of a rose with unknown parentage. Her perfect pink flowers remain cupped until fully open. The petals are unusually soft and silky to the touch.

## Maggie

Maggie enhances perception to see the truth in situations. Hidden aspects can only be seen and felt from the heart. If you listen, the heart will guide you, for it has the capacity to "see" and "feel" what is best for you. The Seat of the Soul is in its rightful place in a peaceful heart, content with all things, lacking in none; Maggie calls on our greatest capacity to see through the masque of the personality to the soul level in every situation.

*I perceive the Truth in every situation.*

Origin: Maggie is a found rose of unknown parentage. It carries the heavy scent of the Bourbon roses. Bourbon roses were originally parented by chance from Old Blush crossing itself with a Damask rose. Maggie is a magenta beauty that favors its Damask parentage.

## Marie Pavie

Marie Pavie encourages us to follow the heart's yearning in love relationships. It is indicated when our thoughts deny what our hearts know is right. The essence may ignite the flame in burned-out relationships. The individual may be recovering from deep disappointments in family relationships causing a feeling of loss and grief. Marie Pavie may encourage recovery from post-viral syndromes with symptoms of aching and malaise, referred to by Oriental healers as dampness in the channels.

*I follow my heart.*

Origin: *Rosa floribunda* is a rose of unknown parentage found by the French in 1888. She is a dainty plant with an abundance of cluster blooms. The flowers range from white to a hint of pink. Floribundas are ever blooming throughout the season.

## Marquis Boccella

Marquis Boccella is the constant bloom of perpetual love. The essence encourages long-term relationships that build intimacy through trust. It is often indicated when we are searching for but not attracting kindred spirits to share our joy. Marquis Boccella also aids those who fall in love with people who are not mutually attracted.

In the body, the essence affects the subtle energy inherent in the nervous system, what is called *sukshma* in Sanskrit. This energy communicates sensory messages to the subtle body and affects the sensory organs. It is especially indicated for those stressed by a busy schedule, replenishing vitality and increasing acuity.

*I am the rose of Perpetual Love.*

Origin: Marquis Boccella is a found rose of unknown parentage, known to the French as "Jacques Cartier." She proudly produces cupped pink flowers that open into short, deeply perfumed petals. It was found in 1868.

## Old Blush

Old Blush enhances our stamina, the ability to keep going. The essence works with the motor pathways of the neuronal system to initiate muscular contraction.

Old Blush originated in China thousands of years ago as an ever-blooming dark pink rose. She will catalyze an inner strength and calm to adapt a creative expression into every aspect of your life and health. Neuronal pathways will be stimulated by renewed willpower. You may accomplish more in your life than you ever thought possible.

*I am the continuous bloom of inner strength.*

Origin: This hybrid of *Rosa chinensis* is an old rose cultivated in China for thousands of years. She arrived in the U.S., then known as Parson's Pink, prior to the American Revolution. Her fragrant abundance of pink blooms made her a favorite in southern gardens. At the end of the American Civil War, Old Blush stood behind General Lee at Appomattox as he surrendered to General Grant.

## Silver Moon

Silver Moon subdues a restless mind, obsessive thoughts, fearful dreams, and constant chattering or "head talk." From the stillness of a quiet mind, pure awareness emerges. Restless energy often affects the heart chakra, causing stuttering and an increased need for personal attention and admiration. An imbalance of the fire element can exaggerate the sense of importance and the need to be "different." Silver Moon encourages us to return to a quiet center and affirm the kingdom of peace.

*From the stillness of a quiet mind pure awareness emerges.*

Origin: *Rosa laevigata* hybrid is a child of Cherokee Rose. In springtime, it bursts into large, fragrant, pure white flowers with golden stamens. Beautiful on a trellis or fence, Silver Moon grows from fifteen to twenty feet in height.

# Viridiflora

Viridiflora grounds our sensory input by mediating impulses between the sensory and motor neurons. It helps those who are very sensitive to their environment by maintaining and aligning power centers. This runs though all chakras and is grounded in earth energy. Viridiflora can enhance personal power by aligning the power centers.

Viridiflora's bronze-green flowers are as unique as her parentage. Her link with the earth magnifies the energy running through our spine and vitalizes every potential neuronal connection. The personality will feel very centered with clarity of purpose.

*I bloom from personal power.*

Origin: *Rosa Viridiflora* is the most mysterious antique rose. The parentage and origin is unknown. It was discovered in 1833 and named "Green rose." The leaves are very obviously of the rose family. Blooms are formed from a multitude of green bracts turning bronze with age. A rose without origin or blooms, it is disease-free, adapting to a variety of soils.

As Vinnie finished with Viridiflora, he quietly stepped aside to allow Spider some time.

"And with Viridiflora, we end a very long series on flower remedies from the garden. This is Spider on assignment in the Garden of Beauty."

"Thank you, Spider, we are looking forward to your return with your assistants, Vinnie and Snake," said the commentator. "This is John Stardust signing off and wishing you a good evening."

## Back in the Land of Thyme

After the series ended, Vinnie, Snake and Spider bid farewell to Faith and packed to return to the Land of Thyme. They could only hope the future would be exciting as the past year in the Garden of Beauty. The knowledge acquired was well received in the fairy community, which welcomed the trio home as heroes.

In the trio's honor, the late-night fairy tale, "The Origin of the Rose," aired upon their return. The fairies gathered in the community building to watch the program. Vinnie, Snake, and Spider sat in the front row as guests of honor, delighted to be home. "The Origin of the Rose" was one of the most popular fairy tales in the Land of Thyme. It began where the flowering of the pine forests left off.

## The Origin of the Rose Fairy Tale

We left the fairies flying all over the world scattering seed for new varieties of blooms. It was paying off. As the plants acclimated to different soil and climates, new and more exotic blooms appeared.

One of the fairies became lost in a forest known to humans as Breceliande. He was wandering from tree to tree looking for a signpost with directions a fairy could read, when he was caught up in a dust storm. No, maybe it was smoke! Suddenly, there was a voice saying something about a Holy Grail to what appeared to be a man-shaped metal sculpture standing close by. For a moment, the fairy got a glimpse of a giant elf, called Merlin, before he disappeared in a billow of smoke. The metal sculpture, calling himself a Knight of the Holy Grail, agreed to obtain this very important item and return to his homeland in Camelot. Soon, the fairy learned this Sacred Grail was a magical cup holding the gift of fertility. Now, that sounded to the fairy like a good place to plant some seeds and it would sure cut down on his travels.

He hitched a ride on the mane of a de-horned unicorn carrying the giant back to a castle in Camelot. The fairy soon realized he confused the tail for the unicorn's mane and was in a very bad mood by the time he arrived.

Camelot turned out to be a bigger place than the fairy imagined. The giant sculpture seemed well received by the inhabitants of the big house. The fairy was shocked when he heard the sculpture speak. Maybe there was a human trapped inside. The king thought so because he engaged in quite a long conversation with the metal sculpture he called Gawain. From this, the fairy learned he had to travel overseas on an ark with sails to find the Holy Grail.

The fairy rode for days on end in an ark with a huge tablecloth tied to a rope catching the wind. The deck was the only place cool enough to sleep. Even the human, Gawain, stepped outside his metal garment during the journey to cool off.

They landed on an island called "The Dead" and were greeted by a pile of bones with very sad faces. The island was strangely devoid of flora. The rocks were sharp and hurt his feet.

Gawain put his metal extensions back on and did battle with numerous foes. The fairy helped him out whenever he could, placing his seeds in a very plain cup for safekeeping. Dragons and monsters of every kind came out to oppose Gawain.

As it turned out, the fighting was directed toward a row of cups, including the plain one holding the seeds. The fairy was busy tying up snakes when what looked like a dragon magically turned into an old, haggard woman. Surely, Gawain wouldn't harm a helpless retired goddess.

To avoid the fatal blows of Gawain's sword, the old woman picked up a dazzling bejeweled cup and turned into a beautiful princess, the like of which no one had seen since the days of Cinderella. She put the cup to her lips, then offered it to the stunned Gawain, who by now had managed to pull off his metal head and stood with his mouth wide open. As he reached out to accept the cup, the fairy realized his seeds were in the plain cup being spirited away by a raven. In an act of heroism, the fairy threw a stone at the raven, which dropped the cup right into Gawain's outstretched hand. Looking a little confused, Gawain replied, "The choice is up to you, princess." With this, the beautiful princess was released from a lifelong spell of indecision on the Island of Death. She smiled and fell into Gawain's arms. He fell in love at first sight of this lovely maiden, thinking she obviously chose him as her lover. Little did he know he almost drank from the cup of indecision and would have been in eternal imprisonment on the Island of Death. Even worse, he almost drank the seeds!

As Gawain caressed the beautiful princess, the fairy went to retrieve the seeds. There were angels everywhere. The cup began to move on its own power as enchanting music filled the air. It emitted a great radiance as an inviting perfume filled the room. The fairy sensed that something really big was about to happen and turned to witness the birth of the most beautiful flower he had ever gardened, growing out of the cup. "Is this the Holy Grail? he asked out loud. To his astonishment, the flower turned and spoke directly to him in a melodious voice.

> *I am the rose, the flower of love, innocence, and unity.*
> *I bloom from the heart of creation, symbolizing perfection and the return of spirituality.*
> *Grow me wherever you desire Paradise to return.*
> *My red petals will ignite joy, passion, and consummation of your desires.*
> *White petals will restore purity to humankind.*
> *Golden yellow petals will unite opposites to attain what seems impossible.*
> *My four-petal flowers represent the elements that enfold Gaia.*
> *Five petals represent the microcosm living in every human.*
> *Six petals denote the macrocosm guarded by every angel.*
> *My stamens are lit by the sun.*
> *My petals are the wheels of life generating the chakras.*
> *My fragrance represents immortality through spiritual rebirth.*
> *I am the gift of the Heart.*

As the program ended, the fairies wiped their eyes, realizing the importance of their work as Mother Nature's flower fairies. They affirmed their desire to manifest perfection and return the Land of Thyme into a Paradise.

# Epilogue

The adventure in the Garden of Beauty changed many lives in the Land of Thyme. The fairies finally became more health conscious on a daily basis as they grew into a self-actualized community. They gradually changed their diets to one with less fat and sugar and plenty of lightly glazed, flavored Melba toast. In time, they became as light as fairies used to be. However, their interest in the news did not change. Spider continued to report breathtaking news stories to the new anchor, Vinnie! Yes, Vinnie's delivery of the antique rose collection not only won him fame, but also a job where he could do what he naturally did the best — talk! He quickly learned to channel his abundant energy for the news media and became a popular newscaster.

His pet and friend, Snake, ran for the office of mayor and won unopposed, becoming a symbol of leadership and wisdom in the garden community. He soon won a reputation for fairness and love of beauty, as Snake developed the Land of Thyme into a virtual wonderland. Gardens were laced with many new varieties of flowers transported from the Garden of Beauty. Every garden was equipped with a distillation unit to make flower essences and essential oils on site. Business boomed as Snake found new markets for the products.

Nimbus and Sweet Tooth became the proud parents of a baby girl they named Kindness. Their lives centered on her well-being and upbringing. The desire to be model parents gave them even more incentive to eat healthy and stay fit. In time, their passion for Kindness became a passion for life.

Flora surprised everyone by adding chakra and flower essence information in her nutrition classes. Her popularity soared after Snake and Vinnie co-hosted a special about her work. The most avid student was no other than the captain, Chief Justice of the Garden. After choosing essences to overcome underlying feelings of insecurity, the captain began studying music after his weight training. It was confirmed by a wise wisteria blooming outside Flora's window that the captain serenaded Flora on a regular basis. In time, the fairy community expected the two lovers to announce their engagement, hopefully after the shy fairy, Jason, popped the question to his true love, Petite.

And Mother Nature? Well, she makes frequent visits with her devoted companion, Apollo. As time dreams on, their love will become the most celebrated in fairydom.

# Supplier List

Bulk Herbs:
Simply Natural
Box 84
Aledo, TX 76008
E-mail: simnat2@yahoo.com

Essential Oils and Flower Essences:
Herbal Health Inc.
Box 330411
Ft. Worth, TX 76163
www.aromahealthtexas.com
E-mail: petitefl@aromahealthtexas.com
Phone: 817-293-5410
Fax: 817-293-3213

Antique Roses, Native Plants, and Seeds
Weston Gardens in Bloom
8101 Anglin Dr.
Ft. Worth, TX 76140
Phone: 817-572-0549
Website: www.westongardens.com
E-mail: weston@westongardens.com

# Bibliography

Baker, Margaret. *Gardener's Magic and Folklore.* New York: Universe Books, 1978.

Bourne, Eleanor. *Heritage of Flowers.* New York: G.P. Putnam Sons, 1980.

Bremness, Lesley. *Herbs.* London: Dorling Kindersley, 1994.

Chin, Wee Yeow and Hsuan King. *An Illustrated Dictionary of Chinese Medicinal Herbs.* California: CRCS Publications, 1990.

Cook, J.D. *Absorption of Food Iron*, Chronicle Books, 1997.

Cooper, J.C. *An Illustrated Encyclopedia of Traditional Symbols.* London: Thames & Hudson, 1978.

Downing, C. *Gods In Our Midst.* New York: Crossroads Publishing Co., 1993.

Flynn, R. and M. Roest. *Your Guide to Standardized Herbal Products.* Prescott, Arizona: One World Press, 1995.

Griffin, J., Dr. *Aromasignatures.* Fort Worth, Texas: Herbal Essence, Inc, 1996.

Griffin, J. Dr. *Mother Nature's Herbal.* St. Paul, Minnesota: Llewellyn Worldwide, 1997.

Griffin, J. Dr. *Herbs For All Seasons.* (Speech) Fort Worth, Texas: Japanese Botanical Garden Festival, October 19, 1996.

King, Eleanor. *Biblical Plants for American Gardens.* New York: Dover Books, 1975.

Mercatante, Anthony S. *The Magic Garden.* New York: Harper and Row, 1976.

Miller, Gloria Bley. *The Thousand Recipe Chinese Cookbook.* New York: Simon and Schuster, Inc., 1966.

Murry, M. and J. Pizzorno. *Encyclopedia of Natural Medicine.* Rockland, California: Prima Publishing, 1991.

Vickery, Roy. *Oxford Dictionary of Plantlore.* New York: Oxford University Press, 1995.

Pickles, Sheila. *The Language of Wild Flowers.* London: Pavilillion Books, Unlimited, 1995.

Reader's Digest Association, Inc. *The Magic and Medicine of Plants.* Pleasantville, New York, 1986.

Rodale. *Rodale's Illustrated Encyclopedia of Herbs.* Emmaus, Pennsylvania: Rodale Press, 1987.

Steinberg, Rafael. *The Cooking of Japan.* Alexandria, Virginia: Time Life Books, 1976.

Stodol, Jiri and Jan Volak. *The Illustrated Book Of Herbs.* New York: Gallery Books, 1985.

Teeguarden, R. *Chinese Tonic Herbs.* Tokyo and New York: Japan Publishing, Inc., 1984.

Titley, Norah and Francis Wood. *Oriental Gardens.* San Francisco, California: Chronicle Books, 1991.

Viscott, D. *Emotionally Free.* Chicago, Illinois: Contemporary Books, 1992.

# Acknowledgements

A special thanks to Linda Stephens for her fine typing skills, Jason Ermis for his patient and thorough editing corrections, Vincent Ermis for poetry, Gina Lima for inspiration and encouragement, Howard and Flamina Palombi for teaching me to love flowers and respect nature, Dorothy Ferguson for typing, Nancy Buchanan for support of every kind, Fran Goreham for initial editing and advice, Erika Lieberman, my editor at Paraview Press, and my copyeditor, Lisa Kaiser.

CPSIA information can be obtained at www.ICGtesting.com
Printed in the USA
BVOW081135071012

302377BV00005B/10/A